# Advances in Neurologic Therapy

*Editor*

JOSÉ BILLER

# NEUROLOGIC CLINICS

www.neurologic.theclinics.com

*Consulting Editor*
RANDOLPH W. EVANS

August 2013 • Volume 31 • Number 3

**ELSEVIER**

1600 John F. Kennedy Boulevard • Suite 1800 • Philadelphia, Pennsylvania, 19103-2899

http://www.theclinics.com

**NEUROLOGIC CLINICS Volume 31, Number 3**
**August 2013 ISSN 0733-8619, ISBN-13: 978-0-323-18611-7**

Editor: Donald Mumford

*Neurologic Clinics* (ISSN 0733-8619) is published quarterly by Elsevier Inc., 360 Park Avenue South, New York, NY 10010–1710. Months of issue are February, May, August, and November. Periodicals postage paid at New York, NY, and additional mailing offices. Subscription prices are $285.00 per year for US individuals, $489.00 per year for US institutions, $140.00 per year for US students, $359.00 per year for Canadian individuals, $586.00 per year for Canadian institutions, $397.00 per year for international individuals, $586.00 per year for international institutions, and $199.00 for Canadian and foreign students/residents. To receive student/resident rate, orders must be accompanied by name of affiliated institution, date of term, and the *signature* of program/residency coordinator on institution letterhead. Orders will be billed at individual rate until proof of status is received. Foreign air speed delivery is included in all *Clinics* subscription prices. All prices are subject to change without notice. **POSTMASTER:** Send address changes to *Neurologic Clinics*, Elsevier Health Sciences Division, Subscription Customer Service, 3251 Riverport Lane, Maryland Heights, MO 63043. **Customer Service: Telephone: 1-800-654-2452 (U.S. and Canada); 314-447-8871 (outside U.S. and Canada). Fax: 314-447-8029. E-mail: journalscustomerservice-usa@elsevier.com (for print support); journalsonlinesupport-usa@elsevier.com (for online support).**

*Reprints.* For copies of 100 or more of articles in this publication, please contact the Commercial Reprints Department, Elsevier Inc., 360 Park Avenue South, New York, New York, 10010-1710; Tel.: (+1) 212-633-3812; Fax: (+1) 212-462-1935, and E-mail: reprints@elsevier.com.

*Neurologic Clinics* is also published in Spanish by Nueva Editorial Interamericana S.A., Mexico City, Mexico.

*Neurologic Clinics* is covered in *Current Contents/Clinical Medicine, MEDLINE/PubMed (Index Medicus), EMBASE/Excerpta Medica, and PsycINFO, and ISI/BIOMED.*

Printed and bound by CPI Group (UK) Ltd, Croydon, CR0 4YY

Transferred to digital print 2012

# Contributors

## CONSULTING EDITOR

**RANDOLPH W. EVANS, MD**
Clinical Professor, Department of Neurology, Baylor College of Medicine, Houston, Texas

## EDITOR

**JOSÉ BILLER, MD, FACP, FAAN, FANA, FAHA**
Professor and Chair, Department of Neurology, Stritch School of Medicine, Loyola University, Maywood, Illinois

## AUTHORS

**MARIA I. AGUILAR, MD**
Associate Professor of Neurology, Division of Cerebrovascular Diseases, Department of Neurology, Mayo Clinic, Phoenix, Arizona

**DOUGLAS ANDERSON, MD**
Professor, Department of Neurologic Surgery, Loyola University Medical Center, Maywood, Illinois

**JORGE J. ASCONAPÉ, MD**
Professor of Neurology, Stritch School of Medicine, Loyola University Chicago, Maywood, Illinois

**JARED R. BROSCH, MD**
Resident, Department of Neurology, Indiana University School of Medicine, Indianapolis, Indiana

**ALICIA C. CASTONGUAY, PhD**
Stroke and Neurointerventional Postdoctoral Fellow, Division of Neurointervention, Department of Neurology, Froedtert Hospital and Medical College of Wisconsin, Milwaukee, Wisconsin

**JOSÉ E. COHEN, MD**
Director of Endovascular Neurosurgery and Interventional Radiology Center, Department of Neurosurgery, Hadassah-Hebrew University Medical Center, Jerusalem, Israel

**ANDREW P. DUKER, MD**
Assistant Professor, Department of Neurology and Rehabilitation Medicine, James J. and Joan A. Gardner Center for Parkinson's disease and Movement Disorders, University of Cincinnati Neuroscience Institute, University of Cincinnati, Cincinnati, Ohio

**ALBERTO J. ESPAY, MD, MSc**
Associate Professor, Department of Neurology and Rehabilitation Medicine, James J. and Joan A. Gardner Center for Parkinson's disease and Movement Disorders, University of Cincinnati Neuroscience Institute, University of Cincinnati, Cincinnati, Ohio

**MARTIN R. FARLOW, MD**
Professor, Department of Neurology, Indiana University School of Medicine, Indianapolis, Indiana

**MURRAY FLASTER, MD, PhD**
Associate Professor of Neurology and Neurosurgery, Department of Neurology, Stritch School of Medicine, Loyola University Chicago, Maywood, Illinois

**WILLIAM D. FREEMAN, MD**
Associate Professor of Neurology, Departments of Neurology, Neurosurgery, and Critical Care, Mayo Clinic College of Medicine, Jacksonville, Florida

**JOAO A. GOMES, MD, FAHA**
Director, Neurointensive Care Fellowship Program, Cerebrovascular Center; Assistant Professor of Medicine, Cleveland Clinic Lerner School of Medicine at Case Western Reserve University, Cleveland Clinic, Cleveland, Ohio

**RICARDO A. HANEL, MD, PhD**
Professor, Department of Neurosurgery, Mayo Clinic College of Medicine, Jacksonville, Florida

**NINITH KARTHA, MD**
Assistant Professor of Neurology, Stritch Medical School, Loyola University Medical Center, Maywood, Illinois

**RUTH S. KUO, PharmD**
Clinical Pharmacy Specialist-Cardiology, Scripps Memorial Hospital, La Jolla, California

**MARC A. LAZZARO, MD**
Assistant Professor of Neurology and Neurosurgery, Division of Neurointervention, Department of Neurology, Froedtert Hospital and Medical College of Wisconsin, Milwaukee, Wisconsin

**RONEN R. LEKER, MD, FAHA**
Director, Comprehensive Stroke Center; Department of Neurology, Hadassah-Hebrew University Medical Center, Jerusalem, Israel

**RIMAS V. LUKAS, MD**
Assistant Professor, Department of Neurology, University of Chicago, Chicago, Illinois

**EDWARD MANNO, MD, FCCM, FAHA, FAAN**
Director, Neurointensive Care Unit, Cerebrovascular Center, Cleveland Clinic, Cleveland, Ohio

**MATTHEW MCCOYD, MD**
Director, Neurology Residency Training Program; Assistant Professor of Neurology, Loyola University Medical Center, Maywood, Illinois

**DAVID A. MILLER, MD**
Assistant Professor, Departments of Neurosurgery and Radiology, Mayo Clinic College of Medicine, Jacksonville, Florida

**SARKIS G. MORALES VIDAL, MD**
Assistant Professor, Department of Neurology, Stritch School of Medicine, Loyola University Chicago, Maywood, Illinois

**MARTIN KELLY NICHOLAS, MD, PhD**
Assistant Professor, Section of Neurosurgery, Departments of Neurology and Radiation and Cellular Oncology, University of Chicago, Chicago, Illinois

**ROBERTA L. NOVAKOVIC, MD**
Assistant Professor, Division of Neuroradiology, Department of Radiology; Department of Neurology, UT Southwestern Medical Center, Dallas, Texas

**ADRIANA SOFIA PLONEDA PERILLA, MA**
Stritch School of Medicine, Loyola University Chicago, Chicago, Illinois

**ALEJANDRO RABINSTEIN, MD**
Professor of Neurology; Director, Regional Acute Stroke Center, Mayo Clinic Health System, Rochester, Minnesota

**SEAN RULAND, DO**
Associate Professor, Department of Neurology, Stritch School of Medicine, Loyola University Chicago, Maywood, Illinois

**MICHAEL J. SCHNECK, MD**
Professor of Neurology and Neurosurgery, Department of Neurology, Stritch School of Medicine, Loyola University Medical Center; Department of Neurosurgery, Stritch School of Medicine, Loyola University Chicago, Chicago, Illinois

**MICHAEL STAR, MD**
Resident in Neurology, Department of Neurology, Stritch School of Medicine, Loyola University Chicago, Maywood, Illinois

**PHILIPP TAUSSKY, MD**
Assistant Professor, Departments of Neurosurgery and Radiology, University of Utah, Salt Lake City, Utah

**RABIH G. TAWK, MD**
Assistant Professor, Department of Neurosurgery, Mayo Clinic College of Medicine, Jacksonville, Florida

**OSAMA O. ZAIDAT, MD, MS**
Professor of Neurology, Radiology, and Neurosurgery; Chief, Division of Neurointervention, Department of Neurology, Froedtert Hospital and Medical College of Wisconsin, Milwaukee, Wisconsin

# Contents

**Preface**                                                                              xiii

José Biller


**Platelet Antiaggregants in Stroke Prevention**                                         633

Sarkis G. Morales Vidal and Sean Ruland

> Antiplatelet agents are one of the main interventions for recurrent ischemic stroke prevention. Their time of use, dosage, and combination of therapy have different effects in terms of stroke risk reduction and adverse effects. This review provides an evidence-based update of the latest on antiplatelet therapy for stroke prevention.

**New Anticoagulants (Dabigatran, Apixaban, Rivaroxaban) for Stroke Prevention in Atrial Fibrillation**                                                                   659

Maria I. Aguilar, Ruth S. Kuo, and William D. Freeman

> New oral anticoagulants have been found to be as efficacious as warfarin and safer in terms of intracranial bleeding. All patients with nonvalvular atrial fibrillation should receive antithrombotic therapy for stroke prevention. For those at low risk, antiplatelet therapy is probably sufficient. For those at intermediate or high risk, anticoagulation is superior to antiplatelet therapy. Four oral anticoagulants are currently approved for stroke and systemic embolism prevention in atrial fibrillation: warfarin, dabigatran, rivaroxaban, and apixaban. Management of bleeding complications while on the new agents remains an area of concern and management is based on anecdotal experience and observational studies.

**Unanswered Questions in Thrombolytic Therapy for Acute Ischemic Stroke**               677

Adriana Sofia Ploneda Perilla and Michael J. Schneck

> This article reviews some of the current literature in support or against extension of the intravenous tissue plasminogen activator window, use of intra-arterial therapy or devices, as well alternative pharmacologic therapies that may extend the window for treatment of patients with acute ischemic stroke, with consideration of the relative risk of thrombolytic complications, factors for worse outcomes, and unclear stroke onset, as seen in patients with wake-up stroke. The issue of newer concomitant antithrombotic therapies as they affect the decision for acute ischemic stroke thrombolytic therapy is also explored.

**New Strategies for Endovascular Recanalization of Acute Ischemic Stroke**              705

José E. Cohen, Ronen R. Leker, and Alejandro Rabinstein

> Although intravenous thrombolysis with recombinant tissue plasminogen activator is a proven effective therapy for acute ischemic stroke, it is often insufficient to achieve recanalization in patients with large intracranial artery occlusions. In these cases, intra-arterial reperfusion techniques

may be useful. Intra-arterial thrombolysis has been largely replaced by mechanical thrombectomy as the preferred endovascular approach. Rapid technological advances have led to the development and refinement of various neurothrombectomy devices. This article reviews the evolution of neuroendovascular approaches for the management of severe acute ischemic stroke, including evidence from the main trials evaluating clinical and angiographic outcomes after neurothrombectomy.

**New Developments in the Treatment of Intracerebral Hemorrhage**    721

Joao A. Gomes and Edward Manno

Understanding of intracerebral hemorrhage (ICH) pathophysiology and technological advances are now providing the opportunity to significantly reduce the morbidity and mortality associated with this debilitating type of stroke. As reviewed in this article, several ongoing clinical trials may transform the way this patient population is treated within the next 5 years. Although more research is needed, a new era for ICH management is beginning.

**New Therapies for Unruptured Intracranial Aneurysms**    737

Philipp Taussky, Rabih G. Tawk, David A. Miller, William D. Freeman, and Ricardo A. Hanel

The concept of flow diversion is based on placing a stent across the neck of an intracranial aneurysm, which then results in flow away from the aneurysm, inducing thrombosis and occlusion of the aneurysm over time. Modern flow diverters, such as the Pipeline embolization device, are currently used for unruptured anterior circulation aneurysm. As the use and application of flow diverters becomes more widespread, some important questions remain relating to the effective treatment of dual antiplatelet therapy, the occurrence of delayed aneurysm ruptures and intraparenchymal hemorrhages, and long-term patency rates.

**The Diagnosis and Management of Brain Arteriovenous Malformations**    749

Roberta L. Novakovic, Marc A. Lazzaro, Alicia C. Castonguay, and Osama O. Zaidat

Although uncommon in the general population, cerebral arteriovenous malformations (AVMs) can pose a significant health risk if a rupture occurs. Advances in noninvasive imaging have led to an increase in the identification of unruptured AVMs, presenting new challenges in management, given their poorly understood natural history. Over the past decade, there have been significant developments in the management and treatment of intracranial AVMs. This article discusses the pathophysiology, natural history, clinical presentations, and current treatment options, including multimodal approaches, for these vascular malformations.

**Advances and Controversies in the Management of Cerebral Venous Thrombosis**    765

Michael Star and Murray Flaster

Cerebral venous thrombosis (CVT) is a rare form of stroke found most often in young women of reproductive age, often associated with oral contraceptive use, genetic or acquired thrombophilia, pregnancy, dehydration, or infection. CVT should be considered in any young patient who presents with an unexplained headache in combination with known hypercoagulable state, focal neurologic deficits, seizure, lobar hemorrhage, or bilateral thalamic or basal ganglionic edema. Acute treatment is with unfractionated heparin or low-molecular-weight heparin. It is important to provide supportive treatment. Outcomes are good compared with other types of stroke. Pediatric patients, excluding neonates, have similar presentation, treatment, and outcomes as adults.

**Epilepsy: New Drug Targets and Neurostimulation**    **785**

Jorge J. Asconapé

Despite advances in the medical and surgical therapy for epilepsy, about 30% of patients do not achieve full seizure control. In the past 5 years new antiepileptic drugs have been approved for clinical use. Some of these drugs have unique, novel mechanisms of action. Overall efficacy of these agents, however, seems similar to other antiepileptic drugs. Vagus nerve stimulation is a well-established palliative therapy for medically resistant epilepsy. Neurostimulation, with newer devices and targets becoming available, is a rapidly expanding field in epileptology. Considerable development and research are still necessary before these newer techniques become the standard of care for the treatment of epilepsy.

**Surgical Treatment of Parkinson Disease: Past, Present, and Future**    **799**

Andrew P. Duker and Alberto J. Espay

Advances in functional neurosurgery have expanded the treatment of Parkinson disease (PD) to targeted electrical stimulation of specific nodes in the basal ganglia circuitry. Deep brain stimulation (DBS), applied to selected patients and difficult-to-manage motor fluctuations, yields substantial reductions in off time and dyskinesia. Emerging concepts in DBS include examination of new targets, such as the potential efficacy of pedunculopontine nucleus stimulation for treatment of freezing and falls, the use of pathologic oscillations in the beta band to construct an adaptive "closed-loop" DBS, and new technologies, including segmented electrodes to steer current toward specific neural populations.

**Deep Brain Stimulation in Nonparkinsonian Movement Disorders and Emerging Technologies, Targets, and Therapeutic Promises in Deep Brain Stimulation**    **809**

Douglas Anderson and Ninith Kartha

This article focuses on the evolution of deep brain stimulation (DBS) targets within the brain, beginning with the discovery of DBS's potential in non–Parkinson disease movement disorders. DBS has gained in popularity and applicability for a growing number of neuropathologic conditions with neural network disorders and dysfunction. Targets within the brain have been based frequently on historical sites used for ablative surgeries in years past, derived from experiment and experience but also have arisen via elucidation of neural networks, transmitter function and location, disease neuropathology, and also, fortuitous discovery.

**Update on Therapeutic Options for Multiple Sclerosis**                    827

Matthew McCoyd

> Multiple sclerosis (MS) is one of the most common neurologic disorders
> that affects young people. The disorder has long been associated with
> clinical relapses and a disabling course. However, there has been a rapid
> expansion in the available treatment options for MS, and new insights into
> existing therapies, as decades of research has begun to produce tangible
> treatment results leading to newly approved an emerging therapies.

**Update in the Treatment of High-grade Gliomas**                    847

Rimas V. Lukas and Martin Kelly Nicholas

> Advances in the molecular classification of high-grade gliomas are laying
> the groundwork for potential changes in the treatment of high-grade glio-
> mas. Currently, a combined modality approach involving surgery, radiation
> therapy, and chemotherapy is most often used in the treatment of high-
> grade gliomas. The authors review recent advances in the treatment of
> these primary brain tumors.

**Immunotherapy for Alzheimer's Disease**                    869

Martin R. Farlow and Jared R. Brosch

> The immune system plays a significant role in Alzheimer disease (AD).
> β-Amyloid deposition in the cortex is thought to be an initiating event in
> AD and the widely believed amyloid hypothesis proposes removal of
> amyloid may delay disease progression. Human trials of active or passive
> immune agents have failed to show benefit and increased adverse events
> of vasogenic edema and microhemorrhages. Evidence suggests the ill-
> ness may be too advanced by the time patients are symptomatic with de-
> mentia. Future directions include better understanding of how and where
> immunotherapies should be targeted and treating patients at earlier stages
> of the illness.

**Index**                    879

# NEUROLOGIC CLINICS

**FORTHCOMING ISSUES**

*October 2013*
**Clinical Neurogenetics**
Brent L. Fogel, MD, *Editor*

*February 2014*
**Neuroimaging**
Lazslo Mechtler, MD, *Editor*

*May 2014*
**Secondary Headache**
Randolph W. Evans, MD, *Editor*

**RECENT ISSUES**

*May 2013*
**Peripheral Neuropathies**
Richard J. Barohn, MD, and
Mazen M. Dimachie, MD, FAAN, *Editors*

*February 2013*
**Spinal Cord Diseases**
Alireza Minagar, MD, FAAN, and
Alejandro A. Rabinstein, MD, FAAN,
*Editors*

*November 2012*
**Sleep Disorders**
Bradley V. Vaughn, MD, *Editor*

**RELATED INTEREST**

*Neuroimaging Clinics of North America*, May 2013, Volume 23, number 2
**Pediatric Demyelinating Disease and its Mimics**
Manohar Shroff, MD, *Editor*

**NOW AVAILABLE FOR YOUR iPhone and iPad**

# NEUROLOGIC CLINICS

FORTHCOMING ISSUES

October 2013
Clinical Neurogenetics
Brent L. Fogel, MD, Editor

February 2014
Neuroimaging
Laszlo Mechtler, MD, Editor

May 2014
Secondary Headache
Randolph W. Evans, MD, Editor

RECENT ISSUES

May 2013
Advances in Neurologic Therapy
Robert J. Barohn, MD, and
Mazen M. Dimachkie, MD, FAAN, Editors

February 2013
Spinal Cord Diseases
Alireza Minagar, MD, FAAN, and
Alejandro A. Rabinstein, MD, FAAN,
Editors

November 2012
Sleep Disorders
Bradley V. Vaughn, MD, Editor

RELATED INTEREST

Neurologic Clinics of North America, February 2012, Volume 22, Issue 1
Chronic Demyelinating Diseases and Dementias
Abuzzahab Sheikh, MD, Editor

# Preface

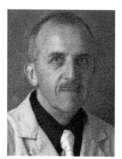

José Biller, MD, FACP, FAAN, FANA, FAHA
*Editor*

Neurology has grown into an exciting and therapeutically oriented discipline. Over the past decades, there has been an explosion of new and innovative host of therapies for a variety of neurologic disorders. Accordingly, it is critical for us to keep abreast of this scientific outpouring. This issue of *Neurologic Clinics* presents 14 articles and has been written with the specific intent of making the information relevant and memorable to the practitioner to whom it is primarily directed.

We have chosen several topical areas we believe will be of interest to the readership of this series, including the latest data on antiplatelet therapy for stroke prevention and new anticoagulants for stroke prevention in atrial fibrillation. Following these 2 introductory articles, the issue focuses on unanswered questions on thrombolytic therapy for acute ischemic stroke, new strategies for endovascular recanalization of acute ischemic stroke, new developments in the treatment of intracerebral hemorrhage, new therapies for unruptured intracranial aneurysms, new and emergent therapies for arteriovenous malformations, and advances in the management of cerebral venous thrombosis. The issue subsequently concentrates on neurostimulation and new drug targets in epilepsy, surgical treatment of Parkinson disease, and deep brain stimulation (DBS) in non-parkinsonian movement disorders and emerging therapeutic promises in DBS. We conclude with new and emerging therapies in multiple sclerosis, updates in the treatment of high-grade gliomas, and immunotherapy for Alzheimer disease.

A special thanks to all of the authors for their scholarly and practical contributions.

I am hopeful this issue of *Neurologic Clinics* is timely and informative and of practical use to those colleagues caring for persons with neurologic disorders, and we

Neurol Clin 31 (2013) xiii–xiv
http://dx.doi.org/10.1016/j.ncl.2013.04.015
0733-8619/13/$ – see front matter © 2013 Published by Elsevier Inc.

**neurologic.theclinics.com**

always welcome their feedback. Finally, there is every reason to believe that future advances in neurologic therapy are sure to come.

José Biller, MD, FACP, FAAN, FANA, FAHA
Professor and Chair
Department of Neurology
Loyola University Chicago
Stritch School of Medicine
2160 South 1st Avenue
Maywood, IL 60153, USA

E-mail address:
jbiller@lumc.edu

# Platelet Antiaggregants in Stroke Prevention

Sarkis G. Morales Vidal, MD[a],*, Sean Ruland, DO[b]

KEYWORDS

- Antiplatelet • Aspirin • Clopidogrel • Dypiridamole • Cilostazol • Stroke
- Hemorrhage

KEY POINTS

- Dual antiplatelet therapy with aspirin + clopidogrel is not more efficacious than monotherapy for recurrent stroke prevention in patients with atrial fibrillation who are not candidates for anticoagulant therapy.
- Dual antiplatelet therapy with aspirin + clopidogrel is inferior to anticoagulant therapy for recurrent stroke prevention in patients with atrial fibrillation.
- Cilostazol is a promising alternative for recurrent stroke prevention in patients with non-cardioembolic strokes but further research is needed before it can be routinely recommended.
- Although newer antiplatelet agents are efficacious for coronary artery disease, increased rates of intracranial hemorrhage (e.g, prasugrel) may limit their role for recurrent stroke prevention.

## INTRODUCTION

Antiplatelet agents are one of the main interventions for recurrent ischemic stroke prevention. Aspirin has been the most studied and is currently the most commonly prescribed antiplatelet agent. Other well-known antiplatelet agents include dypiridamole, clopidogrel, and cilostazol. Over the past 5 years, multiple clinical trials have evaluated the efficacy of these agents in several clinical scenarios. In addition, new agents, such as prasugrel and trifusal, have been studied in patients with a history of stroke or transient ischemic attacks (TIAs). Some of these trials included patients with coronary artery disease and substudies evaluated their respective efficacy in patients with cerebrovascular disease. This review provides a summary of the major clinical trials that support the use of these agents for stroke prevention as well as an update of remarkable studies that may change practice in the near future.

[a] Neurology Department, Stritch School of Medicine, Loyola University Chicago, 2160 South 1st Avenue, Building 105, Room 2700, Maywood, IL 60153, USA; [b] Neurology Department, Stritch School of Medicine, Loyola University Chicago, 2160 South 1st Avenue, Maywood, IL, USA
* Corresponding author.
*E-mail address:* smoralesvidal@lumc.edu

Neurol Clin 31 (2013) 633–657
http://dx.doi.org/10.1016/j.ncl.2013.03.004
0733-8619/13/$ – see front matter © 2013 Elsevier Inc. All rights reserved.

## MECHANISM OF ACTION: REVIEW OF OLD DRUGS AND POTENTIAL TARGETS OF NOVEL AGENTS

Antiplatelet agents act via different mechanisms to inhibit the platelet adhesion and aggregation pathway. Aspirin irreversibly and selectively inhibits acetylation of the cyclooxygenase (COX)-1 hydroxyl group. This renders the enzyme incapable of converting arachidonic acid into prostaglandin $H_2$ (PGH$_2$). Because PGH$_2$ is the precursor to the formation of the platelet aggregation stimulator, thromboxane (TX)A$_2$, the pathway is blocked. Unlike aspirin, which acts intracellularly, the thienopyridines, clopidogrel and ticlopidine, act as irreversible P2Y$_{12}$ adenosine diphosphate (ADP) surface receptor blockers, preventing the binding of fibrinogen by this receptor. This results in the blockade of a cascade of later events that would otherwise stimulate platelet aggregation. Dipyridamole inhibits platelet phosphodiesterase E5, which increases cyclic adenosine monophosphate (cAMP) levels, potentiating the platelet inhibitory actions of prostacyclin.

Cilostazol and ticagrelor are newer antiplatelet agents that have more recently garnered increasing interest. Cilostazol prevents platelet aggregation by inhibiting phosphodiesterase 3, thus increasing cAMP concentrations to reduce the risk of recurrence of cerebral infarction. In addition, cilostazol is reported to have other biological actions, such as vasodilatation, vascular endothelial cell protection, and improvement of lipid metabolism, all which may also ascribe to their antiplatelet activity.[1–4] Ticagrelor blocks P2Y12 ADP receptors. However, unlike clopidogrel, ticagrelor is an allosteric antagonist that binds to a different site on the ADP receptor, making the blockage reversible.

Because each antiplatelet agent is unique in its mechanism of action, it is postulated that they may also provide varying degrees of vascular protection. As a result, combination therapy has become popular among some physicians because it has been perceived to provide greater effectiveness in reducing vascular events despite contrary evidence and safety concerns. Currently, multiple clinical trials are examining the efficacy of these agents for stroke prevention, whether alone or in combination.

### Aspirin

Aspirin remains the most common agent for the prevention of vascular events. It is often prescribed initially because of its affordability, tolerability, and ease of use. A previous meta-analysis by the Antiplatelet-Trialists Collaboration (ATC) studied the efficacy of aspirin from 6 clinical trials conducted between the late 1970s to the mid-1990s.[5] For primary prevention, aspirin yielded a 12% proportional reduction in serious vascular events (0.51% aspirin vs 0.57% control per year) that included myocardial infarction (MI), stroke, and vascular death. However, the reduction was due mainly to a decreased incidence of nonfatal MI and the net effect on stroke risk was nonsignificant. Subsequently, a meta-analysis that included another 9 primary prevention trials from 1998 to 2005 demonstrated a 14% reduction in cardiovascular events with aspirin use, once more primarily driven by a reduction in nonfatal MI.[6] For recurrent stroke prevention, the ATC meta-analysis reported aspirin to be associated with a 1.5% absolute reduction in serious vascular events (6.7% aspirin vs 8.2% control per year) with approximately one-fifth relative reduction in stroke events.

The optimal dose of aspirin remains debatable. The drug has been shown to be similarly effective in preventing recurrent strokes with doses of 30 to 1300 mg daily.[7–11] However, some observational studies and meta-analyses have shown no incremental benefit with higher dosages of aspirin for secondary stroke prevention.[12–17] For example, the Clopidogrel and Aspirin Optimal Dose Usage to Reduce

Recurrent Events-Seventh Organization to Assess Strategies in Ischemic Syndromes (CURRENT-OASIS) was a randomized clinical trial that assigned 25,086 patients with acute coronary syndrome (ACS) to receive either low-dose (75–100 mg per day) or high-dose (300–325 mg per day) for maintenance therapy after an initial loading dose.[18] The study reported no difference in the primary end point of cardiovascular death, MI, or stroke at 30 days between the 2 doses. In addition, several trials have reported increased rates of adverse events such as gastrointestinal hemorrhage associated with higher doses of aspirin.[5–11] Thus, there is no evidence of a net benefit supporting routinely prescribing high doses (>325 mg/d) of aspirin in light of increased bleeding risk.

Cardiomyopathy with decreased ejection fraction is a stroke risk factor.[19,20] Although previous studies have associated aspirin with a lower risk of death in patients with coronary artery disease and heart failure, the evidence for stroke prevention is uncertain as the superiority of anticoagulation therapy over aspirin has not been demonstrated. Despite this, the benefit of anticoagulant therapy has long been applied for stroke prevention in patients with heart failure with ejection fraction less than 35%. The Warfarin versus Aspirin in Patients With Reduced Cardiac Ejection Fraction (WARCEF) trial reported that among patients with reduced left ventricular ejection fraction who were in sinus rhythm, any reduced risk of ischemic stroke with warfarin compared with aspirin was offset by an increased risk of major hemorrhages.[21] However, the WARCEF study enrolled few patients with previous stroke; thus, the findings may not be generalizable for secondary stroke prevention. Conversely, a recently published meta-analysis examining trials of warfarin and aspirin in individuals with low ejection fraction and sinus rhythm found that warfarin was associated with a lower stroke risk compared with aspirin (pooled relative risk [RR], 0.59; 95% confidence interval [CI], 0.41 to 0.85; $P = .004$), no difference in risk for MI and mortality,[15] and no significantly increased risk of intracerebral hemorrhage despite increasing the risk of overall major hemorrhages.[22]

Despite aspirin's relative advantages as an antiplatelet agent, it also has several limitations, including gastrointestinal side effects and occasional allergic reactions. Thus, there have been several other randomized controlled trials comparing the effectiveness of aspirin with other antithrombotic agents (**Table 1**) since the meta-analysis published by the ATC in 2009. The more recent publications do not report findings similar to those of the past: that is, although aspirin has efficacy for stroke prevention, it is nonetheless limited.

For patients with atrial fibrillation, the most powerful predictor of stroke is a history of previous stroke or TIA.[23,24] Vitamin K antagonist therapy has been shown to reduce the relative risk of stroke in atrial fibrillation by two-thirds; however, its use is limited because of various food and drug interactions, a narrow therapeutic window, the need for lifelong coagulation monitoring, and a higher risk for intracranial and systemic bleeding compared with aspirin.[25,26] For patients with atrial fibrillation who are deemed unsuitable for vitamin K antagonist therapy, aspirin is commonly used for stroke prevention. In these cases and for low-risk patients, the American Heart Association (AHA) recommends a dose of 81 to 325 mg aspirin daily. Previously, aspirin has been shown to reduce the risk of stroke by about one-fifth compared with placebo.[26] However, in patients with atrial fibrillation at high risk of stroke, a one-fifth reduction in the relative risk of stroke with aspirin, compared with placebo, is suboptimum. Apixaban is a new competitive inhibitor of factor Xa and may fulfill the need for a more effective anticoagulant for patients with atrial fibrillation at high risk of stroke considered to be at high risk for bleeding with vitamin K antagonist therapy. A subgroup analysis of the Apixaban versus Acetylsalicylic Acid to Prevent Stroke in Atrial Fibrillation

**Table 1**
Comparison of efficacies between antiplatelet therapies for secondary stroke prevention: randomized controlled studies from 2008 to 2012

| Trial, Year | Purpose | Patient Population | Treatment Regimes | Primary End Point and Follow-Up | Outcome | Major Safety and Adverse Events |
|---|---|---|---|---|---|---|
| *Aspirin vs Clopidogrel* | | | | | | |
| Tsai et al,[61] 2010 | Investigate differences in platelet activation markers in stroke patients taking aspirin vs clopidogrel | 70 patients with noncardioembolic stroke | Aspirin (100 mg) daily vs clopidogrel (75 mg) daily | Platelet activation markers (CD62P, CD63, CD40L) measured at <24 h, 7, 30, 90 d after stroke | Platelet activation markers were significantly reduced in the clopidogrel group than in the aspirin group 7 d after stroke. The significance persisted for CD62P and CD63 at 1 mo | Gastrointestinal bleeding was noted in 1 patient in each of the aspirin and clopidogrel groups |
| *Aspirin vs Aspirin + Clopidogrel* | | | | | | |
| Benavente et al,[52] 2012 SPS3 investigators | Examine aspirin vs clopidogrel + aspirin for reduction in vascular events in patients with recent lacunar stroke | 3020 patients with symptomatic lacunar infarcts within the preceding 180 d, identified by magnetic resonance imaging | Aspirin (325 mg) + placebo vs aspirin (325 mg) + clopidogrel | Any recurrent stroke, including ischemic stroke and intracranial hemorrhage; mean follow-up of 3.4 y | Aspirin + clopidogrel combination therapy did not significantly reduce risk of recurrent stroke, recurrent ischemic stroke, or disabling/fatal stroke compared with aspirin alone | Rate of all major hemorrhages was significantly higher among patients receiving dual antiplatelet therapy compared with aspirin alone (2.1% vs 1.1%) |

| Study | Objective | Patients | Intervention | Outcome measure | Results | Bleeding |
|---|---|---|---|---|---|---|
| Hankey et al,[34] 2011 CHARISMA (substudy) | Examine aspirin vs clopidogrel + aspirin (within the first 30 d of stroke) in preventing recurrent stroke | 1331 patients within 30 d of ischemic stroke or TIA | Aspirin (75–162 mg) daily + clopidogrel (75 mg) daily vs aspirin (75–162 mg) daily + placebo | Any stroke during follow-up | Nonsignificant decrease in recurrent stroke in clopidogrel group | Severe bleeding in 1.8% of the entire patient population; no significant difference in occurrence between groups |
| Hankey et al,[49] 2010 CHARISMA (prespecified substudy) | Examine aspirin vs clopidogrel + aspirin in reducing rate and functional severity of recurrent stroke | 436 patients with previous TIAs or ischemic stroke | Aspirin (75–162 mg) daily + clopidogrel (75 mg) daily vs aspirin (75–162 mg) daily + placebo | Functional severity of stroke outcome events via the mRS score at 3 mo | The addition of clopidogrel to acetylsalicylic acid did not significantly alter the rate and functional severity of stroke outcome | None reported |
| Hart et al,[48] 2008 CHARISMA (substudy) | Examine aspirin vs clopidogrel + aspirin in stroke reduction in patients with atrial fibrillation | 593 patients with a history of atrial fibrillation | Aspirin (75–162 mg) daily + clopidogrel (75 mg) daily vs aspirin alone | Stroke event (ischemic and hemorrhagic); median follow-up of 2.3 y | Study does not support the use of combination therapy over aspirin alone in patients with a history of atrial fibrillation | Nonsignificant increase in intracranial bleeds and severe/fatal extracranial hemorrhage in combination therapy group |

(continued on next page)

**Table 1**
*(continued)*

*Clopidogrel vs Aspirin + ERDP*

| Trial, Year | Purpose | Patient Population | Treatment Regimes | Primary End Point and Follow-Up | Outcome | Major Safety and Adverse Events |
|---|---|---|---|---|---|---|
| Sacco et al,[70] 2008 PRoFESS | Compare the efficacy and safety of clopidogrel vs aspirin + ERDP | 20,332 patients with recent ischemic stroke (randomized within <90 d of stroke onset) | Aspirin (25 mg) + ERDP (200 mg) twice daily vs clopidogrel (75 mg) daily | First reoccurrence of stroke; follow-up mean 2.5 y | No difference in the rates of recurrent strokes between the 2 treatment groups | Increased risk of intracranial bleeding (including intracerebral hemorrhages) among patients treated with aspirin + ERDP compared with clopidogrel; also higher rates of medication discontinuation because of headaches, gastrointestinal side effects, and other side effects with combination therapy |

*Aspirin vs Aspirin + ERDP*

| Study | Objective | Population | Intervention | Outcome | Conclusion | Results |
|---|---|---|---|---|---|---|
| Uchiyama et al,[67] 2011 JASAP | Examine efficacy and safety of aspirin vs aspirin + ERDP in secondary stroke prevention | 1294 patients with an ischemic stroke (excluding cardiogenic cerebral embolism) | Aspirin (81 mg) daily vs aspirin (25 mg) + ERDP (200 mg) twice daily | Event rate of recurrent ischemic stroke (fatal or nonfatal) | Inconclusive, difference between treatment groups could not be shown | 0.6% deaths in aspirin + ERDP group, 1.6% deaths in aspirin group |
| Dengler et al,[68] 2010 EARLY | Compare efficacy of early addition of aspirin + ERDP vs aspirin in improving stroke outcomes | 543 patients with acute ischemic stroke, NIHSS score ≤20 | Aspirin (25 mg) + ERDP (200 mg) twice daily vs aspirin alone (100 mg) daily during the first 7 d after stroke. All patients were then given aspirin + ERDP for up to 90 d | mRS at 90 d; vascular adverse events (nonfatal stroke, TIA, nonfatal MI, and major bleeding complications) | Early initiation of aspirin + ERDP 7 d after stroke had no significant benefit to late initiation. Both regimes were safe and effective in preventing disability | Recurrent cerebrovascular events were higher in the late ERDP initiation group than in the early initiation group, but not statistically significant (18% vs 16%) |

*Aspirin vs Cilostazol*

| Study | Objective | Population | Intervention | Outcome | Conclusion | Results |
|---|---|---|---|---|---|---|
| Lee et al,[30] 2011 CAIST | Compare the efficacy of cilostazol vs aspirin in acute stroke | 447 patients with NIHSS score ≤15 within 48 h of stroke onset | Aspirin (300 mg) daily vs cilostazol (200 mg) daily | Functional outcome measured by mRS, score of 0–2 at 90 d | No difference in efficacy between cilostazol and aspirin in functional outcome, stroke recurrence, bleeding | Adverse events more common in cilostazol-treated patients although frequency of drug discontinuation was not significantly different; frequencies of bleeding complications were not different between groups |

(continued on next page)

**Table 1**
*(continued)*

| Trial, Year | Purpose | Patient Population | Treatment Regimes | Primary End Point and Follow-Up | Outcome | Major Safety and Adverse Events |
|---|---|---|---|---|---|---|
| Shinohara et al,[29] 2010 CSPS 2 | Assess safety and efficacy of cilostazol vs aspirin for prevention of stroke in patients with noncardioembolic cerebral infarction | 2757 patients with cerebral infarction within the previous 26 wk | Aspirin (81 mg) daily vs cilostazol (100 mg) twice daily | First occurrence of stroke (cerebral infarction/ hemorrhage, subarachnoid hemorrhage); treatment continued for 1–5 y | Cilostazol group had fewer hemorrhagic events than aspirin group (P = .004) | Cilostazol group had more frequent events of headache, diarrhea, palpitations, dizziness, and tachycardia than the aspirin group |
| Guo et al,[31] 2009 | Compare aspirin vs cilostazol on cerebral arteries, cerebrovascular blood flow in secondary stroke prevention | 68 patients with ischemic stroke within 1–6 mo of recruitment | Aspirin (100 mg) daily vs cilostazol (100 mg) twice daily | Cerebrovascular condition by magnetic resonance angiography and transcranial Doppler ultrasonography; follow-up 12 mo | No difference between drugs in preventing the aggravation of cerebral arteries in secondary prevention of ischemic stroke | Gastrointestinal disturbances, bleeding events (including intracranial cerebral hemorrhage, nasal bleeding, gastrointestinal hemorrhage, fecal occult blood, vaginal bleeding). All bleeding events were in aspirin group |

*Aspirin vs Aspirin + Cilostazol*

| | | | | | | |
|---|---|---|---|---|---|---|
| Nakamura et al,[33] 2012 | Compare efficacy of aspirin vs aspirin + cilostazol in secondary stroke prevention | 76 patients with acute noncardioembolic ischemic stroke | Aspirin (300 mg/d) alone vs aspirin (300 mg/d) + cilostazol (100 mg twice daily) | Frequency of early neurologic deterioration or stroke recurrence within 14 d and 6 mo | Aspirin + cilostazol had less neurologic deterioration and more favorable functional status than aspirin alone | Aspirin alone: 1 patient withdrawn because of a drug eruption, 1 patient withdrawn because of gastrointestinal bleeding. Aspirin + cilostazol: 1 patient withdrawn because of a drug eruption, 2 patients withdrawn because of palpitations |
| Lee et al,[32] 2010 | Investigate whether addition of cilostazol to aspirin in patients with ischemic stroke can reduce aspirin resistance | 244 patients with ischemic stroke who already take aspirin | Cilostazol (100 mg) twice daily vs placebo | Incidence of aspirin resistance, as per aspirin resistance unit (ARU) $\geq$550 after 4-wk treatment | No difference in aspirin resistance between groups | Cilostazol addition to aspirin did not prolong bleeding time |

(continued on next page)

**Table 1**
*(continued)*

*Aspirin vs Other Antiplatelet Therapies*

| Trial, Year | Purpose | Patient Population | Treatment Regimes | Primary End Point and Follow-Up | Outcome | Major Safety and Adverse Events |
|---|---|---|---|---|---|---|
| Zinkstok et al,[91] 2012 ARTIS | Compare early addition of intravenous aspirin + alteplase vs alteplase in reducing reocclusion in patients with acute ischemic stroke | 642 patients with acute ischemic stroke | Alteplase (0.9 mg/kg) alone vs alteplase (0.9 mg/kg) + aspirin (300 mg, intravenous) | Favorable outcome, defined as a score of 0–2 on the mRS at 3 mo | At 3 mo, patients in the aspirin group vs patients in the standard treatment group had a slightly favorable outcome | Trial terminated prematurely because of an excess of symptomatic intracranial hemorrhage events. This occurred significantly more often in the aspirin group than in the standard treatment group ($P = .04$) |
| Diener et al,[27] 2012 AVERROES (subgroup analysis) | Compare efficacy of apixaban vs aspirin in reducing stroke or systemic embolism | 5599 patients with previous stroke/TIA with atrial fibrillation who were at increased risk for stroke but unsuitable for vitamin K antagonist therapy | Apixaban (mg twice daily) vs aspirin (81–324 mg/d) | Stroke or systemic embolism; mean follow-up 1.1 y | Apixaban reduced the risk of stroke comparable with aspirin. Apixaban should be considered for the prevention of stroke when treating patients not suitable for vitamin K antagonist therapy | Bleeding complications were consistent with both treatment groups and more frequent in patients without a history of previous stroke |

| Study | Objective | Population | Intervention | Outcome measure | Results | Adverse events |
|---|---|---|---|---|---|---|
| Wang et al,[37] 2011 FISS-tris | Evaluate the efficacy and safety of LMWH vs aspirin in poststroke outcome | 353 patients with large artery occlusive disease | LMWH (nadroparin calcium 3800 antifactor Xa IU/0.4 mL twice daily) vs aspirin (160 mg/d) | Barthel Index Score dichotomized at 85, 6 mo after stroke | LMWH significantly improved outcome among patient >68 y of age over aspirin ($P = .043$), and with symptomatic posterior circulation arterial disease | None reported |
| Torgano et al,[92] 2010 | Compare efficacy of aspirin vs tirofiban in improving stroke outcome | 150 patients with stroke onset within 6 h; baseline NIHSS score of 5–25 | Aspirin (300 mg) daily by intravenous bolus for 3 d vs tirofiban (0.6 μg/kg/min) for 30 min followed by 0.15 μg/kg/min for 3 d | Proportion of patients with an NIHSS score reduction of ≥4 after 72 h; proportion of patients with mRS score of 0–1 at 3 mo | No difference between treatment groups | Rates of symptomatic intracranial hemorrhage were 1% (tirofiban) and 4% (aspirin); 3 mo mortality rate same for both groups (10.6%) |
| Hao et al,[38] 2008 | To determine the frequency of MES in LMWH vs aspirin treatment | 47 patients with large artery occlusive diseases from the FISS-tris study | LMWH (nadroparin calcium 3800 antifactor Xa IU/0.4 mL twice daily) vs aspirin (160 mg/d) for 10 d | MES detection by transcranial Doppler | No significant difference in frequency of MES between groups | None reported |
| Sprigg et al,[86] 2008 | To compare combination therapy of aspirin, clopidogrel, and dipyridamole vs aspirin alone | 17 patients with ischemic stroke or TIA within the past 5 y | Aspirin (75 mg) daily + clopidogrel (75 mg) daily + dipyridamole (200 mg) twice daily vs aspirin alone | Tolerability to treatment assessed as the number of patients completing randomized treatment | Long-term triple antiplatelet therapy was associated with a significant increase in adverse events and bleeding rates, and their severity, and a trend to increased discontinuations | One patient in the triple therapy group died of acute myeloid leukemia; bleeding events significantly increased in the triple therapy group |

*Abbreviations:* ERDP, extended release dypiridamole; LMWH, low molecular weight heparin; MES, microemboli signal; mRS, modified Rankin Scale; NIHSS, National Institutes of Health Stroke Scale; TIA, transient ischemic attack.

Patients who have Failed or are Unsuitable for Vitamin K Antagonist Treatment (AVERROES) trial, apixaban significantly reduced the risk of stroke or systemic embolism by half without increasing major bleeding or intracranial hemorrhage in patients with atrial fibrillation with at least 1 risk factor for stroke who had failed or were unsuitable for vitamin K antagonist therapy.[27,28]

Recurrent stroke prevention trials of combination therapy using aspirin and cilostazol or clopidogrel have not demonstrated greater effectiveness at reducing vascular events while increasing the occurrence of major bleeding complications.[29–34] However, the AHA suggests considering the addition of clopidogrel to aspirin to reduce the risk of major vascular events in patients with atrial fibrillation in whom oral anticoagulation with warfarin is considered unsuitable because of patient preference or the physician's assessment of the patient's ability to safely sustain anticoagulation.[35,36]

When pertaining to large-vessel stenoocclusive atherosclerotic cerebrovascular disease, a couple of acute treatment trials have tested anticoagulants against aspirin. A subgroup analysis of the Fraxiparin In Stroke Study for ischemic stroke (FISS-tris) concluded that low molecular weight heparin (LMWH) had improved stroke outcome compared with aspirin (160 mg/d) in patients with acute ischemic stroke and large-vessel occlusive disease who were older than 65 years of age.[37] However, another study reported no significant difference in the frequency of microemboli signal (MES) among patients with large-vessel occlusive disease given LMWH versus aspirin.[38] The Warfarin-Aspirin Symptomatic Intracranial Disease (WASID) study compared the efficacy of warfarin with aspirin for the prevention of major vascular events (ischemic stroke, MI, or sudden death) in patients with symptomatic stenosis of a major intracranial artery.[39] Warfarin is not considered superior to aspirin mainly because of increased risk of major hemorrhages. The Warfarin-Aspirin Recurrent Stroke Study (WARSS) examined whether warfarin is efficacious in preventing recurrent noncardioembolic ischemic strokes compared with aspirin. Although it was reported that both warfarin and aspirin can be regarded as reasonable therapeutic alternatives, the sample size was small and WARSS was neither designed nor powered to study equivalence. Thus, the WARSS trial could be interpreted as warfarin lacking superiority over aspirin, although this can only be generalized to patients with recent noncardioembolic ischemic stroke who do not have high-grade symptomatic cervical carotid stenosis.[40] Given all the findings and despite the advent of several newer antithrombotic agents, aspirin continues to be the number 1 prescribed antithrombotic agent for the prevention of recurrent stroke in patients with large-vessel disease.

### Clopidogrel

Clopidogrel is a prodrug with insufficient metabolism; only 15% of the drug reaches its target receptor after undergoing hepatic biotransformation by cytochrome (CY) P450 enzymes. Recently, several reports indicate that certain polymorphisms of CYP450s are associated with an excess of vascular events. Patients who are carriers of a loss of function of a CYP2C19 allele may have a reduced rate of converting clopidogrel to its active metabolite, resulting in decreased efficacy of the drug.[41] However, a recent analysis of 5059 patients with ACS or atrial fibrillation showed that response to clopidogrel compared with placebo was consistent irrespective of CYP2C19 loss-of-function carrier status.[42] Thus, it is possible that CYP2C19 variants do not directly alter the efficacy and safety of clopidogrel. Several drugs metabolized by the CYP450 pathway can compete with clopidogrel for metabolism, thereby, attenuating its antiplatelet activity. For example, data from a recent 2012 systemic review reported that proton pump inhibitors (PPIs) were found to reduce the efficacy of clopidogrel through competitive inhibition of CYP2C19 in 70% of laboratory studies examining healthy volunteers.[43] For patients, this was observed in 61% of studies.[43] However, data pertaining to clinical studies showed significant heterogeneity in observed outcomes. Thus, the clinical consequences of concomitant clopidogrel and PPI use remain controversial.[43]

The Clopidogrel versus Aspirin in Patients at Risk of Ischemic Events (CAPRIE) trial was 1 of the earliest clinical trials showing modest benefit in efficacy of clopidogrel over aspirin for the prevention of cardiovascular events in patients with a variety of atherothrombotic ischemic diseases including stroke.[44] Subsequently, the Clopidogrel in Unstable Angina to Prevent Recurrent Events (CURE) study was published a few years later demonstrating a reduction in MI in patients presenting with ACS with the addition of clopidogrel to aspirin.[16,45] However, subsequently, the Clopidogrel for High Atherothrombotic Risk and Ischemic Stabilization, Management and Avoidance (CHARISMA) study raised safety concerns of this strategy by reporting no benefit of combination therapy in the overall study population and increased bleeding risk.[46] Similar concerns had been raised by the Management of Atherothrombosis with Clopidogrel in High Risk Patients with Recent Transient Ischemic Attacks or Ischemic Stroke (MATCH trial).[47] The MATCH study failed to show that combination therapy of aspirin plus clopidogrel was more effective than clopidogrel alone in patients with a recent TIA or ischemic stroke. Furthermore, combination therapy was associated with increased frequency of major bleeding events than with monotherapy.

More recent randomized controlled trials comparing combination therapy with aspirin and clopidogrel with aspirin monotherapy for recurrent stroke prevention have not shown any consistent benefit despite similar bleeding rates to earlier studies (see **Table 1**). In patients with atrial fibrillation, more recent CHARISMA substudies reported no significant benefit of combination therapy of aspirin and clopidogrel.[48] In addition, combination therapy did not reduce the rate and functional severity of recurrent stroke at follow-up,[26] even when implemented early.[34,49] Comparisons of aspirin plus clopidogrel versus aspirin alone in patients with atrial fibrillation deemed unsuitable for warfarin, either because of risk of bleeding, physician judgment, or patient preference, was examined in the Atrial Fibrillation Clopidogrel Trial With Irbesartan for Prevention of Vascular Events-A (ACTIVE-A) study.[50] Although combination therapy reduced the rate of major vascular events compared with aspirin alone, any therapeutic benefit was hampered by a high incidence of systemic and intracranial hemorrhage. The ACTIVE-W trial assessed whether clopidogrel plus aspirin was noninferior to warfarin therapy for the prevention of vascular events.[51] Warfarin was found to be superior to clopidogrel plus aspirin for prevention of vascular events in patients with atrial fibrillation at high risk of stroke, especially in those already taking oral anticoagulation therapy. The same pattern of insignificant net benefit coupled with increased bleeding risk was also reported in the Stroke Prevention in Small Subcortical Stroke (SPS3) trial, in which more than 3020 patients with a recent lacunar stroke were randomized to the combination of clopidogrel with aspirin or aspirin alone.[52] Combination therapy was also found to increase mortality.

Patients with 70% to 99% intracranial arterial stenosis who have experienced a stroke or TIA in the past 30 days are at significantly increased risk of recurrent stroke.[53] Building on these findings, the Stenting versus Aggressive Medical Management for Preventing Recurrent stroke in Intracranial Stenosis (SAMMPRIS) study showed that combined used of aspirin and clopidogrel for 90 days followed by aspirin alone, coupled with intensive management of stroke risk factors, achieved impressive results in these high-risk patients.[54] The results were notable for a reduced rate of recurrent stroke and death in the medical arm group compared with the control group, suggesting that short-term combination therapy may be efficacious in these cases. However, it cannot be discounted that the lower-than-expected recurrent stroke rate may be attributed to aggressive treatment of hypertension and the use of statins in the medical arm group rather than the introduction of dual antiplatelet therapy.

Compared with other antiplatelet therapies, clopidogrel has not shown differences in rates of cerebral infarction, MI, and vascular death compared with ticlopidine or ticagrelor.[55,56] However, clopidogrel is better tolerated than ticlopidine, including fewer occurrences of hematologic disorders (leukopenia, neutropenia, thrombocytopenia) and hepatic dysfunction (increased alanine aminotransferase, aspartate aminotransferase, γ-glutamyl transpeptidase, and bilirubin levels). Compared with ticagrelor, no significant differences in bleeding rates for clopidogrel have been reported.

There is no evidence that clopidogrel doses higher than 75 mg daily decrease the risk of recurrent ischemic cerebrovascular events. After endovascular stent placement, clopidogrel is typically used at a maintenance dose of 75 mg daily. A conventional loading dose of 300 mg or more is commonly given, particularly in patients undergoing endovascular interventions. Mechanistic studies have demonstrated greater suppression of platelet aggregation with 900 mg and 600 mg loading doses, although absorption may be saturated at 600 mg.[57,58] For maintenance therapy, 2 studies have shown that doubling the dose from 75 mg to 150 mg daily increases platelet inhibition and reduce inflammation and endothelial dysfunction.[59,60] However, even at the typical dose of 75 mg, clopidogrel has been shown to decrease platelet activation markers (CD62P, CD63, CD40L) compared with aspirin.[61]

## Cilostazol

The first clinical trial examining the efficacy of cilostazol for stroke prevention was the Cilostazol Stroke Prevention Study (CSPS). Cilostazol was found to lower the rate of recurrent cerebral infarction without increasing the occurrence of cerebral hemorrhage compared with placebo.[62] In a subsequent CSPS subanalysis, cilostazol's benefit was particularly noted for diabetic patients who were at high risk for stroke recurrence.[63]

Subsequently,[18] the CSPS 2 study enrolled 2757 Japanese patients within 26 weeks of cerebral infarction who were randomized to be given either 81 mg aspirin daily or 100 mg cilostazol daily for up to 5 years.[29] The primary end point was the first occurrence of stroke (including cerebral infarction and intracranial hemorrhage). At a mean follow-up of 29 months, the yearly rates of recurrent stroke (infarction or hemorrhage) for cilostazol and aspirin were 2.7% and 3.7%, respectively. Furthermore, the annual rates of hemorrhagic events (intracerebral hemorrhage, subarachnoid hemorrhage, or other hemorrhage requiring hospitalization) were lower with cilostazol than with aspirin. The investigators concluded that cilostazol is noninferior and might be superior to aspirin for prevention of stroke after an ischemic stroke, and cilostazol was associated with fewer hemorrhagic events. In contrast, the Cilostazol in Acute Ischemic Stroke Treatment (CAIST) study showed no difference between cilostazol and aspirin in functional outcome, stroke recurrence, and bleeding risk in patients with recent ischemic stroke.[30] Furthermore, nonbleeding adverse events, with headache being the most common, were more common in patients treated with cilostazol similar to the CSPS 2 study. However, the frequency of drug discontinuation was not significant between groups.

The CSPS studies support the efficacy and safety of cilostazol for secondary stroke prevention only in selective populations. There remains limited to no high-quality data regarding the use of cilostazol for secondary stroke prevention in non-Asian ethnic groups. Future studies examining the safety and efficacy of cilostazol in non-Asian ethnic groups is warranted.

Clinical trials comparing aspirin with aspirin plus cilostazol are few and require further research. One pilot study reported that such combination therapy reduced neurologic deterioration with more favorable functional status than aspirin alone.[33] Another study reported that the addition of cilostazol to aspirin failed to reduce the frequency of aspirin resistance.[32] Indeed, such combination therapies are suggested in part to combat concerns of aspirin resistance. Such concerns were raised in part to the variable response of patients to the Dual Antiplatelet Therapy (DAPT) study. Data from meta-analyses conducted in the past 6 years suggest that 5% to 65% of patients could be hyporesponsive to aspirin, a phenomenon backed by biochemical evidence that these patients may experience persistent platelet activation in their bodies, as measured by platelet function tests. However, no standardized definition of such tests currently exists.[64] A few studies have attempted to quantify the clinical and pharmacologic resistance of aspirin, but the reported data are hampered by internal and external validity concerns including small sample sizes, lack of agreement between different platelet function tests, different dose regimens and nonadherence, and insufficient information about measurement stability over time. Because of its multifactorial nature and the absence of a general consensus regarding how to treat patients with this phenomenon, there is currently no indication to screen patients for aspirin resistance.

### Aspirin + Extended Release Dypiridamole

The combination of low-dose aspirin and extended release dypiridamole (ERDP) has been available for more than a decade. Studies comparing this combination with aspirin alone for recurrent stroke prevention have reported relative risk reductions of 20% to 23% for stroke prevention.[10,65,66] The European/Australian Stroke Prevention in Reversible Ischaemia Trial (ESPRIT) and European Stroke Prevention Study 2 (ESPS-2) trials reported similar benefits for combination therapy over aspirin amongst patients with a wide range of stroke severity.[10,65,66] However, the more recently published Japanese Aggrenox Stroke Prevention versus Aspirin Programme (JASAP) reported no benefit for aspirin plus ERDP over aspirin alone in Japanese patients with recent noncardioembolic ischemic stroke (see **Table 1**).[67] The EARLY trial reported no benefit in early initiation of aspirin plus ERDP within 7 days after stroke compared with aspirin alone.[68] Although the early initiation group had fewer recurrent cerebrovascular events overall, the results were nonsignificant.

The effectiveness of aspirin plus ERDP has also been compared with that of clopidogrel. The Prevention Regimen for Effectively Avoiding Second Strokes (PRoFESS) study[47,48] randomized 20,332 patients within less than 90 days of ischemic stroke onset to aspirin plus ERDP or clopidogrel.[69,70] No difference in the rate of recurrent strokes was found between the groups and a slightly higher rate of intracranial bleeding events was seen in the aspirin plus ERDP group. In addition, higher rates of discontinuation because of headaches, gastrointestinal side effects, and other side effects were associated with aspirin plus ERDP.

There is conflicting evidence between the results of the CAPRIE, ESPRIT and ESPS-2, and PRoFESS studies. Because aspirin plus ERDP was shown to be substantially more effective than aspirin alone in ESPRIT and ESPS-2, and clopidogrel was only slightly more effective than aspirin in CAPRIE, indirect comparison suggested that aspirin plus ERDP should be more effective than clopidogrel for recurrent stroke prevention. However, this was not the case in the PRoFESS study and underscores the need for direct comparisons in head-to-head randomized clinical trials before making assertions about comparative effectiveness.

### Ticagrelor

Ticagrelor is an oral cyclopentyl-triazolo-pyrimidine that is a direct reversible inhibitor of the P2Y12 receptor. Compared with clopidogrel, ticagrelor is a newer P2Y12 inhibiting antiplatelet agent with a more favorable pharmacokinetic and pharmacodynamic profile. There have been no reported influences on its effects by genetic polymorphisms to date. Previously, varying effects on platelet inhibition have been noted with clopidogrel use because its metabolism requires biotransformation of the CYP enzymes where several genetic variants have been discovered. In contrast, ticagrelor does not undergo CYP biotransformation but acts as a direct ADP antagonist.[71,72]

The Platelet Inhibition and Patient Outcomes (PLATO) study was one of the first clinical trials that examined the effectiveness of ticagrelor in the prevention of vascular events.[73] In PLATO, 18,624 patients with ACS were randomly assigned to receive ticagrelor (180 mg loading does followed by 90 mg twice daily) or clopidogrel (300–600 mg loading dose, followed by 75 mg daily) against a background of aspirin therapy. Ticagrelor was superior to clopidogrel for the prevention of cardiovascular death, MI, or stroke without increasing overall major bleeding. However, ticagrelor was associated with more intracranial bleeding, including fatal intracranial bleeding. Patients with a previous history of stroke or TIAs had a lower relative risk reduction of recurrent ischemic events in the ticagrelor group. Conversely, a 50% relative risk reduction in mortality was reported for those randomized to ticagrelor compared with clopidogrel among those undergoing coronary artery bypass graft (CABG) surgery.[74] Given its reversible affinity for the P2Y12 receptor, it is possible that ticagrelor might redistribute to new platelets that enter the circulation before administration of the next dose, accounting for its comparative benefits.

However, ticagrelor is associated with bradyarrythmias and dyspnea and decreased creatinine and uric acid clearance. The PLATO study also reported that the ticagrelor arm had significantly more cases of intracranial bleeding compared with the clopidogrel arm. Ticagrelor presented with a better efficacy and safety profile in European test centers compared with US centers, leading to its approval by the European Commission in 2010. In contrast, the US Food and Drug Administration postponed its approval to better understand why these differences in data existed between European and US centers. It was theorized that the inconsistency was in part due to the aspirin dose: the median dose of aspirin in the US patients was 325 mg daily compared with 100 mg daily in the non-US patients. Patients treated with 100 mg or less of aspirin had a better outcome on ticagrelor compared with patients taking 300 mg or more. With this new knowledge in mind, ticagrelor was finally approved in the United States in July 2011, with an indication to reduce the rate of thrombotic cardiovascular events in patients with ACS. When coadministered with aspirin, low doses no greater than 100 mg are recommended. A subgroup analysis of the PLATO study that included 1152 patients with history of stroke or TIAs reported a net benefit of ticagrelor over clopidogrel for the prevention of recurrent vascular event and reduced mortality.[56] Currently, ticagrelor is not recommended for the sole purpose of stroke prevention.

### NOVEL ANTIPLATELET AGENTS

Although aspirin, clopidogrel, and the combination of aspirin plus ERDP are the only FDA-approved medications for recurrent stroke prevention after noncardioembolic stroke and are commonly prescribed, potential serious adverse effects, the existence of genetic polymorphisms that adversely influence effects, and limited overall benefits create a need for more efficacious therapies. Potential novel candidate agents are described in this section.

## Prasugrel

As mentioned previously, newer P2Y12 antiplatelet therapies are more favorable than clopidogrel because they do not seem to be affected by any known genetic polymorphism. Prasugrel is an irreversible thienopyridine that is efficiently metabolized and offers more rapid, consistent, and robust platelet inhibition with less interindividual variability than clopidogrel.[75] The Trial to Assess Improvement in Therapeutic Outcomes by Optimizing Platelet Inhibition with Prasugrel Thrombolysis in Myocardial Infarction (TRITON-TIMI 38) was a head-to-head comparative trial of prasugrel (60 mg loading dose followed by 10 mg per day) versus clopidogrel (300 mg loading dose followed by 75 mg per day) in patients with ACS undergoing revascularization.[76] During 15 months of follow-up, prasugrel was found to have a 19% relative risk reduction ($P<.001$) in death, nonfatal MI, or stroke compared with clopidogrel, although this came at the expense of more life-threatening major and fatal bleeding in non-CABG patients. However, intracranial bleeding was not increased significantly with prasugrel.

However, there is a practical concern that limits the uniform use of prasugrel in all patients presenting with ACS. Among the patients in the TRITON-TIMI study, the rate of major bleeding in the prasugrel group was more than 4 times that in the clopidogrel group (13.4% vs 3.2%) for those undergoing CABG surgery. Thus, prasugrel should be discontinued at least 7 days before the planned CABG surgery. Moreover, the elderly (age >75 years) and those who are underweight (<60 kg) may be at highest risk for bleeding. Prasugrel is approved in Europe and the United States for patients with ACS undergoing percutaneous coronary intervention procedures. Prasugrel is contraindicated in patients with a previous history of stroke or TIAs.

## Cangrelor

Cangrelor and elinogrel are also novel P2Y12 inhibitors that have been compared with clopidogrel. Cangrelor is an ATP analogue that directly and reversibly inhibits the receptor within minutes after infusion. However, the Cangrelor versus Standard Therapy to Achieve Optimal Management of Platelet Inhibition (CHAMPION) study failed to report the drug to be more efficacious than clopidogrel at reducing incidences of death, MI, or revascularization at 48 hours in patients with ACS who were undergoing percutaneous coronary intervention (PCI).[77] Elinogrel is a direct, reversible, competitive inhibitor of the P2Y12 receptor. Compared with clopidogrel (300–600 mg loading dose followed by 75 mg per day maintenance), elinogrel (120 mg bolus/100 mg twice daily or 120 mg bolus/150 mg twice-daily maintenance) was found to have more robust and rapid platelet inhibitory activity with comparable clinical effectiveness in 652 randomized patients undergoing PCI.[78] In addition, no excess major bleeding was reported with elinogrel. These agents may be of interest in future clinical trials evaluating their efficacy for stroke prevention.

## Triflusal

Triflusal is a newer COX-1 inhibitor that is currently under investigation. Previously, it has demonstrated similar efficacy to aspirin for the prevention of recurrent vascular events in patients with previous MI or stroke, with less intracerebral bleeding.[79] The Comparison of Triflusal and Clopidogrel Effect in Secondary Prevention of Stroke Based on the Cytochrome P450 2C19 Genotyping (MAESTRO) trial is an ongoing clinical trial comparing the effectiveness of triflusal with clopidogrel for recurrent stroke prevention among patients with CYP2C19 polymorphisms. Triflusal is not currently approved for use in the United States.

## Sarpogrelate

Another novel agent is sarpogrelate, an antiplatelet agent that decreases 5-hydroxy-tryptamine (5-HT) levels in platelets via blockade of 5-HT2 receptors, and has been studied in patients with peripheral arterial disease.[80] One clinical trial previously performed a double-blind, controlled, clinical study to investigate the antiplatelet efficacy of sarpogrelate in patients with ischemic stroke. Forty-seven patients with cerebral infarction were given sarpogrelate 3 times daily in doses of 15, 25, or 100 mg for 7 days to evaluate its dose-response effects on platelet aggregation.[81] The investigators concluded that sarpogrelate treatment inhibited platelet aggregation dose dependently in patients with ischemic stroke, with the greatest effect on platelet aggregation observed in those receiving 100 mg. Shortly after, the Sarpogrelate-Aspirin Comparative Clinical Study for Efficacy and Safety in Secondary Prevention of Cerebral Infarction (S-ACCESS), a randomized double-blind trial, compared the relative efficacy of sarpogrelate (100 mg 3 times daily) to aspirin (81 mg once daily) in 1510 patients with recent cerebral infarction.[82] Patients were followed for 0.9 to 3.5 years. The primary end point was recurrent stroke and relative safety. The investigators reported that sarpogrelate was not noninferior to aspirin for prevention of recurrence of cerebral infarction, and bleeding events were significantly fewer with sarpogrelate than with aspirin (11.9% vs 17.3%, respectively).

## Vorapaxar and Atopaxar

A novel class of antiplatelet therapy is under development. Vorapaxar (previously SCH-530348) and atopaxar (previously E5555) are 2 investigational, protease-activated, receptor 1 (PAR-1) antagonists that selectively target thrombin-induced platelet activation, the most potent pathway in platelet aggregation. Vorapaxar was under investigation in 1 phase III trial in patients with ACS.[83] The addition of vorapaxar versus placebo to standard therapy did not significantly reduce the primary end points of death from cardiovascular causes, MI, stroke, recurrent ischemia with rehospitalization, or urgent coronary revascularization. Furthermore, vorapaxar increased the risk of intracranial bleeding, halting the clinical trial in January 2011. Atopaxar has demonstrated rapid-onset antiplatelet activity and fewer ischemic events without increasing major bleeding compared with placebo.[84] Clinical trials will be necessary to determine the role, if any, in recurrent stroke prevention of all novel agents before they are approved for this use.

## ONGOING CLINICAL TRIALS

There are several ongoing trials investigating available antiplatelet agents as well as novel therapies for stroke prevention. The Triple Antiplatelets for Reducing Dependency After Ischaemic Stroke (TARDIS) study aims to examine if triple antiplatelet therapy of aspirin, clopidogrel and dipyridamole will be more effective than aspirin plus dipyridamole in patients at high risk for stroke recurrence.[85] A previous study had examined the same combination of triple antiplatelet therapy in 17 patients (see **Table 1**). Triple therapy was found to be associated with more severe adverse events including bleeding compared with aspirin alone.[86]

Other studies aim to determine whether or not adding anticoagulant agents to current antiplatelet therapies is more efficacious than antiplatelet therapy alone. For example, The Warfarin and Antiplatelet Vascular Evaluation (WAVE) study is an international, multicenter, randomized clinical trial comparing moderate-intensity warfarin (target internationalized normalized ratio of 2.4–3.0) added to antiplatelet therapy with antiplatelet therapy alone in reducing serious cardiovascular events. The study targets patients at high risk for peripheral vascular disease.[87]

Cilostazol is being studied in the Preventlon of CArdiovascular Events in iSchemic Stroke Patients With High Risk of Cerebral HemOrrhage (PICASSO) study where investigators are set to test the hypothesis that cilostazol alone or with probucol, an antihyperlipidemic drug that lowers the level of cholesterol in the bloodstream by increasing the rate of low-density lipoprotein catabolism, will reduce the risk of cerebral hemorrhage without similar ischemic cardiovascular events compared with aspirin in patients with recent ischemic stroke and evidence of previous symptomatic or asymptomatic cerebral hemorrhage.[88] Other studies include the Clopidogrel and the Optimization of Gastrointestinal Events (COGENT-1) trial developed to determine whether clopidogrel plus omeprazole compared with clopidogrel alone is safe and effective in reducing gastrointestinal bleeding and symptomatic peptic ulcer disease in the setting of concomitant aspirin therapy.[89] In the Second Prevention Trial for Ischemic Stroke With Deng Zhan ShengMai Capsule (SPIRIT-DZSM-1), the investigators seek to determine the preventative effect of the Deng Zhan ShengMai capsule on stroke recurrence, cardiovascular events, and peripheral arterial events.[90]

---

**Case study**

A 55-year-old woman with a history of diabetes and hypertension presented with a chief complaint of a stuttering onset of sensory loss over the right side of her face, arm, and leg that started 6 hours ago. She had no loss of motor function except that she could not hold objects with her right hand. On examination, blood pressure was 150/94 mm Hg, pulse 72 bpm, no cardiac murmur or bruits in her neck. Her speech and language functions were normal. There was no motor weakness or abnormal muscle stretch reflexes. Sensation was diminished to a pin on the right side of her face, arm, and leg. Magnetic resonance imaging of the brain showed restricted diffusion of the right thalamus. Magnetic resonance angiography of the extracranial and extracranial circulation were unremarkable. An echocardiogram showed left ventricular hypertrophy. She was given 325 mg of aspirin within 12 hours of onset of symptoms. She was offered participation in a clinical trial evaluating the benefit of aspirin + clopidogrel versus aspirin + placebo but she refused.

---

## REFERENCES

1. Kohda N, Tani T, Nakayama S, et al. Effect of cilostazol, a phosphodiesterase III inhibitor, on experimental thrombosis in the porcine carotid artery. Thromb Res 1999;96(4):261–8.
2. Tanaka K, Gotoh F, Fukuuchi Y, et al. Effects of a selective inhibitor of cyclic AMP phosphodiesterase on the pial microcirculation in feline cerebral ischemia. Stroke 1989;20(5):668–73.
3. Kim KY, Shin HK, Choi JM, et al. Inhibition of lipopolysaccharide-induced apoptosis by cilostazol in human umbilical vein endothelial cells. J Pharmacol Exp Ther 2002;300(2):709–15.
4. Tani T, Uehara K, Sudo T, et al. Cilostazol, a selective type III phosphodiesterase inhibitor, decreases triglyceride and increases HDL cholesterol levels by increasing lipoprotein lipase activity in rats. Atherosclerosis 2000;152(2):299–305.

5. Baigent C, Blackwell L, Collins R, et al. Aspirin in the primary and secondary prevention of vascular disease: collaborative meta-analysis of individual participant data from randomised trials. Lancet 2009;373(9678):1849–60.
6. Bartolucci AA, Tendera M, Howard G. Meta-analysis of multiple primary prevention trials of cardiovascular events using aspirin. Am J Cardiol 2011;107(12):1796–801.
7. A comparison of two doses of aspirin (30 mg vs 283 mg a day) in patients after a transient ischemic attack or minor ischemic stroke. The Dutch TIA Trial Study Group. N Engl J Med 1991;325(18):1261–6.
8. Swedish Aspirin Low-Dose Trial (SALT) of 75 mg aspirin as secondary prophylaxis after cerebrovascular ischaemic events. The SALT Collaborative Group. Lancet 1991;338(8779):1345–9.
9. Antithrombotic Trialists' Collaboration. Collaborative meta-analysis of randomised trials of antiplatelet therapy for prevention of death, myocardial infarction, and stroke in high risk patients. BMJ 2002;324(7329):71–86.
10. Diener HC, Cunha L, Forbes C, et al. European Stroke Prevention Study. 2. Dipyridamole and acetylsalicylic acid in the secondary prevention of stroke. J Neurol Sci 1996;143(1–2):1–13.
11. Sze PC, Reitman D, Pincus MM, et al. Antiplatelet agents in the secondary prevention of stroke: meta-analysis of the randomized control trials. Stroke 1988;19(4):436–42.
12. Berger JS, Brown DL, Burke GL, et al. Aspirin use, dose, and clinical outcomes in postmenopausal women with stable cardiovascular disease: the Women's Health Initiative Observational Study. Circ Cardiovasc Qual Outcomes 2009;2(2):78–87.
13. Steinhubl SR, Bhatt DL, Brennan DM, et al. Aspirin to prevent cardiovascular disease: the association of aspirin dose and clopidogrel with thrombosis and bleeding. Ann Intern Med 2009;150(6):379–86.
14. Jolly SS, Pogue J, Haladyn K, et al. Effects of aspirin dose on ischaemic events and bleeding after percutaneous coronary intervention: insights from the PCI-CURE study. Eur Heart J 2009;30(8):900–7.
15. Joyal D, Freihage JH, Cohoon K, et al. The influence of low (81 mg) versus high (325 mg) doses of ASA on the incidence of sirolimus-eluting stent thrombosis. J Invasive Cardiol 2007;19(7):291–4.
16. Peters RJ, Mehta SR, Fox KA, et al. Effects of aspirin dose when used alone or in combination with clopidogrel in patients with acute coronary syndromes: observations from the Clopidogrel in Unstable angina to prevent Recurrent Events (CURE) study. Circulation 2003;108(14):1682–7.
17. Topol EJ, Easton D, Harrington RA, et al. Randomized, double-blind, placebo-controlled, international trial of the oral IIb/IIIa antagonist lotrafiban in coronary and cerebrovascular disease. Circulation 2003;108(4):399–406.
18. Mehta SR, Tanguay JF, Eikelboom JW, et al. Double-dose versus standard-dose clopidogrel and high-dose versus low-dose aspirin in individuals undergoing percutaneous coronary intervention for acute coronary syndromes (CURRENT-OASIS 7): a randomised factorial trial. Lancet 2010;376(9748):1233–43.
19. Massie BM, Collins JF, Ammon SE, et al. Randomized trial of warfarin, aspirin, and clopidogrel in patients with chronic heart failure: the Warfarin and Antiplatelet Therapy in Chronic Heart Failure (WATCH) trial. Circulation 2009;119(12):1616–24.
20. Pullicino P, Thompson JL, Barton B, et al. Warfarin versus aspirin in patients with reduced cardiac ejection fraction (WARCEF): rationale, objectives, and design. J Card Fail 2006;12(1):39–46.

21. Homma S, Thompson JL, Pullicino PM, et al. Warfarin and aspirin in patients with heart failure and sinus rhythm. N Engl J Med 2012;366(20):1859–69.
22. Kumar G, Goyal MK. Warfarin versus aspirin for prevention of stroke in heart failure: a meta-analysis of randomized controlled clinical trials. J Stroke Cerebrovasc Dis 2012. http://dx.doi.org/10.1016/j.jstrokecerebrovasdis.2012.09.015.
23. Stroke Risk in Atrial Fibrillation Working Group. Independent predictors of stroke in patients with atrial fibrillation: a systematic review. Neurology 2007;69(6):546–54.
24. Hart RG, Pearce LA, Aguilar MI. Meta-analysis: antithrombotic therapy to prevent stroke in patients who have nonvalvular atrial fibrillation. Ann Intern Med 2007;146(12):857–67.
25. Wann LS, Curtis AB, January CT, et al. 2011 ACCF/AHA/HRS focused update on the management of patients with atrial fibrillation (updating the 2006 guideline): a report of the American College of Cardiology Foundation/American Heart Association Task Force on Practice Guidelines. J Am Coll Cardiol 2011;57(2):223–42.
26. Mant J, Hobbs FD, Fletcher K, et al. Warfarin versus aspirin for stroke prevention in an elderly community population with atrial fibrillation (the Birmingham Atrial Fibrillation Treatment of the Aged Study, BAFTA): a randomised controlled trial. Lancet 2007;370(9586):493–503.
27. Diener HC, Eikelboom J, Connolly SJ, et al. Apixaban versus aspirin in patients with atrial fibrillation and previous stroke or transient ischaemic attack: a predefined subgroup analysis from AVERROES, a randomised trial. Lancet Neurol 2012;11(3):225–31.
28. Connolly SJ, Eikelboom J, Joyner C, et al. Apixaban in patients with atrial fibrillation. N Engl J Med 2011;364(9):806–17.
29. Shinohara Y, Katayama Y, Uchiyama S, et al. Cilostazol for prevention of secondary stroke (CSPS 2): an aspirin-controlled, double-blind, randomised non-inferiority trial. Lancet Neurol 2010;9(10):959–68.
30. Lee YS, Bae HJ, Kang DW, et al. Cilostazol in Acute Ischemic Stroke Treatment (CAIST Trial): a randomized double-blind non-inferiority trial. Cerebrovasc Dis 2011;32(1):65–71.
31. Guo JJ, Xu E, Lin QY, et al. Effect of cilostazol on cerebral arteries in secondary prevention of ischemic stroke. Neurosci Bull 2009;25(6):383–90.
32. Lee JH, Cha JK, Lee SJ, et al. Addition of cilostazol reduces biological aspirin resistance in aspirin users with ischaemic stroke: a double-blind randomized clinical trial. Eur J Neurol 2010;17(3):434–42.
33. Nakamura T, Tsuruta S, Uchiyama S. Cilostazol combined with aspirin prevents early neurological deterioration in patients with acute ischemic stroke: a pilot study. J Neurol Sci 2012;313(1–2):22–6.
34. Hankey GJ, Johnston SC, Easton JD, et al. Effect of clopidogrel plus ASA vs ASA early after TIA and ischaemic stroke: a substudy of the CHARISMA trial. Int J Stroke 2011;6(1):3–9.
35. Fuster V, Rydén LE, Cannom DS, et al. ACC/AHA/ESC 2006 guidelines for the management of patients with atrial fibrillation: a report of the American College of Cardiology/American Heart Association Task Force on Practice Guidelines and the European Society of Cardiology Committee for Practice Guidelines (Writing Committee to Revise the 2001 Guidelines for the Management of Patients With Atrial Fibrillation): developed in collaboration with the European Heart Rhythm Association and the Heart Rhythm Society. Circulation 2006;114(7):e257–354.

36. Wann LS, Curtis AB, January CT, et al. 2011 ACCF/AHA/HRS focused update on the management of patients with atrial fibrillation (updating the 2006 guideline): a report of the American College of Cardiology Foundation/American Heart Association Task Force on Practice Guidelines. Circulation 2011;123(1):104–23.

37. Wang QS, Chen C, Chen XY, et al. Low-molecular-weight heparin versus aspirin for acute ischemic stroke with large artery occlusive disease: subgroup analyses from the Fraxiparin in Stroke Study for the treatment of ischemic stroke (FISS-tris) study. Stroke 2012;43(2):346–9.

38. Hao Q, Chang HM, Wong MC, et al. Frequency of microemboli signal in stroke patients treated with low molecular weight heparin or aspirin. J Neuroimaging 2008;20(2):118–21.

39. Chimowitz MI, Kokkinos J, Strong J, et al. The Warfarin-Aspirin Symptomatic Intracranial Disease Study. Neurology 1995;45(8):1488–93.

40. Hankey GJ. Warfarin-Aspirin Recurrent Stroke Study (WARSS) trial: is warfarin really a reasonable therapeutic alternative to aspirin for preventing recurrent noncardioembolic ischemic stroke? Stroke 2002;33(6):1723–6.

41. Shuldiner AR, O'Connell JR, Bliden KP, et al. Association of cytochrome P450 2C19 genotype with the antiplatelet effect and clinical efficacy of clopidogrel therapy. JAMA 2009;302(8):849–57.

42. Paré G, Mehta SR, Yusuf S, et al. Effects of CYP2C19 genotype on outcomes of clopidogrel treatment. N Engl J Med 2010;363(18):1704–14.

43. Jaspers Focks J, Brouwer MA, van Oijen MG, et al. Concomitant use of clopidogrel and proton pump inhibitors: impact on platelet function and clinical outcome- a systematic review. Heart 2013;99(8):520–7.

44. CAPRIE Steering Committee. A randomised, blinded, trial of clopidogrel versus aspirin in patients at risk of ischaemic events (CAPRIE). CAPRIE Steering Committee. Lancet 1996;348(9038):1329–39.

45. Mehta SR, Yusuf S, Peters RJ, et al. Effects of pretreatment with clopidogrel and aspirin followed by long-term therapy in patients undergoing percutaneous coronary intervention: the PCI-CURE study. Lancet 2001;358(9281):527–33.

46. Bhatt DL, Topol EJ. Clopidogrel added to aspirin versus aspirin alone in secondary prevention and high risk primary prevention: rationale and design of the Clopidogrel for High Atherothrombotic Risk and Ischemic Stabilization, Management, and Avoidance (CHARISMA) trial. Am Heart J 2004;148(2):263–8.

47. Diener HC, Bogousslavsky J, Brass LM, et al. Aspirin and clopidogrel compared with clopidogrel alone after recent ischaemic stroke or transient ischaemic attack in high-risk patients (MATCH): randomised, double-blind, placebo-controlled trial. Lancet 2004;364(9431):331–7.

48. Hart RG, Bhatt DL, Hacke W, et al. Clopidogrel and aspirin versus aspirin alone for the prevention of stroke in patients with a history of atrial fibrillation: subgroup analysis of the CHARISMA randomized trial. Cerebrovasc Dis 2008;25(4):344–7.

49. Hankey GJ, Hacke W, Easton JD, et al. Effect of clopidogrel on the rate and functional severity of stroke among high vascular risk patients: a prespecified substudy of the Clopidogrel for High Atherothrombotic Risk and Ischemic Stabilization, Management and Avoidance (CHARISMA) trial. Stroke 2010;41(8): 1679–83.

50. ACTIVE Investigators, Connolly SJ, Pogue J, Hart RG, et al. Effect of clopidogrel added to aspirin in patients with atrial fibrillation. N Engl J Med 2009;360(20): 2066–78.

51. ACTIVE Writing Group of the ACTIVE Investigators, Connolly S, Pogue J, Hart R, et al. Clopidogrel plus aspirin versus oral anticoagulation for atrial fibrillation in

the Atrial fibrillation Clopidogrel Trial with Irbesartan for prevention of Vascular Events (ACTIVE W): a randomised controlled trial. Lancet 2006;367(9526): 1903–12.

52. SPS3 Investigators, Benavente OR, Hart RG, McClure LA, et al. Effects of clopidogrel added to aspirin in patients with recent lacunar stroke. N Engl J Med 2012;367(9):817–25.

53. Chimowitz MI, Lynn MJ, Howlett-Smith H, et al. Comparison of warfarin and aspirin for symptomatic intracranial arterial stenosis. N Engl J Med 2005; 352(13):1305–16.

54. Chimowitz MI, Lynn MJ, Derdeyn CP, et al. Stenting versus aggressive medical therapy for intracranial arterial stenosis [Erratum appears in N Engl J Med 2012;367(1):93]. N Engl J Med 2011;365(11):993–1003.

55. Uchiyama S, Fukuuchi Y, Yamaguchi T. The safety and efficacy of clopidogrel versus ticlopidine in Japanese stroke patients: combined results of two phase III, multicenter, randomized clinical trials. J Neurol 2009;256(6):888–97.

56. James SK, Storey RF, Khurmi NS, et al, PLATO Study Group. Ticagrelor versus clopidogrel in patients with acute coronary syndromes and a history of stroke or transient ischemic attack. Circulation 2012;125(23):2914–21.

57. von Beckerath N, Taubert D, Pogatsa-Murray G, et al. Absorption, metabolization, and antiplatelet effects of 300-, 600-, and 900-mg loading doses of clopidogrel: results of the ISAR-CHOICE (Intracoronary stenting and antithrombotic regimen: choose between 3 high oral doses for immediate clopidogrel effect) Trial. Circulation 2005;112(19):2946–50.

58. Patti G, Colonna G, Pasceri V, et al. Randomized trial of high loading dose of clopidogrel for reduction of periprocedural myocardial infarction in patients undergoing coronary intervention: results from the ARMYDA-2 (Antiplatelet therapy for Reduction of MYocardial Damage during Angioplasty) study. Circulation 2005;111(16):2099–106.

59. Patti G, Grieco D, Dicuonzo G, et al. High versus standard clopidogrel maintenance dose after percutaneous coronary intervention and effects on platelet inhibition, endothelial function, and inflammation results of the ARMYDA-150 mg (antiplatelet therapy for reduction of myocardial damage during angioplasty) randomized study. J Am Coll Cardiol 2011;57(7):771–8.

60. von Beckerath N, Kastrati A, Wieczorek A, et al. A double-blind, randomized study on platelet aggregation in patients treated with a daily dose of 150 or 75 mg of clopidogrel for 30 days. Eur Heart J 2007;28(15):1814–9.

61. Tsai NW, Chang WN, Shaw CF, et al. Serial change in platelet activation markers with aspirin and clopidogrel after acute ischemic stroke. Clin Neuropharmacol 2010;33(1):40–5.

62. Gotoh F, et al. Cilostazol stroke prevention study: a placebo-controlled double-blind trial for secondary prevention of cerebral infarction. J Stroke Cerebrovasc Dis 2000;9(4):147–57.

63. Shinohara Y, Gotoh F, Tohgi H, et al. Antiplatelet cilostazol is beneficial in diabetic and/or hypertensive ischemic stroke patients. Subgroup analysis of the cilostazol stroke prevention study. Cerebrovasc Dis 2008;26(1):63–70.

64. Krasopoulos G, Brister SJ, Beattie WS, et al. Aspirin "resistance" and risk of cardiovascular morbidity: systematic review and meta-analysis. BMJ 2008; 336(7637):195–8.

65. Halkes PH, van Gijn J, Kappelle LJ, et al. Aspirin plus dipyridamole versus aspirin alone after cerebral ischaemia of arterial origin (ESPRIT): randomised controlled trial. Lancet 2006;367(9523):1665–73.

66. Halkes PH, van Gijn J, Kappelle LJ, et al. Medium intensity oral anticoagulants versus aspirin after cerebral ischaemia of arterial origin (ESPRIT): a randomised controlled trial. Lancet Neurol 2007;6(2):115–24.

67. Uchiyama S, Ikeda Y, Urano Y, et al. The Japanese aggrenox (extended-release dipyridamole plus aspirin) stroke prevention versus aspirin programme (JASAP) study: a randomized, double-blind, controlled trial. Cerebrovasc Dis 2011;31(6): 601–13.

68. Dengler R, Diener HC, Schwartz A, et al. Early treatment with aspirin plus extended-release dipyridamole for transient ischaemic attack or ischaemic stroke within 24 h of symptom onset (EARLY trial): a randomised, open-label, blinded-endpoint trial. Lancet Neurol 2010;9(2):159–66.

69. Diener HC, Sacco RL, Yusuf S, et al. Effects of aspirin plus extended-release dipyridamole versus clopidogrel and telmisartan on disability and cognitive function after recurrent stroke in patients with ischaemic stroke in the Prevention Regimen for Effectively Avoiding Second Strokes (PRoFESS) trial: a double-blind, active and placebo-controlled study. Lancet Neurol 2008;7(10): 875–84.

70. Sacco RL, Diener HC, Yusuf S, et al. Aspirin and extended-release dipyridamole versus clopidogrel for recurrent stroke. N Engl J Med 2008;359(12):1238–51.

71. Mega JL, Close SL, Wiviott SD, et al. Genetic variants in ABCB1 and CYP2C19 and cardiovascular outcomes after treatment with clopidogrel and prasugrel in the TRITON-TIMI 38 trial: a pharmacogenetic analysis. Lancet 2010;376(9749): 1312–9.

72. Wallentin L, James S, Storey RF, et al. Effect of CYP2C19 and ABCB1 single nucleotide polymorphisms on outcomes of treatment with ticagrelor versus clopidogrel for acute coronary syndromes: a genetic substudy of the PLATO trial. Lancet 2010;376(9749):1320–8.

73. Cannon CP, Harrington RA, James S, et al. Comparison of ticagrelor with clopidogrel in patients with a planned invasive strategy for acute coronary syndromes (PLATO): a randomised double-blind study. Lancet 2010;375(9711): 283–93.

74. Held C, Asenblad N, Bassand JP, et al. Ticagrelor versus clopidogrel in patients with acute coronary syndromes undergoing coronary artery bypass surgery: results from the PLATO (Platelet Inhibition and Patient Outcomes) trial. J Am Coll Cardiol 2010;57(6):672–84.

75. Bhatt DL. Intensifying platelet inhibition–navigating between Scylla and Charybdis. N Engl J Med 2007;357(20):2078–81.

76. Wiviott SD, Braunwald E, McCabe CH, et al. Prasugrel versus clopidogrel in patients with acute coronary syndromes. N Engl J Med 2007;357(20):2001–15.

77. Bhatt DL, Lincoff AM, Gibson CM, et al. Intravenous platelet blockade with cangrelor during PCI. N Engl J Med 2009;361(24):2330–41.

78. Leonardi S, Rao SV, Harrington RA, et al. Rationale and design of the randomized, double-blind trial testing INtraveNous and Oral administration of elinogrel, a selective and reversible P2Y(12)-receptor inhibitor, versus clopidogrel to eVAluate Tolerability and Efficacy in nonurgent Percutaneous Coronary Interventions patients (INNOVATE-PCI). Am Heart J 2010;160(1):65–72.

79. Costa J, Ferro JM, Matias-Guiu J, et al. Triflusal for preventing serious vascular events in people at high risk. Stroke 2006. [Epub ahead of print].

80. Miyazaki M, Higashi Y, Goto C, et al. Sarpogrelate hydrochloride, a selective 5-HT2A antagonist, improves vascular function in patients with peripheral arterial disease. J Cardiovasc Pharmacol 2007;49(4):221–7.

81. Uchiyama S, Ozaki Y, Satoh K, et al. Effect of sarpogrelate, a 5-HT(2A) antagonist, on platelet aggregation in patients with ischemic stroke: clinical-pharmacological dose-response study. Cerebrovasc Dis 2007;24(2–3):264–70.

82. Shinohara Y, Nishimaru K, Sawada T, et al. Sarpogrelate-Aspirin Comparative Clinical Study for Efficacy and Safety in Secondary Prevention of Cerebral Infarction (S-ACCESS): a randomized, double-blind, aspirin-controlled trial. Stroke 2008;39(6):1827–33.

83. Tricoci P, Huang Z, Held C, et al. Thrombin-receptor antagonist vorapaxar in acute coronary syndromes. N Engl J Med 2012;366(1):20–33.

84. O'Donoghue ML, Bhatt DL, Wiviott SD, et al. Safety and tolerability of atopaxar in the treatment of patients with acute coronary syndromes: the lessons from antagonizing the cellular effects of Thrombin–Acute Coronary Syndromes Trial. Circulation 2011;123(17):1843–53.

85. Bath P. Triple Antiplatelets for Reducing Dependency after Ischaemic Stroke(TARDIS). Available at: http://clinicaltrials.gov/show/NCT01661322. Accessed June 10, 2013.

86. Sprigg N, Gray LJ, England T, et al. A randomised controlled trial of triple antiplatelet therapy (aspirin, clopidogrel and dipyridamole) in the secondary prevention of stroke: safety, tolerability and feasibility. PLoS One 2008;3(8):e2852.

87. Sonia A. Warfarin and Antiplatelet Vascular Evaluation (WAVE) study. Available at: http://clinicaltrials.gov/show/NCT00125671. Accessed June 10, 2013.

88. Kwon SU. Prevention of CArdiovascular Events in iSchemic Stroke Patients With High Risk of Cerebral HemOrrhage (PICASSO). Available at: http://clinicaltrials.gov/show/NCT01013532. Accessed June 10, 2013.

89. Lapuerta P. Clopidogrel and the Optimization of Gastrointestinal Events (COGENT-1). Available at: http://clinicaltrials.gov/show/NCT00557921. Accessed June 10, 2013.

90. Huang Y. The Second Prevention Trial for Ischemic Stroke With Dengzhan Shengmai Capsule (SPIRIT-DZSM-1). Available at: http://clinicaltrials.gov/show/NCT00548223. Accessed June 10, 2013.

91. Zinkstok SM, Roos YB, ARTIS investigators. Early administration of aspirin in patients treated with alteplase for acute ischaemic stroke: a randomised controlled trial. Lancet 2012 Aug 25;380(9843):731–7.

92. Torgano G, Zecca B, Monzani V, et al. Effect of intravenous tirofiban and aspirin in reducing short-term and long-term neurologic deficit in patients with ischemic stroke: a double-blind randomized trial. Cerebrovasc Dis 2010 Feb;29(3):275–81.

# New Anticoagulants (Dabigatran, Apixaban, Rivaroxaban) for Stroke Prevention in Atrial Fibrillation

Maria I. Aguilar, MD[a],*, Ruth S. Kuo, PharmD[b],
William D. Freeman, MD[c,d,e]

## KEYWORDS

- Anticoagulation • Stroke • Atrial fibrillation • Reversal • Direct thrombin inhibitors
- Factor Xa inhibitors • Dabigatran • Rivaroxaban • Apixaban • Edoxaban

## KEY POINTS

- Patients with atrial fibrillation have an annual ischemic stroke risk of 5% without thromboprophylaxis.
- The $CHADS_2$ (congestive heart failure; hypertension; age 75 years or older; diabetes mellitus; and prior stroke, transient ischemic attack, or thromboembolism) and $CHA_2D_2$-VASc (atrial fibrillation risk factors where C = congestive heart failure [CHF], H = hypertension, A = age [age <65 = points, 65–75 = 1 point, age >75 = 2 points], D = diabetes [absent = 0 point, present = 1 point], S = Stroke or TIA history = 2 points, absent = 0 points. Other risk factors like CHF or hypertension are given 1 point if present, 0 if absent. V = Vascular disease [prior myocardial infarction, peripheral artery disease, or aortic plaque] = 1 point) scores are tools to estimate stroke risk and help guide therapy.
- For more than 50 years, warfarin has been the mainstay of oral anticoagulation for stroke prevention in patients with atrial fibrillation.
- The US Food and Drug Administration has recently approved the use of an oral direct thrombin inhibitor, dabigatran, and the factor Xa inhibitors rivaroxaban and apixiban, to reduce the risk of stroke and systemic embolism in patients with nonvalvular atrial fibrillation.
- Dabigatran, rivaroxaban, apixaban, and edoxaban are new anticoagulants that have more predictable pharmacokinetic profiles and do not require routine monitoring.
- Dabigatran, rivaroxaban, and apixaban were just as efficacious as warfarin, and in some cases superior to warfarin.

*Continued*

---

Funding Sources and Conflicts of Interest: None.
[a] Division of Cerebrovascular Diseases, Department of Neurology, Mayo Clinic, 5777 East Mayo Boulevard, Phoenix, AZ 85054, USA; [b] Department of Pharmacy, Scripps Memorial Hospital, 9888 Genesse Avenue, La Jolla, CA 92037, USA; [c] Department of Neurology, Mayo Clinic, 4500 San Pablo Road, Cannaday 2 East Neurology, Jacksonville, FL 32224, USA; [d] Department of Neurosurgery, Mayo Clinic, 4500 San Pablo Road, Cannaday 2 East Neurology, Jacksonville, FL 32224, USA; [e] Department of Critical Care, Mayo Clinic, 4500 San Pablo Road, Cannaday 2 East Neurology, Jacksonville, FL 32224, USA
* Corresponding author.
*E-mail address:* aguilar.maria@mayo.edu

Neurol Clin 31 (2013) 659–675
http://dx.doi.org/10.1016/j.ncl.2013.03.001
0733-8619/13/$ – see front matter © 2013 Elsevier Inc. All rights reserved.

**neurologic.theclinics.com**

*Continued*

- All three anticoagulants have lower risks of intracranial hemorrhage, but extracranial bleeding, as well as ways to reverse this bleeding in the setting of life-threatening extracranial or intracranial bleeding, are the main concerns with these agents.

- Expert guidelines on how to best manage bleeding events with newer anticoagulants, such as drug discontinuation and anticoagulation reversal methods, need to be researched to optimize future management of these patients.

- There are still no prospective randomized trials in humans studying antidotes for these newer anticoagulants, problems with interpreting coagulation assays, and conflicting data on whether newer hemostatic agents such as prothrombin complex concentrates (PCCs) and recombinant factor VIIa (rFVIIa) are effective in reversing these newer anticoagulants.

---

**Case study**

A 72-year-old man with nonvalvular paroxysmal atrial fibrillation (PAF) presents to the emergency department after a 10-minute episode of expressive aphasia. Other vascular risk factors include hypertension (well controlled on lisinopril) and diabetes mellitus type 2 (well controlled on metformin). His neurologic examination is nonfocal. He has been on warfarin 5 mg per day for 3 months since he was diagnosed with PAF, because he was deemed to be in the high-risk group (CHADS$_2$ score $\geq$2) in terms of future stroke and systemic embolism. After this event (transient ischemic attack [TIA]) his CHADS$_2$ score became 4. His carotids have no significant stenosis, and his low-density lipoprotein is 68 mg/dL. On brain magnetic resonance imaging he has small-vessel ischemic changes and no evidence of acute or recent ischemia. No microhemorrhages on T2 gradient echo sequences are noted. His International Normalization Ratio (INR) is 1.7, and he reports difficulties maintaining a therapeutic INR. Renal function is normal (creatinine 1.0 mg/dL and creatinine clearance [CrCl] 73 mL/min, weight 78 kg). Liver function tests are normal. He has a history of peptic ulcer disease but no gastrointestinal bleeding. He does not have coronary artery disease. Because of all these factors, apixaban 5 mg twice per day was considered as the optimal anticoagulant for future prevention of stroke and systemic embolism, but at the time the patient was seen, it was not yet approved by the US Food and Drug Administration (FDA) (FDA approved in December 2012). Therefore, the patient was given the option of dabigatran 150 mg twice per day or rivaroxaban 20 mg daily; he chose the latter agent because of its once-daily dosing. Compared with warfarin, which is less expensive but requires frequent blood draws in some patients and, over time, expensive laboratory monitoring for some, what are the risks and benefits of newer anticoagulants, the mechanism of action, and the laboratory and drug metabolism of these agents, as well as the risks of intracranial and extracranial bleeding compared with warfarin? This case shows a patient with likely noncompliance or complex genomic phenotype to warfarin (resistance), which makes management of the patient problematic for stroke prevention. This article reviews and compares with warfarin 3 newly FDA-approved anticoagulants for stroke prevention.

---

## INTRODUCTION

Cardioembolic stroke accounts for 20% of all ischemic strokes, and its frequency has increased over time, reflecting increased longevity of the population as well as improvements in cardiac imaging. The most common source of cardiac embolism in adults is atrial fibrillation (AF).[1] Evidence supports the use of antithrombotic therapy for most patients who have AF; oral anticoagulants are more effective but also carry higher risk of hemorrhagic complications than antiplatelet agents.[2] For more than 5 decades, warfarin has been the only oral agent available for chronic outpatient management of AF. However, warfarin has continued to be underused for stroke prevention because of its narrow therapeutic window, unpredictable response, and multiple food and drug interactions. In 2010, the FDA approved an oral direct thrombin inhibitor (DTI), dabigatran (Pradaxa), for prevention of stroke and systemic embolism in patients with nonvalvular AF (NVAF). An oral factor Xa inhibitor, rivaroxaban (Xarelto), was approved for the same indication the following year (2011). Apixiban was recently approved for stroke prevention by the FDA (December 2012), which has a trade name Eliquis and is another oral factor Xa inhibitor.

These new anticoagulants target specific factors in the common coagulation pathway, unlike warfarin, which affects factors in the extrinsic, intrinsic, and protein C and S pathways of the coagulation cascade. Factor X is known as Stuart factor. Factor Xa promotes the conversion of prothrombin (II) to thrombin (IIa) via the common pathway. This step in the coagulation pathway is the convergence point of the extrinsic and intrinsic pathways and is a key step that mitigates the propagation of thrombin. Each molecule of factor Xa can potentiate the formation of more than 1000 molecules of thrombin (IIa), making factor Xa inhibitors very potent.[3] DTIs target the last step in the cascade, binding to the thrombin (IIa) molecules and preventing the conversion of fibrinogen (factor I) to fibrin (Ia). Because DTIs target the final step of the coagulation cascade, it preserves some hemostatic mechanisms and may have lower bleeding risks compared with other anticoagulants.[4] Both factor Xa and thrombin play a central role in the coagulation pathway, and the inhibition of these factors prevents thrombus formation (**Fig. 1**).[5,6]

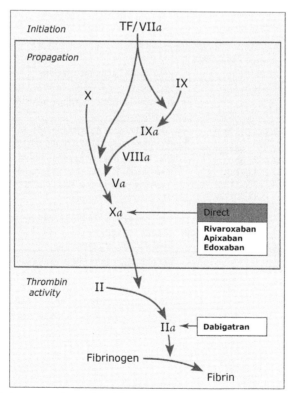

**Fig. 1.** Coagulation cascade and inhibitory drugs. TF, Tissue Factor. (*Adapted from* De Caterina R, Husted S, Wallentin L, et al. New oral anticoagulants in atrial fibrillation and acute coronary syndromes: ESC Working Group on Thrombosis-Task Force on Anticoagulants in Heart Disease position paper. J Am Coll Cardiol 2012;59:1414; with permission.)

## PATIENT EVALUATION OVERVIEW

Patients with AF are placed on chronic oral anticoagulants when they are at risk for developing stroke. The $CHADS_2$ (congestive heart failure, hypertension, age $\geq 75$ years, diabetes mellitus, prior stroke or TIA) score is commonly used to estimate stroke risk and to help guide clinicians in determining which patients would benefit from anticoagulation therapy. Patients with a $CHADS_2$ score of 2 or more are considered high risk, and the American College of Chest Physicians (ACCP) guidelines[1] recommend that chronic oral anticoagulation therapy be initiated (grade 1A). Although there is little debate that high-risk patients benefit from anticoagulation therapy in terms of stroke prevention, assuming there is no contraindication, there is much to consider in patients with intermediate ($CHADS_2 = 1$) to low risk ($CHADS_2 = 0$). The ACCP guidelines[1] also suggest that patients with a $CHADS_2$ score of 1 may also benefit from oral anticoagulation rather than no therapy (grade 1B) or antiplatelet therapy (grade 2B). In addition, independent stroke risk factors, such as gender and vascular disease, are not included in the $CHADS_2$ score, which has prompted some to propose a new tool, the $CHA_2DS_2$-VASc (congestive heart failure, hypertension, age $\geq 75$ y [double weight], diabetes, prior stroke or TIA [double weight], vascular disease, age 65–74 y, female sex category) score, to more accurately predict stroke risk.[7,8] **Table 1**[9,10] provides the risk stratification of the two scores and the current

**Table 1**
Estimating stroke risk using $CHADS_2$ and $CHA_2DS_2$-VASc scores with ACCP recommendations for antithrombotic therapy

| $CHADS_2$ Score | Annual Stroke Risk (95% CI) | 2012 ACCP Recommendations |
|---|---|---|
| 0 | 1.9 (1.2–3.0) | No therapy is safer than antithrombotic therapy (2B) If antithrombotic therapy is selected, use ASA or combo (2B) |
| 1 | 2.8 (2.0–3.8) | OAC outweighs no therapy (1B), ASA, or combo (2B) If OAC is not selected, combo is better than ASA (2B) |
| 2 | 4.0 (3.1–5.1) | OAC outweighs no therapy (1A), ASA, or combo (1B) |
| 3 | 5.9 (4.6–7.3) | Dabigatran is OAC of choice, rather than VKA (2B) |
| 4 | 8.5 (6.3–11.1) | If OAC is not selected, combo is better than ASA (1B) |
| 5 | 12.5 (8.2–17.5) | |
| 6 | 18.2 (10.5–17.4) | |

| $CHA_2DS_2$-VASc Score | Adjusted Annual Stroke Risk | 2010 ESC Recommendations |
|---|---|---|
| 0 | 0 | No therapy is safer than antithrombotic therapy If antithrombotic therapy is selected, use ASA |
| 1 | 1.3 | OAC or ASA is recommended, but OAC is preferred OAC recommendation: VKA or dabigatran |
| 2 | 2.2 | OAC is recommended: VKA or dabigatran |
| 3 | 3.2 | |
| 4 | 4 | |
| 5 | 6.7 | |
| 6 | 9.8 | |
| 7 | 9.6 | |
| 8 | 6.7 | |
| 9 | 15.2 | |

*Abbreviations:* ASA, aspirin; CI, confidence interval; combo, aspirin plus clopidogrel; ESC, European Society of Cardiology; OAC, oral anticoagulant; VKA, vitamin K antagonist (warfarin).

recommendations for antithrombotic therapy. A modeling analysis on dabigatran, rivaroxaban, and apixaban was performed to predict net clinical benefit of the new oral anticoagulants compared with warfarin.[11] Net clinical benefit is a quantitative method of estimating risk-benefits of ischemic stroke versus intracranial hemorrhage, with assessment based on the $CHADS_2$, $CHA_2DS_2$-VASc, and HAS-BLED (H = Hypertension [systolic blood pressure >160 mm Hg], A = abnormal renal and liver function, S = stroke, B = bleeding tendency/predisposition, L = labile INRs [if on Warfarin], E = elderly [eg. age >65 y], D = Drugs or alcohol [1 point each]) scores.[12] In patients with low to moderate risk of stroke and high risk of bleeds, apixaban and dabigatran seem to be superior. In patients with high risk of stroke and high risk of bleeds, the net clinical benefits of dabigatran, rivaroxaban, and apixaban were greater than those of warfarin. Physicians are now challenged with finding whether or not patients with lower stroke risk will benefit from long-term anticoagulation with factor Xa inhibitors or from DTIs, because they have more predicable effects and a lower risk of intracranial hemorrhage than warfarin.

## PHARMACOLOGIC TREATMENT OPTIONS
### Dabigatran

Dabigatran etexilate is a prodrug that, once metabolized to its active form, dabigatran, directly inhibits free and clot-bound thrombin and modulates thrombus formation. It has poor bioavailability and is coated with tartaric acid to aid absorption. Once absorbed, it has a rapid onset of action and peak levels are achieved within 1 to 2 hours of ingestion; the half-life of the drug is 14 to 17 hours. The medication is 80% cleared through the kidneys, and dabigatran exposure is increased 3-fold in patients with creatinine clearance (CrCl) of 30 mL/min. The remaining drug is metabolized hepatically, but bypasses the cytochrome P450 enzymes, thereby minimizing drug interactions. Other than bleeding, the major adverse effect was dyspepsia, which is attributed to the acidic coating on the capsule (Boehringer Ingelheim Pharmaceuticals; www.Pradaxa.com) (**Table 2**).

In the Randomized Evaluation of Long-Term Anticoagulation Therapy (RE-LY) trial,[4] dabigatran was compared with warfarin in 18,133 patients with NVAF and a mean $CHADS_2$ score of 2.1. Dabigatran was dosed at 110 mg or 150 mg twice daily, and warfarin was dose adjusted to an INR of 2 to 3. The primary outcome was stroke and systemic embolism. Dabigatran 110 mg twice daily was noninferior to warfarin, and had lower rates of major hemorrhage. Dabigatran 150 mg twice daily was superior to warfarin with similar risk of major hemorrhage, although gastrointestinal bleeding was observed in the dabigatran arm. Because the safety and efficacy of warfarin are based on INRs in the therapeutic range, a subsequent analysis[13] further characterized patients treated with warfarin, whose INRs remained within therapeutic range greater than 72.6% of the time, as noninferior to dabigatran 150 mg twice daily for prevention of stroke and systemic embolism. However, dabigatran 150 mg twice daily was superior to warfarin when INRs were in therapeutic range less than 72.6% of the time.

Based on these results, the FDA approved the use of dabigatran 150 mg twice daily for the reduction of ischemic stroke and systemic embolism in patients with NVAF who have good renal function (CrCl >30 mL/min). In patients with renal impairment (CrCl 15–30 mL/min), dosing is decreased to 75 mg twice daily, although this dosing was never included in clinical trials. Dabigatran has quickly gained acceptance since its approval because of its good pharmacokinetic profile, few drug interactions, and lack of routine monitoring. It received a class 1B recommendation as a useful alternative to warfarin in patients with NVAF from the 2011 American College of Cardiology

**Table 2**
Comparison of the new anticoagulants

| | Dabigatran | Rivaroxaban | Apixaban | Edoxaban |
|---|---|---|---|---|
| Mechanism of Action | DTI | Direct factor Xa inhibitor | Direct factor Xa inhibitor | Direct factor Xa inhibitor |
| FDA-approved indication(s) | Reduction of stroke and systemic embolism in patients with NVAF | Reduction of stroke and systemic embolism in patients with NVAF Treatment and prevention of thromboembolism | Reduction of stroke and systemic embolism in patients with NVAF | Not FDA approved |
| Dosing for NVAF | 150 mg orally bid 75 mg orally bid in renal impairment (CrCl 15–30 mL/min) | 20 mg orally once a day 15 mg orally once a day in renal impairment (CrCl 15–50 mL/min) | 5 mg orally bid 2.5 mg orally bid in patients with at least 2 of the following: renal impairment (SCr ≥1.5 mg/dL), age ≥80 y, weight <60 kg | 60 mg orally once a day 30 mg orally once a day in renal impairment |
| Bioavailability (%) | 3–7, not affected by food | 66 (in fasted state) and higher with food | 56, not affected by food | 50,[a] not affected by food |
| Time to peak (h) | 1–2, delayed when taken with food | 2–4 | 1–3 | 1–2 |

|  |  |  |  |  |
| --- | --- | --- | --- | --- |
| Half-life (h) | 12–17, longer in renally impaired | 5–9, 11–13 in elderly | 12 | 8–10 |
| Distribution | 35% protein bound<br>Vd = 50–70 L | 92%–95% protein bound<br>Vd = 50 L | 87% protein bound<br>Vd = 21 L | 40%–59% protein bound<br>Vd >300 L |
| Elimination (%) | 80 renal<br>20 hepatic (non-CYP450 pathway) | 33 renal<br>67 hepatic through CYP450 pathways | ~25 renal<br>~75 hepatic through CYP450 pathways | 35–39 renal<br>61–65 hepatic through CYP450 pathways |
| Major drug interactions | P-glycoprotein inhibitors or inducers | CYP450 3A4 inhibitors and inducers, P-glycoprotein inducers or inhibitors | CYP450 3A4 inhibitors and inducers, P-glycoprotein inducers or inhibitors | CYP450 3A4 inhibitors and inducers, P-glycoprotein inducers or inhibitors |
| Most common ADRs other than bleeding | Dyspepsia, gastritislike symptoms (>15%) | No significant ADRs |  | — |

*Abbreviations:* ADRs, adverse drug reactions; bid, twice a day; CrCl, creatinine clearance; CYP450, cytochrome P450; FDA, US Food and Drug Administration; Vd, volume of distribution.

[a] Based on animal studies.

*Adapted from* De Caterina R, Husted S, Wallentin L, et al. New oral anticoagulants in atrial fibrillation and acute coronary syndromes: ESC Working Group on Thrombosis-Task Force on Anticoagulants in Heart Disease position paper. Journal of the American College of Cardiology 2012;59:1416; with permission.

Foundation, American Heart Association, Heart Rhythm Society (ACCF/AHA/HRS) guideline update on management of AF.[14] In addition, the more recent 2012 ACCP guidelines[1] suggest that dabigatran should be selected rather than warfarin as the oral anticoagulant of choice in NVAF.

## Rivaroxaban

Rivaroxaban is a competitive factor Xa inhibitor with high affinity to both free and clot-bound factor Xa, and does not require antithrombin III for activity. It is readily absorbed, with food enhancing absorption, and achieves peak levels in 2 to 4 hours. The half-life is 5 to 9 hours, but it is 95% protein bound, which allows less frequent dosing. Rivaroxaban has a dual mode of elimination with one-third of the drug being eliminated unchanged in the urine. The remaining two-thirds of the drug is then metabolized by the CYP3A4/5 and CYP2J2 hepatic enzymes, and it is then renally excreted. Rivaroxaban is the first orally active factor Xa inhibitor to be approved by the FDA for prevention of stroke and systemic embolism in patients with NVAF. It is the only new anticoagulant that is dosed once daily. Rivaroxaban is dosed 20 mg once daily with the evening meal in patients with CrCl greater than 50 mL/min, and 15 mg daily in patients with CrCl of 15 to 50 mL/min (Janssen Pharmaceuticals www.xalerto-us.com) (see **Table 2**).

The approval of rivaroxaban was largely a result of the Rivaroxaban Once Daily Oral Direct Factor Xa Inhibition Compared with Vitamin K Antagonism for Prevention of Stroke and Embolism Trial in Atrial Fibrillation (ROCKET AF) study (**Table 3**).[15] More than 14,000 patients with NVAF, with a mean CHADS$_2$ score of 3.5, were assigned to either rivaroxaban 15 or 20 mg daily, or warfarin. Warfarin was adjusted to an INR of 2 to 3, and time in therapeutic range was approximately 55%. The primary end point was stroke, ischemic or hemorrhagic, or systemic embolism, in which rivaroxaban was noninferior to warfarin ($P<.001$). The risk of major and nonmajor clinical bleeding events was similar in both groups, but the risk of intracranial hemorrhages ($P = .02$), and therefore fatal bleeding ($P = .003$), was significantly reduced in the rivaroxaban group.

In a subgroup analysis of the ROCKET AF trial,[16] efficacy and safety of rivaroxaban and warfarin in patients with previous stroke or TIA were compared with those without previous events. The number of events per 100 person-years for stroke or systemic embolism was higher in the patients with previous stroke or TIA (2.87%) compared with those without previous events (1.66%), regardless of treatment choice. Bleeding events were lower in patients with previous stroke or TIA (13.31% rivaroxaban vs 13.87% warfarin) compared with those without (16.69% rivaroxaban vs 15.19% warfarin). Safety and efficacy were comparable between rivaroxaban and warfarin among patients with initial or recurrent stroke or TIA, but a greater benefit may be seen in patients with secondary stroke prevention than primary stroke prevention.

## Apixaban

Apixaban (Eliquis) is another orally active factor Xa inhibitor. It is readily bioavailable, with plasma concentrations peaking within 3 to 4 hours, and a plasma half-life of 8 to 15 hours. The drug is predominantly eliminated via hepatic CYP450 3A4 metabolism, with about 25% renally excreted.[17] Apixiban is the most recent factor Xa inhibitor to be FDA approved for prevention of stroke and systemic embolism in AF. The Apixaban versus Acetylsalicylic Acid to Prevent Stroke in Atrial Fibrillation Patients Who Have Failed or Are Unsuitable for Vitamin K Antagonist Treatment (AVERROES) and Apixaban for Reduction in Stroke and Other Thrombotic Events in Atrial Fibrillation (ARISTOTOLE) trials were the two studies reviewed.

The AVERROES study[18] comprised approximately 5600 patients with AF who were at risk for stroke and for whom warfarin therapy was unsuitable. Patients received apixaban 2.5 or 5 mg twice daily, or aspirin 81 to 324 mg once a day. Patients were followed for a little longer than a year before the study was terminated because of overwhelming results showing apixaban (1.6% event rate/y) to be superior to aspirin (3.7% event rate/y) in prevention of stroke or systemic embolism ($P<.001$). Major bleeding rates, including intracranial bleeding, were comparable between groups. The conclusion of the trial was that apixaban reduced the risk of stroke or systemic embolism by 55%, without significantly increasing the risk of major bleeding or intracranial hemorrhage.

The much larger ARISTOTLE trial[19] with more than 18,201 patients with NVAF, and a mean $CHADS_2$ score was 2.1, compared apixaban 2.5 mg or 5 mg twice daily with warfarin adjusted to an INR of 2 to 3. Patients in the warfarin group had INRs maintained in the target range an average of 62.2% of the time. Apixaban was superior to warfarin, with a rate of stroke or systemic embolism of 1.27% per year in the apixaban group compared with 1.60% per year in the warfarin group ($P<.001$ for noninferiority, $P = .01$ for superiority). Major bleeding was significantly lower in the apixaban group (2.13%/y) compared with the warfarin group (3.09%/y) ($P<.001$), with the rate of hemorrhagic stroke lower in the apixaban group. Rates of death from any cause were 3.52% in the apixaban group and 3.94% in the warfarin group ($P = .047$). In conclusion, apixaban was superior to warfarin in preventing stroke or systemic embolism, caused less bleeding, and resulted in lower mortality.

In a subsequent subgroup analysis of the ARISTOTLE trial,[20] safety and efficacy of apixaban and warfarin in patients with prior history of stroke and TIA were compared with those without prior event. There were no differences in safety or efficacy in the two patient groups, regardless of prior history of stroke or TIA. Patients with prior history of stroke or TIA had higher absolute rates of stroke and systemic embolism, therefore the benefit of apixaban may be greater in secondary stroke prevention.

### Edoxaban

Edoxaban (Lixiana) is the newest oral factor Xa inhibitor on the market seeking approval for prevention of stroke caused by AF. It has been commercially available in Japan since 2011 for prevention of venous thromboembolism after major orthopedic surgery. Edoxaban is rapidly absorbed, reaching peak concentrations in 1 to 2 hours, and having a half-life of 8 to 10 hours. Edoxaban is primarily eliminated by renal excretion and is a substrate for P-glycoprotein.[3,5]

It is currently undergoing a phase III, randomized, double-blind, double-dummy, multinational, noninferiority study titled Effective Anticoagulation with Factor Xa Next Generation in Atrial Fibrillation–Thrombolysis In Myocardial Infarction study 48 (ENGAGE AF-TIMI 48; phase III trial, results not reported at time of publication).[21] Approximately 20,500 patients are expected to be randomized to edoxaban 30 mg or 60 mg daily (adjusted for renal function), or warfarin dosed to a target INR of 2 to 3. Patients are included if they have a diagnosis of AF from less than or equal to 12 months and a $CHADS_2$ score greater than or equal to 2. The primary objective is to determine whether edoxaban is noninferior to warfarin for the prevention of stroke and systemic embolism. The primary safety end point is major bleeding events. Median follow-up is 24 months with anticipated study completion in early 2013.

There are no head-to-head trials yet comparing the efficacy and safety of these new anticoagulants. Based on indirect comparisons[22] in patients with $CHADS_2$ score greater than or equal to 3, dabigatran 150 mg twice a day, apixaban 5 mg twice a day, and rivaroxaban 20 mg daily resulted in statistically similar rates of stroke and systemic embolism, but apixaban had 30% lower risk of major hemorrhage compared with dabigatran (hazard ratio, 0.70; 95% confidence interval, 0.57–0.86) and rivaroxaban.

**Table 3**
**Summary of clinical trials for prevention of AF**

| | RE-LY | ROCKET AF | AVERROES | ARISTOTLE | ENGAGE AF-TIMI 48 |
|---|---|---|---|---|---|
| Treatment Groups | Dabigatran 110 mg bid or 150 mg bid vs dose-adjusted warfarin[a] | Rivaroxaban 20 mg/d vs dose-adjusted warfarin[a] | Apixaban 5 mg/d vs aspirin 81–324 mg/d | Apixaban 5 mg/d vs dose-adjusted warfarin[a] | Edoxaban 30 mg/d or 60 mg/d vs dose-adjusted warfarin[a] |
| Number of patients | 18,113 | 14,246 | 5559 | 18,201 | 20,500 |
| Design | Open-labeled, noninferiority, randomized controlled trial | Double-blind, double-dummy, noninferiority, randomized controlled trial | Double-blind, double-dummy, superiority, randomized controlled trial | Double-blind, double-dummy, noninferiority, randomized controlled trial | Double-blind, double-dummy, noninferiority, randomized controlled trial |
| Inclusion criteria | NVAF with 1 or more risk factors for stroke | NVAF with 2 or more risk factors for stroke | NVAF with 1 or more risk factors for stroke Patients who have failed or are unsuitable for warfarin | NVAF with 1 or more risk factors for stroke | NVAF within past 12 mo and a CHADS$_2$ score $\geq 2$ |
| Median follow-up (y) | 2 | 1.9 | 1.1 | 1.8 | 2 (anticipated) |
| Mean patient's age (y) | 72 | 73 | 70 | 70 | 72[b] |
| Average CHADS$_2$ score | 2.2 | 3.5 | 2.1 | 2.1 | 81% with score of 2–3[b] 19% with score of 4–6[b] |
| Prior stroke, TIA, or systemic embolism (%) | 20 | 55 | 14 | 19 | NR |

| | | | | | |
|---|---|---|---|---|---|
| Time in therapeutic range, INR 2–3 (%) | 64 | 55 | 63 | 66 | NR |
| Primary end point: stroke or systemic embolism (%) | 1.11 vs 1.69[c] (P<.001) | 2.12 vs 2.42 | 1.6 vs 3.7 (P<.001) | 1.27 vs 1.6 (P = .01) | NR |
| Rates of hemorrhagic stroke (%) | 0.1 vs 0.38[c] (P<.001) | 0.926 vs 0.44 (P = .024) | 0.2 vs 0.3 | 0.97 vs 1.05 (P<.001) | NR |
| Rates of ischemic stroke (%) | 0.92 vs 1.2[c] (P = .03) | 1.34 vs 1.42 | 1.1 vs 3 (P<.001) | 0.97 vs 1.05 | NR |
| Primary safety end point: rates of major bleeding (%) | 3.11 vs 3.36[c] (P = .003) | 3.6 vs 3.45 | 1.4 vs 1.2 | 2.13 vs 3.09 (P<.001) | NR |
| Rates of intracranial hemorrhage (%) | 0.3 vs 0.74[c] (P<.001) | 0.49 vs 0.74 (P = .019) | 0.4 vs 0.4 | 0.33 vs 0.8 (P<.001) | NR |
| All-cause mortality (%) | 3.64 vs 4.13[c] | 1.87 vs 2.21 | 3.5 vs 4.4 | 3.52 vs 3.94 (P = .046) | NR |

Risk factors for stroke include: previous stroke or TIA, CHF as defined by EF <40% or New York Heart Association class II or higher, hypertension, coronary artery disease, or be an age at least 75 years or 65–74 years with diabetes mellitus.

*Abbreviations:* ARISTOTLE, Apixaban for Reduction in Stroke and Other Thrombotic Events in Atrial Fibrillation; AVERROES, Apixaban Versus Acetylsalicylic Acid to Prevent Stroke in Atrial Fibrillation Patients Who Have Failed or Are Unsuitable for Vitamin K Antagonist Treatment; ENGAGE AF-TIMI 48, Effective Anticoagulation with factor Xa Next Generation in Atrial Fibrillation–Thrombolysis In Myocardial Infarction study 48; NR, Not Reported; NVAF, Nonvalvular Atrial Fibrillation; RE-LY, Randomized Evaluation of Long-Term Anticoagulation Therapy.

[a] Adjusted to INR 2 to 3.
[b] Based on the initial 15,000 patients enrolled.
[c] Results based on the arm receiving 150 mg twice daily.

*Adapted from* De Caterina R, Husted S, Wallentin L, et al. New oral anticoagulants in atrial fibrillation and acute coronary syndromes: ESC Working Group on Thrombosis-Task Force on Anticoagulants in Heart Disease position paper. J Am Coll Cardiol 2012;59:1413–25; with permission.

Intention-to-treat results were used for efficacy end points, and on-treatment analyses for safety end points.

### Complications

A recent meta-analysis by Miller and colleagues[23] compared efficacy and safety of new oral anticoagulants with those of warfarin in patients with AF. Data regarding intracranial bleeding favored the use of new anticoagulants rather than warfarin, but data regarding major bleeding and gastrointestinal bleeding were inconclusive **Table 4**.

### Managing bleeding complications

The main problem with the new anticoagulants is the lack of specific antidotes and consensus guidelines on the management of bleeding. In addition, many of the recommended coagulation assays used in studies, such as the ecarin clotting time (ECT) for measuring residual DTI effect[24] and plasma thrombin-antithrombin complex (TAT) levels or thrombin generation time (TGT) for measuring factor Xa effect[25] are unavailable in many US institutions. The available coagulation assays, prothrombin time (PT), activated partial thromboplastin time (aPTT), activated clotting time (ACT), and thrombin time (TT) all have limitations in clinical usefulness and results should be interpreted with caution.

There are several published expert opinions on the management of bleeding complications.[24,26] The Thrombosis and Hemostasis Summit of North America (THSNA) also formulated recommendations on the management of bleeding caused by the new anticoagulants.[27] General strategies include discontinuing the anticoagulant and providing routine supportive care, such as maintaining diuresis to aid in drug elimination in renally cleared medication, using mechanical compression when

**Table 4**
**Meta-analysis of safety of new oral anticoagulants (NOA) versus warfarin in patients with AF**

|  | Trial | Favors NOA | Favors Warfarin | RR (95% CI) |
|---|---|---|---|---|
| **Major Bleeding** | | | | |
| Dabigatran | RE-LY | x | — | 0.94 (0.82–1.07) |
| Rivaroxaban | ROCKET AF | — | x | 1.03 (0.89–1.18) |
| Apixaban | ARISTOTLE | xx | — | 0.70 (0.61–0.81) |
| Subtotal | — | x | — | 0.88 (0.71–1.09) |
| **Intracranial Bleeding** | | | | |
| Dabigatran | RE-LY | xxx | — | 0.41 (0.28–0.60) |
| Rivaroxaban | ROCKET AF | xx | — | 0.66 (0.47–0.92) |
| Apixaban | ARISTOTLE | xxx | — | 0.42 (0.31–0.59) |
| Subtotal | — | xx | — | 0.49 (0.36–0.66) |
| **GI Bleeding** | | | | |
| Dabigatran | RE-LY | — | xx | 1.50 (1.20–1.89) |
| Rivaroxaban | ROCKET AF | — | xx | 1.46 (1.19–1.78) |
| Apixaban | ARISTOTLE | x | — | 0.88 (0.68–1.14) |
| Subtotal | — | — | x | 1.25 (0.91–1.72) |

*Abbreviations:* GI, gastrointestinal; NOA, new oral anticoagulant; RR, relative risk.

*Adapted from* Miller CS, Grandi SM, Shimony A, et al. Meta-analysis of efficacy and safety of new oral anticoagulants (dabigatran, rivaroxaban, apixaban) versus warfarin in patients with atrial fibrillation. Am J Cardiol 2012;110:458; with permission.

possible, and giving blood product transfusions if required (**Fig. 2**). Other ways of eliminating drug are through the use of activated charcoal, if drug ingestion was within a couple of hours, and hemodialysis. Hemodialysis was successful at removing up to 68% of dabigatran because of low protein binding,[24] but is not likely effective for the rivaroxaban and apixaban because of their high protein binding, and is uncertain in edoxaban. In practice, the time it takes to initiate emergent dialysis often deters the clinician managing the bleed. Nonetheless, in patients with poor renal function who may have delayed drug clearance, hemodialysis should be considered and nephrologists should be consulted immediately to aid in management. Guidelines[27] do not support using fresh frozen plasma (FFP) for reversal because it would have to directly antagonize and overwhelm the effects of either thrombin or Xa to be effective. Replacing the depleted factor's concentration, as in the case of vitamin K antagonist reversal, would not be as effective. Also, studies with FFP were in mouse models and not in humans, so usefulness is not clear. The more controversial use of PCC (activated and nonactivated) and rFVIIa are not yet recommended because of conflicting data that is discussed later.

### Reversing DTI effect with hemostatic agents

Van Ryn and colleagues[24] presented limited, experimental data that evaluated both activated and nonactivated PCCs. Initial results showed that activated PCC, factor

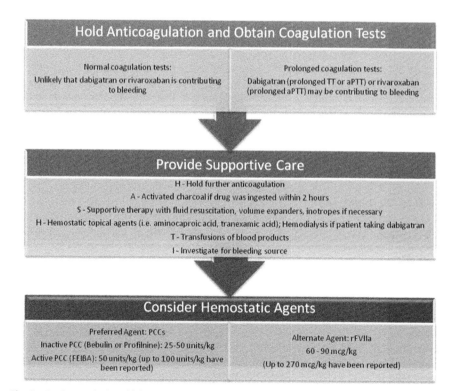

**Fig. 2.** Anticoagulation (dabigatran and rivaroxaban) algorithm for bleeding. FEIBA, factor VIII inhibitor bypassing activity. (*From* Cushman M, Lim W, Zakai NA. 2011 Clinical practice guide on anticoagulant dosing and management of anticoagulant-associated bleeding complications in adults. American Society Hematology 2011; with permission.)

VIII inhibitor bypassing activity (FEIBA), was effective at achieving hemostasis in a rat-tail model evaluating bleeding times, followed by complete reversal in an in vitro study using human plasma. The nonactivated PCC, Beriplex, also had positive results that showed a reduction in bleeding time in animal models. However, in vivo data by Eerenberg and colleagues[28] showed opposite results. Eerenberg and colleagues[28] conducted a randomized, placebo-controlled, crossover trial in 12 healthy male patients. Patients received either dabigatran or rivaroxaban for 2.5 days and, on the third day, received a transfusion of PCC (Cofact, nonactivated) or saline placebo. Blood samples were obtained 24 hours after transfusion. After a washout period, the same process was followed with the other medication. Reversal of anticoagulant effect was successful in patients taking rivaroxaban, but not in patients taking dabigatran.

Recombinant FVIIa has had inconsistent findings with other DTIs in the past, most notably with ximalegatran, an oral DTI used in Europe that has since been withdrawn from the market. It is a commonly used reversal agent for patients undergoing cardiopulmonary bypass surgery with IV DTIs, although, even in many of those cases, the dosing varied and patients required multiple doses of rVIIa. Warkentin and colleagues[29] presented a case from the RE-LY trial in which a 79-year-old male patient with chronic renal insufficiency (CrCl 36 mL/min) underwent cardiothoracic surgery with unintentional therapeutic levels of dabigatran. The patient subsequently developed a massive postoperative bleed that required a series of high-dose rVIIa (total dose 270 μg/kg) and 6 hours of high flux hemodialysis before the patient was able to regain hemostasis. In contrast, Garber and colleagues[30] reported a neurosurgical complication caused by dabigatran that resulted in a catastrophic hemorrhage not reversed by rFVIIa. However, the dosing of rFVIIa was much lower at 75 μg/kg (dosing information not reported, information obtain from direct communication with the author). There was also a case in which an 86-year-old man was admitted to our care with a left subdural hematoma after being on dabigatran and clopidogrel.[31] The drug was stopped immediately and supportive care (ie, fluids, platelets, blood) was provided. The patient deteriorated rapidly, and an emergent craniotomy was performed after administration of rFVIIa 60 μg/kg. The subdural hematoma was successfully evacuated, and the patient did not require any additional blood products after surgery. These conflicting cases are consistent with earlier findings that the use of rFVIIa is variable, and in some cases may require high doses to be successful.

### Reversing FXa inhibitors

The same year rivaroxaban was approved in the United States, the study by Eerenberg and colleagues[28] on reversing the drug's effect was published, giving some hope that rivaroxaban would be easier than dabigatran to manage in the event of a life-threatening bleed. A more recent study[25] examined the reversal effects of edoxaban using PCC (PPSB-HT), activated PCC (FEIBA), or recombinant factor VIIa (NovoSeven). The reversal effect of the hemostatic agent was determined based on PT prolongation in vitro using pooled human plasma at therapeutic and excess concentrations of edoxaban. Template bleeding times were also evaluated in rats receiving intensive anticoagulation with edoxaban, followed by addition of FEIBA or rFVIIa for reversal. All three hemostatic agents shortened PT in the pool human plasma analysis, with rFVIIa showing the most potential for reversing edoxaban, followed by FEIBA, then PPSB-HT. In the rat template bleeding time analysis, FEIBA and rFVIIa were also able to neutralize the activity of edoxaban. At the June 2012 AHA Emerging Science Series, Dr Escolar (Ecolar and colleagues[32]) presented results on an in vitro study with apixaban. Blood from healthy volunteers was mixed with apixaban at 200 ng/mL, which is double the expected drug concentration at normal treatment. rFVIIa at 270 μg/kg, activated

PCC (FEIBA) at 75 U/kg, and PCC (Beriplex) at 50 IU/kg were tested in a variety of coagulation assays. All three hemostatic agents were able to compensate for or reverse the effects of apixaban, although responses to these factors varied. The newest trial, Reversal of the Antithrombotic Action of New Oral Anticoagulants (REVANT; www.clinicaltrials.gov, trial identifier NCT01478282) is currently underway. The research will be performed ex vivo in blood samples obtained from healthy volunteers taking dabigatran and rivaroxaban at therapeutic doses and the ability of PCCs and rFVIIa to reverse the effects will be evaluated.

### Clinical usefulness of hemostatic agents

The clinical usefulness of hemostatic agents in most hospitals depends on availability of products. rFVIIa (NovoSeven) is likely the most accessible agent, but efficacy has been variable among DTIs and FXa inhibitors, and THSNA guidelines have not recommended routine use of rFVIIa because of the conflicting data. It is also expensive. PCCs may also be hard for all hospitals to obtain, or to obtain all the variants of PCCs with differing amounts of factors described later. Furthermore, the PCCs used in several of the clinical studies (Cofact, Beriplex, PPSB-HT) may be more potent because they contain all 4 factors (II, VII, IX, and X), albeit in inactivated forms. In the United States, only 3-factor (II, IX, and X) PCCs are commercially available (ie, Bebulin VH, Profilnine SD). Even among the 2 types of inactive PCCs, components of each factor may vary, and because of the lack of clinical studies, comparative efficacy is unknown. If a PCC is chosen, the activated PCC (FEIBA) is commercially available, and may be effective at mitigating the anticoagulant effects of both DTIs and factor Xa inhibitors. Experts[27] have cautiously recommended the use of PCCs if a hemostatic agent is chosen, but no consensus has been reached. Until in vivo studies are done in patients taking therapeutic doses of oral DTIs or FXa inhibitors with these factor antagonists, reversing effects of the new anticoagulants will continue to be challenging.

### SUMMARY

The new oral anticoagulants have been found to be as efficacious as warfarin (all stroke and systemic embolism, ischemic stroke) and safer in terms of intracranial bleeding. Data regarding major bleeding in general and gastrointestinal bleeding are inconclusive and concerning. The findings are based on meta-analysis because no head-to-head trials are available to date.

All patients with NVAF should receive antithrombotic therapy. For those at low risk (CHADS = 0) antiplatelet therapy is probably sufficient. For those at intermediate (CHADS$_2$ = 1) or high risk (CHADS$_2$ $\geq$2), anticoagulation is superior to antiplatelet therapy.

Four oral anticoagulants currently carry FDA approval for stroke and systemic embolism prevention in AF: warfarin, dabigatran, rivaroxaban, and apixaban. Older subjects ($\geq$75 years), those with impaired renal function (CrCl <30 mL/min), and those with symptomatic peptic ulcer disease or at a higher risk of gastrointestinal bleeding are probably best managed with warfarin.

For subjects already on warfarin and doing well, there is no indication to switch to one of the new agents.

Management of bleeding complications while on the new agents remains an area of concern and management is based on anecdotal experience and observational studies.

Anticoagulation is evolving rapidly, making it difficult for clinicians to be comfortable using the multiple new agents. As clinical experience is gained and head-to-head trials are conducted, the existing uncertainties should settle. Until then, best clinical judgment, educated decisions in conjunction with patients and their families, and current practice guidelines are the available tools supporting the difficult decision of which is the optimal anticoagulant agent.

## REFERENCES

1. You JJ, Singer DE, Howard PA, et al. Antithrombotic therapy for atrial fibrillation: antithrombotic therapy and prevention of thrombosis, 9th edition: American College of Chest Physicians Evidence-Based Clinical Practice Guidelines. Chest 2012;141: e531S–75S.
2. Freeman WD, Aguilar MI. Stroke prevention in atrial fibrillation and other major cardiac sources of embolism. Neurol Clin 2008;26:1129–60, x–xi.
3. Camm AJ, Bounameaux H. Edoxaban: a new oral direct factor Xa inhibitor. Drugs 2011;71:1503–26.
4. Connolly SJ, Ezekowitz MD, Yusuf S, et al. Dabigatran versus warfarin in patients with atrial fibrillation. N Engl J Med 2009;361:1139–51.
5. De Caterina R, Husted S, Wallentin L, et al. New oral anticoagulants in atrial fibrillation and acute coronary syndromes: ESC Working Group on Thrombosis-Task Force on Anticoagulants in Heart Disease position paper. J Am Coll Cardiol 2012;59:1413–25.
6. Lam YY, Ma TK, Yan BP. Alternatives to chronic warfarin therapy for the prevention of stroke in patients with atrial fibrillation. Int J Cardiol 2011;150:4–11.
7. Lip GY, Nieuwlaat R, Pisters R, et al. Refining clinical risk stratification for predicting stroke and thromboembolism in atrial fibrillation using a novel risk factor-based approach: the Euro Heart Survey on Atrial Fibrillation. Chest 2010; 137:263–72.
8. Olesen JB, Torp-Pedersen C, Hansen ML, et al. The value of the CHA2DS2-VASc score for refining stroke risk stratification in patients with atrial fibrillation with a CHADS2 score 0-1: a nationwide cohort study. Thromb Haemost 2012;107: 1172–9.
9. European Heart Rhythm Association, European Association for Cardio-Thoracic Surgery, Camm AJ, Kirchhof P, Lip GY, et al. Guidelines for the management of atrial fibrillation: the Task Force for the Management of Atrial Fibrillation of the European Society of Cardiology (ESC). Eur Heart J 2010;31:2369–429.
10. Garcia DA. Benefits and risks of oral anticoagulation for stroke prevention in nonvalvular atrial fibrillation. Thromb Res 2012;129:9–16.
11. Banerjee A, Lane DA, Torp-Pedersen C, et al. Net clinical benefit of new oral anticoagulants (dabigatran, rivaroxaban, apixaban) versus no treatment in a 'real world' atrial fibrillation population: a modelling analysis based on a nationwide cohort study. Thromb Haemost 2012;107:584–9.
12. Lane DA, Lip GY. Use of the CHA(2)DS(2)-VASc and HAS-BLED scores to aid decision making for thromboprophylaxis in nonvalvular atrial fibrillation. Circulation 2012;126:860–5.
13. Wallentin L, Yusuf S, Ezekowitz MD, et al. Efficacy and safety of dabigatran compared with warfarin at different levels of international normalised ratio control for stroke prevention in atrial fibrillation: an analysis of the RE-LY trial. Lancet 2010;376:975–83.
14. Wann LS, Curtis AB, Ellenbogen KA, et al. 2011 ACCF/AHA/HRS focused update on the management of patients with atrial fibrillation (update on dabigatran): a report of the American College of Cardiology Foundation/American Heart Association Task Force on practice guidelines. Circulation 2011;123:1144–50.

15. Patel MR, Mahaffey KW, Garg J, et al. Rivaroxaban versus warfarin in nonvalvular atrial fibrillation. N Engl J Med 2011;365:883–91.
16. Hankey GJ, Patel MR, Stevens SR, et al. Rivaroxaban compared with warfarin in patients with atrial fibrillation and previous stroke or transient ischaemic attack: a subgroup analysis of ROCKET AF. Lancet Neurol 2012;11:315–22.
17. Potpara T, Polovina M, Licina M, et al. Novel oral anticoagulants for stroke prevention in atrial fibrillation: focus on apixaban. Adv Ther 2012;29:491–507.
18. Connolly SJ, Eikelboom J, Joyner C, et al. Apixaban in patients with atrial fibrillation. N Engl J Med 2011;364:806–17.
19. Granger CB, Alexander JH, McMurray JJ, et al. Apixaban versus warfarin in patients with atrial fibrillation. N Engl J Med 2011;365:981–92.
20. Easton JD, Lopes RD, Bahit MC, et al. Apixaban compared with warfarin in patients with atrial fibrillation and previous stroke or transient ischaemic attack: a subgroup analysis of the ARISTOTLE trial. Lancet Neurol 2012;11:503–11.
21. Ruff CT, Giugliano RP, Antman EM, et al. Evaluation of the novel factor Xa inhibitor edoxaban compared with warfarin in patients with atrial fibrillation: design and rationale for the Effective aNticoaGulation with factor xA next GEneration in Atrial Fibrillation-Thrombolysis in Myocardial Infarction study 48 (ENGAGE AF-TIMI 48). Am Heart J 2010;160:635–41.
22. Schneeweiss S, Gagne JJ, Patrick AR, et al. Comparative efficacy and safety of new oral anticoagulants in patients with atrial fibrillation. Circ Cardiovasc Qual Outcomes 2012;5:480–6.
23. Miller CS, Grandi SM, Shimony A, et al. Meta-analysis of efficacy and safety of new oral anticoagulants (dabigatran, rivaroxaban, apixaban) versus warfarin in patients with atrial fibrillation. Am J Cardiol 2012;110:453–60.
24. van Ryn J, Stangier J, Haertter S, et al. Dabigatran etexilate–a novel, reversible, oral direct thrombin inhibitor: interpretation of coagulation assays and reversal of anticoagulant activity. Thromb Haemost 2010;103:1116–27.
25. Fakuda T, Honda Y, Kamisato C, et al. Reversal of anticoagulant effects of edoxaban, an oral, direct factor Xa inhibitor, with haemostatic agents. Thromb Haemost 2012;107:253–9.
26. Crowther MA, Warkentin TE. Managing bleeding in anticoagulated patients with a focus on novel therapeutic agents. J Thromb Haemost 2009;7(Suppl 1):107–10.
27. Kaatz S, Kouides PA, Garcia DA, et al. Guidance on the emergent reversal of oral thrombin and factor Xa inhibitors. Am J Hematol 2012;87(Suppl 1):S141–5.
28. Eerenberg ES, Kamphuisen PW, Sijpkens MK, et al. Reversal of rivaroxaban and dabigatran by prothrombin complex concentrate: a randomized, placebo-controlled, crossover study in healthy subjects. Circulation 2011;124:1573–9.
29. Warkentin TE, Margetts P, Connolly SJ, et al. Recombinant factor VIIa (rFVIIa) and hemodialysis to manage massive dabigatran-associated postcardiac surgery bleeding. Blood 2012;119:2172–4.
30. Garber ST, Sivakumar W, Schmidt RH. Neurosurgical complications of direct thrombin inhibitors–catastrophic hemorrhage after mild traumatic brain injury in a patient receiving dabigatran. J Neurosurg 2012;116:1093–6.
31. Kuo RS, Freeman WD, Tawk RG. Anticoagulation [letter to the editor]. J Neurosurg 2013;118(2):483–4.
32. Escolar G, Arellano-Rodrigo E, Reverter JC, et al. Reversal of apixaban induced alterations of hemostasis by different coagulation factor concentrates: studies in vitro with circulating human blood. Circulation 2012;126(4):520–1.

# Unanswered Questions in Thrombolytic Therapy for Acute Ischemic Stroke

Adriana Sofia Ploneda Perilla, MA[a], Michael J. Schneck, MD[b,c],*

KEYWORDS

- Stroke • Intravenous thrombolysis • Intra-arterial thrombolysis • Perfusion mismatch
- Time factors

KEY POINTS
## UNANSWERED QUESTIONS TO BE ELUCIDATED IN THIS ARTICLE

- What are the current data and literature in support or against the extension of the time window for tissue plasminogen activator (tPA)?
- Are there other modalities that can be used to determine the benefit of thrombolysis treatment beyond 3 to 4.5 hours (consideration for whom tPA will and will not help)?
- What are the implications of these findings for patients with wake-up stroke?
- Are there other agents/therapies that can be used that will allow the time window to be extended?
- Is endovascular therapy an effective and beneficial alternative to intravenous thrombolysis.
- What are the effects of anticoagulants/antiplatelet drugs on thrombolytic therapy?
- What are the effects of other selection criteria, such as age or stroke location, on the decisions regarding thrombolytic therapy?

## INTRODUCTION

Every 40 seconds, someone in the United States is affected by a stroke, 87% of which are ischemic in nature.[1] With such a high incidence, stroke has retained its title as the leading cause of disability in the United States, as well as the third and fourth leading cause of death in women and men, respectively.[1] Great efforts have been made to ensure that patients receive both prompt and the most appropriate and effective

[a] Stritch School of Medicine, Loyola University Chicago, Chicago, IL, USA; [b] Department of Neurology, Stritch School of Medicine, Loyola University Medical Center, Loyola University Chicago, Suite 2700, Maguire Building, Maywood, IL 60153, USA; [c] Department of Neurosurgery, Stritch School of Medicine, Loyola University Chicago, Chicago, IL, USA
* Corresponding author. Department of Neurology, Loyola University Medical Center, Suite 2700, Maguire Building, Maywood, IL 60153.
E-mail address: mschneck@lumc.edu

Neurol Clin 31 (2013) 677–704
http://dx.doi.org/10.1016/j.ncl.2013.03.006
0733-8619/13/$ – see front matter © 2013 Elsevier Inc. All rights reserved.

**neurologic.theclinics.com**

medical care that provides the best clinical outcome.[1] Significant progress has been made in the treatment of acute ischemic strokes (AIS), particularly with regard to thrombolytic therapy. In 1995, the National Institutes of Neurologic Disorders and Stroke (NINDS) published the results for use of intravenous (IV) alteplase (tissue plasminogen activator [tPA]) for AIS leading to the approval by the US Food and Drug Administration (FDA) of tPA for selected patients with AIS in 1996 within a defined treatment window of 3 hours from onset of stroke symptoms.[2] Since this landmark study, other studies have focused on the feasibility of extending the time window using tPA beyond 3 hours, as well as other pharmacologic or procedural options to extend the time window for AIS intervention (**Table 1**). Subsequent trials sought to further define the benefit of tPA, particularly its benefit beyond this 3-hour time window, leading to the recent ECASS-III study, suggesting a benefit of IV tPA up to 4.5 hours after stroke onset.[3–6] This study led in 2009 to a modification of the American Heart Association (AHA) guidelines for stroke thrombolytic therapy recommending extension of the IV tPA window up to 4.5 hours from symptom onset, although this extended window is still not accepted by the FDA.[7]

Although the opportunity for an extended time window is desirable because it would allow for treatment of more patients with AIS who present later than 3 hours after symptom onset, few studies have convincingly shown the benefit of an expanded window. In this article, the current data on benefits and potential complications of an extended time window for IV tPA treatment are reviewed.

Questions are also explored about treatment modalities other than IV tPA that might further extend the IV thrombolysis window, mechanical devices are considered with regards to their safety and efficacy as endovascular devices for use in patients with AIS, and whether arterial thrombolysis is a better option for selected patients with AIS is discussed. In addition, the use of thrombolytic therapy with concomitant antiplatelet (AP) and anticoagulant (AC) drugs is considered.

| Table 1 | |
|---|---|
| **List of acronyms for trial studies discussed in this article** | |
| NINDS | National Institutes of Neurologic Disorders and Stroke |
| ECASS | European Cooperative Acute Stroke Study |
| ATLANTIS | Alteplase Thrombolysis for Acute Noninterventional Therapy in Ischemic Stroke |
| SITS-ISTR | Safe Implementation of Thrombolysis in Stroke-International Stroke Thrombolysis Registry |
| SITS-MOST | Safe Implementation of Thrombolysis in Stroke-Monitoring Study |
| DEFUSE | DWI Evolution for Understanding Stroke Etiology |
| DIAS | Desmoteplase in Acute Ischemic Stroke |
| DEDAS | Dose Escalation of Desmoteplase for Acute Ischemic Stroke |
| EPITHET | Echoplanar Imaging Thrombolysis Evaluation Trial |
| MERCI | Mechanical Embolus Removal in Cerebral Ischemia |
| PROACT | Prolyse in Acute Cerebral Thromboembolism |
| ASPECTS | Alberta Stroke Program Early CT Score |
| IMS studies | Interventional Management of Stroke (IMS-I, IMS-II, or IMS-III) |
| SYNTHESIS-EXP | Intra-Arterial vs Systemic Thrombolysis for Acute Ischemic Stroke |
| MR-RESCUE | Mechanical Retrieval and Recanalization of Stroke Clots Using Embolectomy |

Although many advances have been made in both pharmacologic and mechanical treatment of patients with AIS (**Table 2**), the time window for treatment and the relative benefit of the various treatment options remains a work in progress. The proper medical management of a AIS patient with AIS presenting for emergent thrombolytic therapy has yet to be clearly defined.

---

**Case study**

An 84-year-old woman with a history of nonobstructive coronary artery disease, an aortic valve, and mitral valve replacement 6 months previously with course complicated by postoperative atrial fibrillation controlled with amiodarone, and a pacemaker, was admitted for cardiac catheterization as a result of worsening dyspnea and lower extremity edema. She underwent a cardiac catheterization via a transseptal approach. The procedure lasted 2 hours and immediately after completion, she was found to be aphasic and with a right hemiparesis. She was evaluated by the Acute Stroke Team and her National Institutes of Health Stroke Scale (NIHSS) score was 24 approximately 130 minutes from when last seen normal. The activated clotting time (ACT) at that time was 161 (130 = normal). The presumption was that the patient had a cardioembolic stroke caused by a calcific embolus. A computed tomography (CT) scan was obtained, limited by motion artifact, but with no acute blood or large infarct changes.

The patient was taken for catheter cerebral angiography with consideration of possible mechanical thrombolysis or intra-arterial (IA) tPA. A complete left TIMI (thrombolysis in myocardial infarction) mid-M1 segment middle cerebral artery (MCA) occlusion was visualized (**Fig. 1**). The patient received IA tPA with no recanalization and a Solitaire stent retriever device (Covidien) was then deployed. Using the Solitaire device, the M1 segment of the left MCA and the M2 segment containing the inferior division of the left MCA were recanalized, but recanalization of the superior M2 segment was unsuccessful. Thereafter, a MERCI retrieval device (Concentric Medical, Inc, Mountain View, CA) was deployed, but the M2 superior division segment remained occluded.

Postprocedure CT showed a left frontoparietal mixed hyperdensity lesion in the MCA territory (**Fig. 2**). In addition, air fluid levels were noted within the densities. CT of the chest/abdomen/pelvis showed evidence of what appeared to be complex ascites with mixed hyperdensity. The postprocedural course was complicated by anemia requiring blood transfusions, abdominal ascites related to the patient's known heart failure, and contrast dye-induced nephropathy, which resolved over time without the need for dialysis.

At discharge to a subacute rehabilitation facility, approximately 10 days after stroke, the patient was able to swallow and eat a pureed diet, follow simple commands and say "Yes" or "No", but otherwise had a severe aphasia, right central facial drop, and right hemiparesis. Modified Rankin scale (mRS) score was 3 and NIHSS score was 17.

Particular points of interest for this case study are:

1. Postcardiac catheterization ischemic stroke

2. Onset of symptoms was less than 3 hours but with increased ACT and high NIHSS score, it was considered that an endovascular approach was preferable to IV tPA

3. Various interventional treatment modalities were used, with little change in final outcome, showing that even despite an aggressive interventional approach with recanalization, the outcome is often less than desirable.

---

## PATIENT EVALUATION OVERVIEW

To ensure effective treatment of AIS, prompt recognition of symptom onset should occur followed immediately by a quick response with the most beneficial medical intervention. Through the ensuing 1 to 2 decades since introduction of IV tPA, public awareness and recognition of the most common symptoms and signs of stroke have

**Table 2**
Thrombolytic options depending on the risk of surgical bleeding

|  | IV Thrombolysis, <3 h | IA Thrombolysis, <6 h | Mechanical Thrombolysis, <8 h |
|---|---|---|---|
| Low-risk surgery (muscle biopsy, digit amputation, skin grafting, arthroscopy, endoscopy, dental procedures) | Yes[a] | Yes | Yes |
| Medium-risk surgery (gastrointestinal/colonic surgery, coronary artery bypass graft, carotid endarterectomy, or carotid stent) | No | Yes | Yes |
| High-risk surgery (craniotomy, transplant surgery) | No | No | Yes |

[a] In selected patients when IA and mechanical thrombolysis are unavailable.

increased. If recanalization of the occluded cerebral artery and subsequent reperfusion fail to occur within a certain time frame, with either IV thrombolytic or endovascular therapy, irreversible damage of brain cells occurs, because glucose, oxygen, and adenosine triphosphate are depleted, leading to mitochondrial damage.[8] As ischemic injury continues, intracellular sodium and calcium concentrations increase, causing anoxic depolarization and release of excitotoxic levels of glutamate, release of oxidative stress factors, and cytotoxic edema.[8] Reperfusing cells at this stage of irreversible injury increases the risk for reperfusion injury, causing more harm than benefit.[9] Defining the point at which harm outweighs benefit has been a driving force of

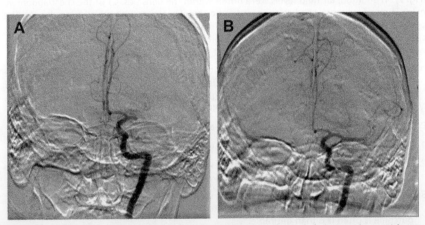

**Fig. 1.** Case study. (*A*) Digital subtraction angiography of the left internal carotid artery (ICA) shows a grossly normal course, caliber, and configuration of the petrous, cavernous, paraclinoid, and supraclinoid segments of the ICA. The A1 and distal segments of the anterior cerebral artery appear normal. The proximal M1 MCA segment appears grossly normal but there is a sharp cutoff at the mid-M1 segment, proximal to the take-off of the anterior temporal branch, and there was no antegrade flow beyond this point. (*B*) Revascularization of the left M1 MCA segment, including the anterior temporal branch and the lenticulostriate vessels, with partial revascularization of the left inferior division of the M2 but persistent occlusion of the superior division of the left MCA.

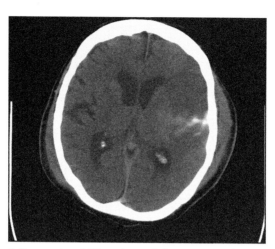

**Fig. 2.** Case study. Follow-up head CT performed the morning after cerebral angiography, showing a large area of low attenuation in the left MCA territory. There is a hyperdense focus (decreased from the immediate postprocedure head CT) of the left basal ganglion, head of the caudate, and left frontal and temporal lobe cortical regions, reflecting contrast stasis with extravasated dye within the left Sylvian fissure as well as minimal hemorrhage in the ventricular occipital horns.

many of the post-1995 NINDS stroke studies. In an attempt to provide a clear outline of how these time windows might be approached, current treatment options with regards to time of stroke onset are summarized in **Fig. 3**.

## PHARMACOLOGIC TREATMENT OPTIONS
### Landmark Studies and the 3-Hour Time Window for IV tPA (Alteplase) Thrombolysis

The 1995 NINDS study was the first trial to report the benefit of administering IV tPA to patients with AIS within 3 hours of stroke onset (**Table 3**).[2] Although this trial would become known as the landmark study that defined the clinical application of tPA, it was set in motion only after the published results of 2 previous pilot studies.[10,11] These 2 pilot studies had reported 2 critical factors that shaped the NINDS trial: (1) patients treated with thrombolytic therapy had higher rates of intracerebral hemorrhage (ICH) and (2) better outcomes were seen in patients treated early. The NINDS investigators modified their trial around these findings by decreasing the administered dose of tPA to 0.9 mg/kg and enrolling only patients with a known stroke onset of less than 3 hours. Results showed a more favorable outcome in the PA group at 3 months, as determined by an absolute increase in the percentage of patients with the lowest NIHSS, mRS, and Glasgow Outcome Scale or highest Barthel Index (BI), compared with the placebo group.[2] In addition, the NINDS study also made the important observation that, despite an increased incidence for ICH in the thrombolysis group (absolute percent value of 7% in the tPA group vs 1% in placebo, $P<.001$), there were no significant differences in mortality compared with the placebo group (absolute percent value of 17% in the tPA group vs 21%, in placebo, $P = .30$). Although seemingly minor at the time, this fact guided the design of many future trials seeking to define the therapeutic window.

In addition to the NINDS study, the ATLANTIS and ECASS trials described the outcomes of patients with onset of stroke symptoms within 5 or 6 hours, respectively. Outcomes from pooled analyses of the ATLANTIS, ECASS, and NINDS trials supported the conclusion that administration of tPA within 3 hours of stroke onset led to improved

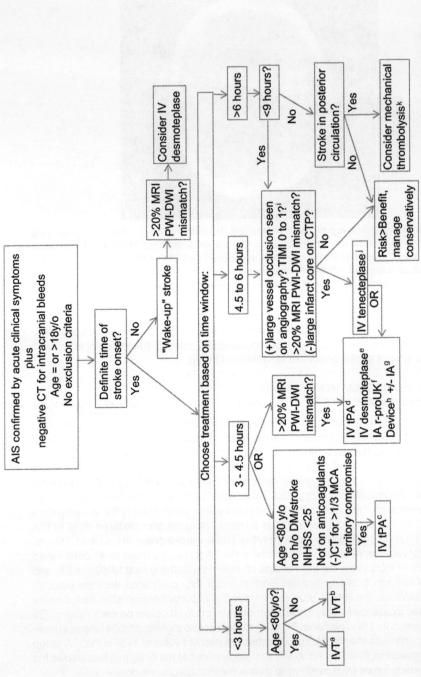

Fig. 3. Management of patients with AIS with consideration of time windows. [a] NINDS, [b] IST-3, [c] ECASS-III and SITS-ISTR, [d] EPITHET and DEFUSE (up to 6 hours), [e] DIAS and DEDAS (nonsignificant upward trend for benefit), [f] suggested within 6 hours by the potential benefit noted in PROACT-II, [g] MERCI-1 (MERCI + IA tPA) and Multi-MERCI trial (L5 Retriever + IA tPA), [h] FDA-approved MERCI, Penumbra, or Solitaire device up to 8 hours, [i] Fiebach and colleagues[26] concluded better 90-day outcome with desmoteplase, benefit to be confirmed by DIAS-3 and 4, [j] Parsons and colleagues[28] for up to 6 hours, [k] suggested with consideration of risk, cost, and potential benefit as determined by clinician and patient/patient's family. Time window unclear (≤24 hours?).

| Table 3 | | | | |
|---|---|---|---|---|
| **Common medical interventions considered with regard to time windows** | | | | |
| Time Window (h) | 0–3 | 3–4.5 | 4.5–6 | >6 |
| Medical Intervention | IVT[a] | IVT[c] | IAT | ED (≤8 h)[b] |
| | IAT | IAT | ED[b] | |
| | ED[b] | ED[b] | | |

*Abbreviations:* ED, endovascular device; IAT, IA thrombolysis; IVT, IV thrombolysis.
[a] FDA approved use of tPA (alteplase) in 1996.
[b] FDA approved use of MERCI Concentric Retriever (2004) and Penumbra device (2008).
[c] AHA stroke guideline recommendations (2007).

clinical outcomes as determined by mRS (0 or 1), BI (95 or 100), and NIHSS scores (0 or 1) at 3 months.[3,5] The early pooled analysis revealed a favorable odds ratio at 3 months for patients within the 3-hour to 4.5-hour treatment time frame (odds ratio [OR] 2.81 [1.75–4.50] for <90 minutes, OR 1.55 [1.12–2.15] for 91–180 minutes, OR 1.40 [1.05–1.85] for 181–270 minutes).[4] A favorable odds ratio was not found for the >4.5 hour treatment group [OR 1.15 (0.90–1.47)]. Similar results were also seen with regards to the increased risk of hemorrhagic transformation (spontaneous ICH [sICH] or parenchymal hemorrhage) in the tPA-treated group without an increase in mortality. Furthermore, this analysis showed that the increased rate of hemorrhagic conversion was not associated with an increase in treatment time ($P = .71$) or baseline NIHSS ($P = .10$), but rather was associated with increased age ($P = .0002$). Particular to the ECASS-II trial, parenchymal hemorrhages were seen in 19.7% of the patients between the ages of 71 to 80 years compared with 11.1% in ages 61 to 70 years and 7.1% in ages 51 to 60 years (for tPA-by-age interaction, OR 1.07, 95% confidence interval [CI] 0.99–1.15, $P = .05$).[12] In addition to this tPA-by-age interaction, the ECASS-II trial also noted a tPA-by-aspirin interaction, in which a higher percentage of parenchymal hemorrhages (24.1% vs 2.1% in the placebo with aspirin group and 8.8% in the tPA no-aspirin group) and sICH (18.9% vs 0% in the placebo with aspirin group and 8.8% in the no-aspirin tPA group) were present in the tPA group who had been using aspirin before their stroke (OR 4.99, 95% CI 0.91–27.4, $P = .06$ with $P \leq 0.06$ with on-treatment criteria). However, despite the increased rate of hemorrhagic transformations in the tPA group, regardless of AP status, the odds for a worsened outcome were lower in the tPA group versus placebo. The results of the ECASS-II study with regard to the interaction of aspirin with tPA brings up one of the unanswered questions expanded on later: What effects do AP drugs and AC drugs have on thrombolysis, and are these effects enough to maintain the current exclusion criteria for patients on these medications?

### Defining the Therapeutic Time Windows for IV tPA (Alteplase) Thrombolysis

**Unanswered question:**
- What are the therapeutic time limits of IV tPA thrombolysis?
- Is there benefit beyond 3 hours? 4.5 hours? 6 hours?

### The 3-hour to 4.5-hour time window: ECASS-III and SITS-ISTR, and SITS-MOST
In the years after the ECASS-I and ECASS-II, NINDS, and ATLANTIS Part A and B trials, additional studies looked at the possibility of an extended time window beyond

3 hours for IV thrombolysis. From 2002 to 2008, the ECASS-III, SITS-MOST (Safe Implementation of Thrombolysis in Stroke-Monitoring Study) and SITS-ISTR (Safe Implementation of Thrombolysis in Stroke-International Stroke Thrombolysis Registry) observational study, together suggested a potential benefit for treatment with IV tPA in an extended 4.5-hour time window.[4,5,13-15]

The ECASS-III trial showed improved 3-month functional outcome (defined as mRS 0 or 1) in patients treated with tPA between 3 and 4.5 hours of onset of stroke symptoms versus placebo (OR 1.34; 95% CI, 1.02–1.76, $P = .04$).[4] Like preceding trials, ECASS-III also noted an increased risk of sICH (2.4% vs 0.2% in placebo, $P = .008$) without an increased rate of mortality (7.7% vs 8.4% in placebo, $P = .68$).

The SITS-ISTR observational study corroborated the findings of ECASS-III.[14] However, by contrast with ECASS-III, the SITS-ISTR investigators did not find a significantly increased risk of sICH in this cohort compared with patients treated within 3 hours. This finding was true for all 3 definitions of sICH as provided by the NINDS (8% vs 7.3%, $P = .46$), ECASS-II (5.3% vs 4.8%, $P = .54$), and SITS-MOST (2.2% vs 1.6%, $P = .24$) trials.[15]

As a result of these positive findings, the AHA/American Stroke Association (ASA) revised their guidelines for IV tPA in the management of AIS and recommended consideration of IV tPA treatment of patients with AIS who present up to 4.5 hours from symptom onset.[7] Although these changes seem to be positive, the new extended time window has not yet been approved by the FDA. This situation may reflect the reality that, although some patients have benefited from treatment in the extended window, there is still uncertainty as to the risk versus benefit for many of these patients. Also, most of the patients in ECASS-III were treated in the early time window for the study, and the results of ECASS-III were not confirmed in the previous ATLANTIS study; ATLANTIS had shown no additional harm with an extended time window up to 5 hours but also showed no additional benefit.[6] Furthermore, there were certain limitations in ECASS-III with regards to the particular age group enrolled (average age 64.9 years). A younger average age of enrollment was also present in the NINDS trial (average age 67 years) and in the SITS-ISTR analysis (average age 65 years), bringing up the unanswered question as to whether treatment would be both safe and effective for patients at an older age, particularly octogenarians, who make up almost 30% of all patients with AIS.[16]

### The 6-hour time window: EPITHET and IST-3
Using pooled data from the NINDS 1 and 2, ECASS-I and ECASS-II, and ATLANTIS A and B trials, Lansberg and colleagues[17] calculated the number needed to treat to benefit (NNTB) and number needed to harm (NNTH) of patients treated with IV tPA thrombolysis in 4 90-minute treatment time intervals. Saver and colleagues[15] made similar arguments regarding NNTB and NNTH from a direct analysis of ECASS-III alone. Lansberg and colleagues[17] suggested that in the 4.5-hour to 6-hour time window, the NNTH was less than the NNTB as determined by 7-strata, 6-strata, and median expert calculations (14.0 and 19.3, 16.1 and 19.4, and 13 and 17, respectively). The number of patients harmed outnumbered those who benefited from IV tPA thrombolysis in the 4.5-hour to 6-hour time window. With regards to the 0 to 90, 91 to 180, and 181 to 270 treatment windows, their results show that as the time window increased, the NNTB trended upwards and the NNTH trended down, with NNTH remaining greater than NNTB.

Although at first these calculated NNTH and NNTB values create the impression that IV tPA thrombolysis beyond 4.5 hours of stroke onset is unpromising, there were some individuals who did seem to benefit from treatment in the analysis. The evidence that tPA could provide benefit to a subset of patients beyond 4.5 hours was the driving force to subsequent investigations. In 2008, the EPITHET investigators suggested that mismatch in perfusion-weighted magnetic resonance imaging (MRI) (PWI) and diffusion-weighted MRI (DWI) could be used as a tool to identify specific patients who would benefit in a 3-hour to 6-hour window.[18] MRI PWI-DWI mismatch was used in 2 ways: (1) to identify initial infarct size and subsequent growth and (2) to assess the degree of reperfusion after either alteplase or placebo administration. The study results showed that in patients with mismatch, a significant association was seen between reperfusion rates (defined as >90% reduction between baseline and 3-day PWI volumes) and successful treatment with tPA versus placebo (56% vs 26%, $P = .010$).[18] In subsequent analyses, a significant association was present between successful reperfusion and better neurologic (NIHSS <1, $P<.001$) and functional (mRS <2 at 90 days, $P = .007$) outcome, as well as a significantly decreased geometric mean ($P = .001$) and median relative infarct growth ($P<.0001$) compared with the group without reperfusion. When analyzing the effects of tPA treatment as a whole in all mismatch patients, a similar decrease in geometric mean (1.24 vs 1.78, $P = .239$) or median relative infarct growth (1.18 vs 1.79, $P = .054$) was not seen despite the higher rates of successful reperfusion. However, a follow-up analysis by Nagakane and colleagues[19] did show a significant correlation with alteplase treatment and mean geometric infarct growth, compared with placebo (1.02 vs 1.77, respectively, $P = .0459$), when DWI/PWI coregistration was used to better quantify the initial penumbral size. This finding is critical in that it emphasizes the beneficial correlates of using MRI to assess penumbra size for patient selection as to the likely benefit of tPA thrombolysis beyond 4.5 hours.

IST-3 (International Stroke Trial 3) also looked at the potential benefit of IV tPA within 6 hours of stroke onset (n = 3035).[20] The original approval of tPA in Europe was for patients younger than 80 years with symptom onset up to 3 hours. IST-3 then explored patients who would otherwise be ineligible under the European license for tPA and included 1617 patients older than 80 years. IST-3 showed no significant benefit for the primary end point of the proportion of patients alive and independent 6 months after stroke. Although a slightly higher percentage of patients treated with IV tPA had a better 6-month outcome compared with placebo, results were not statistically significant (37% vs 35%, respectively; $P = .181$). More deaths occurred within 7 days in the tPA versus control groups (11% vs 7% adjusted OR 1.60 with 95% CI 1.22–2.08). However, there was benefit regarding the level of independent function, especially for those patients treated within 3 hours, and patients older than 80 years had as much benefit as younger patients. When comparing the adjusted effect of treatment in the age group older than 80 years with the age group younger than 80 years, the IST-3 investigators calculated an OR of 1.35 (0.97–1.88), which indicated a greater benefit in the former group compared with the latter ($P = .027$). The IST-3 trial addressed one of the unanswered questions pertaining to the management of octogenerations.

Although in IST-3 enrollment was limited to 6 hours, the calculated average time of onset was 4.2 hours. In a pooled meta-analysis, in which the IST-3 was a major component, the evidence suggested that tPA administered within 6 hours increased the odds of being alive and independent (defined as mRS scale score of 0–2) compared with controls (46% vs 42% OR 1.17; 95% CI 1.06–1.29) but again the benefit was greater the earlier tPA was given.[21]

Although thrombolysis with IV tPA has been shown to be possibly beneficial within a 6-hour window, it is beneficial to only a subset of patients. A reliable manner in which to select out this subset of patients has yet to be found. Whether imaging modalities may help definition of particular subsets of patients who might benefit beyond the classic time window remains indeterminate.

### Alternate Thrombolytic Therapy (Desmoteplase and Tenecteplase)

> **Unanswered question:**
> • Are there other agents that can be used that allow us to extend the time window?

### The 9-hour time window

In addition to using imaging modalities to better select the patients who will benefit from IV tPA in an extended window, exploration of alternative thrombolytic agents might also allow for an extended time window. One of these drugs is a novel fibrin-specific thrombolytic called desmoteplase. The pharmacology of this new agent seems promising in 2 respects: (1) desmoteplase uses fibrin as a cofactor, and thus its activity is enhanced in the presence of fibrin, and (2) administration of desmoteplase, unlike tPA, does not result in excessive fibrinogen depletion, possibly resulting in a lower bleeding risk.[22] DIAS and DEDAS were phase 2 trials to assess the therapeutic potential of desmoteplase. DIAS was a 2-part, randomized trial open to patients with a 3-hour to 9-hour stroke onset who had an apparent MRI PWI-DWI mismatch. Part 1 analyzed the effects of fixed doses of desmoteplase (25 mg, 37.5 mg, or 50 mg) compared with placebo. This phase was terminated early because there was more sICH within the treated group (up to 30.8% in the 37.5/50-mg group vs 0% in placebo).[23] Part 2 was then initiated with administration of a lower weight-adjusted desmoteplase dose (62.5 μg/kg, 90 μg/kg, and 125 μg/kg). In part 2, desmoteplase proved to be both safe, with lower sICH rates (highest percentage in 90-μg/kg group, 6.7% vs 0.0% in the placebo and 62.5-μg/kg or 125-μg/kg groups), as well as effective. Significant independent reperfusion rates were seen in the 90-μg/kg and 125-μg/kg groups (46.7% with $P = .0349$ and 71.4% with $P = .0012$, respectively), and a favorable 90-day clinical outcome was calculated as significant in the 125-μg/kg group (60.0% vs 22.2% in total placebo, $P = 0090$). Overall analysis showed a significant correlation between a favorable 90-day outcome and successful reperfusion ($P = .0028$, favorable clinical outcome in 52.5% of the reperfused group vs 24.6% without reperfusion).

These results were further supported by the subsequent DEDAS trial. Results of the DEDAS trial showed an upward, nonsignificant trend in both reperfusion percentage (53.3% in the 125-μg/kg group, 18.2% in the 90-μg/kg group) and favorable 90-day clinical outcome (60.0% in the 125-μg/kg group, 28.6% in the 90-μg/kg group) if IV desmoteplase was administered within 3 to 9 hours after stroke onset.[24]

However, results of the phase 3 DIAS-2 trial failed to show a beneficial outcome in patients treated with 90 or 125 μg/kg IV desmoteplase versus placebo within the 3-hour to 9-hour time window.[25] Posited reasons for the failure of the DIAS-2 trial included statistically significant differences in such baseline characteristics as core lesion volume ($P<.0001$), mismatch volume in cubic centimeters ($P = .008$), mismatch volume in percent ($P = .002$), and vessel occlusion as determined by the TIMI score ($P = .001$). Furthermore, among the differences between the DIAS-2 trial and the DIAS and DEDAS trials that may have influenced the results was that in all 3 groups the DIAS-2 trial enrolled more patients with a smaller mismatch volume ($cm^3$, $P = .008$; %, $P = .002$) and a lower association with vessel occlusion ($P = .0001$). Taking these differences into consideration, Fiebach and colleagues[26] conducted an analysis of the pooled data for all 3 trials assessing whether degree of vessel occlusion was associated with a positive therapeutic effect of desmoteplase administration and found a favorable 90-day clinical response with desmoteplase treatment in patients with TIMI scores of 0 or 1 ($P = .010$).

As a follow-up to these studies, 2 additional randomized, double-blind phase 3 prospective trials were started in 2009 (DIAS-3 and DIAS-4), with prospective completion dates between 2013 and 2014.[27] These 2 trials seem promising in defining the therapeutic benefits of desmoteplase in that, unlike in the previous 3 trials, DIAS-3 and 4 are enrolling patients only with known vessel occlusion or high-grade stenosis (TIMI 0–1) in proximal cerebral arteries.[27] The treatment window will remain within 3 to 9 hours after stroke onset and only a single IV dose of desmoteplase (90 µg/kg) will be administered. Final 90-day outcome measures will remain similar to the previous DIAS trials with mRS 0–2.

Tenecteplase is another thrombolytic agent that seems promising for patients with onset of stroke symptoms within an extended time window. Although it is FDA approved for use only in acute myocardial infarction, a recent randomized trial showed better reperfusion rates and clinical outcomes in patients treated with tenecteplase (0.1 mg/kg or 0.25 mg/kg) compared with patients treated with a 0.9-mg/kg dose of TPA.[28] Similar to the DIAS-3 and DIAS-4 trials, enrollment was limited to patients with large-vessel occlusions and a large perfusion lesion without a large infarct core as determined by CT perfusion and CT angiographic imaging. The study suggested that in the tenecteplase group, there were better reperfusion outcomes at 24 hours ($P = .004$), more patients with an excellent to good recovery at 90 days (mRS 0–2, $P = .02$), and more mismatch salvage at 90 days, as determined by follow-up MRI ($P = .003$), when compared with the tPA group.

## IA Thrombolysis as an Alternative to IV Thrombolysis

**Unanswered question:**

- Is IA thrombolysis an effective and beneficial alternative to IV thrombolysis?

### PROACT-II and IMS-III trials

Around the time of IV tPA pilot trials, various investigators began to advocate the benefits of local IA thrombolysis with either streptokinase or urokinase.[29,30] Mori and colleagues[30] showed that IA urokinase was both safe and effective for MCA occlusions as shown by reduced infarction volume and a better functional outcome after successful recanalization. A decade later, the PROACT-II study reported improved 90-day clinical outcomes in patients with MCA occlusions who had been given IA recombinant prourokinase (r-proUK) within 6 hours of stroke onset.[31] Nonetheless, the PROACT-II study did not lead to approval of r-proUK. Possible reasons were that the study was conducted on a small subset of patients (n = 180) who had only MCA occlusions out of a larger number of screened patients, and the statistical benefit did not meet prespecified end points ($P = .04$ for positive outcome). Furthermore, the outcomes in the control group were believed by the FDA to be worse than previously reported historical controls; regulators were concerned whether the significant improvement of the treated group was real versus falsely increased because of the poorer outcome in the control group. There were concerns about the effects of r-proUK in the context of concurrent heparin administration. In the PROACT-I study, concurrent use of heparin, most especially high-dose heparin, resulted in a nonsignificant but upward trending incidence of ICHs compared with the placebo group (20.0% with low dose, 72.7% with high dose, vs 0.0% and 20.0% in respective placebo groups, $P>.100$).[32] Although low-dose heparin was used in the PROACT-II study, the regulators were apparently unwilling to license prourokinase without further investigations of the drug in the absence of heparin. Nevertheless, PROACT-I and PROACT-II were landmark studies, because they validated the proof of concept that IA pharmacologic thrombolysis might be beneficial in AIS.

After the PROACT-II study, pharmacologic endovascular thrombolysis remained popular with clinicians using tPA on an off-label use to treat patients who were otherwise ineligible for IV tPA. Another paradigm for off-label endovascular pharmacologic thrombolysis for patients with large strokes encompassed the idea of bridging therapy for patients who did not immediately respond to IV tPA.[33–38] The idea that a combined IV/IA recanalization therapy would be beneficial was investigated in the IMS-I and IMS-II studies, which showed lower 3-month mortality (16% vs 21% in NINDS tPA group) and a significantly better 3-month outcome in the IMS-II patients compared with patients in the NINDS placebo (OR, 2.78; 95% CI, 1.46, 5.31) and IV tPA groups (BI 95–100; OR, 2.29; 95% CI, 1.24, 4.23).[34,35] The IMS-III trial, a phase 3, randomized, multicenter trial, was then initiated to evaluate if the combination of IV tPA with IA therapy in patients with moderate-to-large acute strokes (NIHSS $\geq$10, onset 3 hours or less) had better outcomes compared with the standard 0.9-mg/kg IV tPA dose alone.[36,37] IMS-III allowed for the use of several of either the MERCI Retriever device, EKOS Micro-Infusion Catheter (EKOS Corporation, Bothell, WA) penumbra device (Penumbra, Inc, Alameda, CA), or Solitaire stent retriever device (Covidien, Inc, Mansfield, MA) or a standard microcatheter with local tPA infusion (to a maximum of 22 mg IA tPA with a maximum of 2-mg–4-mg bolus and infusion at 10 mg/h) for clot dissolution in the IV/IA treated group. The randomized allocation scheme was defined such that one-third of patients received standard-of-care therapy and two-thirds of patients received either mechanical or pharmacologic IA thrombolysis, with intervention started within 5 hours and completed within 7 hours of symptom onset.[37] The plan was that patients randomized to the endovascular arm would receive two-thirds of the standard dose, but late in the study, the trial was amended in 2011, so that patients could receive full-dose IV tPA before endovascular therapy. Although no specific safety concerns were noted, the study was recently terminated early, after enrollment of 656 patients (of a planned maximum of 900 patients). An interim analysis of the study failed to show an absolute benefit difference of 10% (defined by mRS at 3 months) in the IV/IA treated group compared with the IV tPA group.[37,38] IMS-II failed to show a significant difference between the endovascular therapy and IV tPA groups in the overall proportion of patients with an mRS of 2 or less (40.8% vs 28.7% (95% CI, −6.1 to 9.1). There was also no significant difference in the prespecified subgroups of patients with severe stroke (NIHSS >19), in whom there was a trend to benefit in favor of the endovascular group (relative risk [RR] reduction, 1.37; 95% CI, 0.63–2.99) with a difference of 6.8% (95% CI, −3.3 to 18.1) or in the prespecified group of patients with NIHSS 8 to 19 for whom IV tPA was slightly more favorable (RR, 1.01 (0.78–1.31) with a difference of 1% in favor of IV tPA (95% CI, −10.8 to 8.8). Patients who underwent endovascular therapy who had better reperfusion rates as measured by Thrombolysis in Cerebral Infarction (TICI) grade 2 to 3 (partial or complete recanalization) were more likely to have an mRS of 2 or less at 90 days (12.7% for TICI [Thrombolysis in Cerebral Infarction] = 0; 27.6% for TICI = 1; 34.3% for TICI = 2a; 47.9% for TICI = 2b; and 71.4% for TICI = 3 ($P<.001$). There were no statistical differences in mortality for the endovascular group versus iv tPA alone (19.1% vs 21.6; $P = .52$) or sICH (6.2% vs 5.9%; $P = .83$), although asymptomatic ICH was greater in the endovascular group than in the IV tPA alone group (27.4% vs 18.9%; $P = .01$). In the IV tPA group, as assessed by magnetic resonance angiography (MRA) or transcranial Doppler (TCD) ultrasonography, the degree of recanalization in the M1 occlusions was only 40%, whereas partial or complete reperfusion (measured as TICI 2–3) was 81% in the endovascular group. Despite the greater revascularization rates after endovascular therapy in this subgroup, there were no significant clinical benefits of endovascular therapy versus IV TPA alone. Thus, revascularization was an insufficient surrogate measure of clinical benefit in this study. The other dilemma of IMS-III reflects the therapeutic choices available during the study. The investigators used higher-dose IV tPA or stent retriever devices as part of endovascular therapy only toward the end of IMS-III. Whether the putative higher revascularization rates associated with these newer strategies would be associated with better outcomes is unknown.

The SYNTHESIS-EXP study, which was published in the same issue of the *New England Journal of Medicine* as the IMS-III trial, was a study funded by the Italian Medicines Agency that similarly randomized patients to either IV tPA or endovascular therapy.[39] In this study, 362 patients were randomly assigned, within 4.5 hours of symptom onset, to the specified intervention, with benefit measured as a primary outcome of disability-free survival (mRS, 0 or 1) at 3 months. Median time to treatment was 1 hour later with endovascular therapy compared with IV tPA (3.75 vs 2.75 hours; $P<.001$). At 3 months, 55 of 181 patients (30.4%) in the endovascular group and 63 of 181 patients (34.8%) in the IV tPA group were alive without disability (adjusted OR, 0.71; 95% CI, 0.44–1.14; $P = .15$). Fatal or nonfatal sICH at 7 days after treatment was 6% in both treatment arms. However, unlike the IMS-III trial, patients assigned to the endovascular arm did not receive IV tPA before angiography. Once the diagnostic angiogram was completed, the patient could undergo IA tPA, mechanical embolectomy, or a combination of both therapeutic interventions. If the patient was to receive IA tPA, a high IA dose of 0.9 mg/kg (to a maximum of 90 mg) was given within the first hour of endovascular therapy to either the maximum dose or recanalization of the vessel. Another significant difference between IMS-III and SYNTHESIS-EXP was that SYNTHESIS patients randomized to endovascular therapy who had neurologic deficits but no significant large-vessel occlusion after diagnostic angiogram still received IA tPA (0.9 mg/kg to a maximum dose of 90 mg) given into the presumptive affected vascular territory based on clinical symptoms. Subgroup analysis did not reveal any differences based on time to treatment, stroke subtype, age, type of center (high vs low volume), or disease severity. The investigators also performed a subgroup analysis excluding protocol deviations. The investigators withdrew 1 center from the study after enrollment of 12 patients for multiple protocol violations. In addition, there were 8 other patients (5 of whom were in the endovascular arm) with major protocol violations. The SYNTHESIS investigators performed a post hoc sensitivity analysis on the primary outcome and reported that the results were not qualitatively different (OR, 0.7; 95% CI, 0.43–1.14; $P = .15$). The overall results were reported as intention to treat; for a variety of reasons, including technical issues, only 163 of 181 patients received the assigned endovascular therapy, whereas 178 of 181 patients assigned to the IV tPA arm received IV tPA (1 patient in this arm had spontaneous resolution of symptoms before treatment and 2 patients assigned to IV tPA underwent mechanical thrombectomy). As in the IMS-III study, newer devices such as the Solitaire stent retriever were not widely used in this study.

In an accompanying editorial to the IMS-III, SYNTHESIS, and MR-RESCUE studies, Chimowitz[38] emphasized that "IV thrombolysis should continue to be the first-line treatment for patients with acute ischemic stroke within 4.5 hours after stroke onset, even if imaging shows an occluded major intracranial artery." Despite the promising conceptual approach that was suggested by the randomized PROACT studies, pharmacologic IA thrombolysis remains of unproven benefit compared with IV TPA.

## SURGICAL/NONPHARMACOLOGIC TREATMENT OPTIONS

**Unanswered question:**

- Does the data support mechanical thrombolysis as an effective and beneficial alternative to IV thrombolysis?
- What is the role of sonothrombolysis as an adjunct to IV thrombolysis?

### Endovascular Thrombectomy as an Alternative to IV Thrombolysis

In 2004, the MERCI-1 safety trial described benefits of thrombus retrieval in patients who presented within 8 hours from stroke onset, or who presented within 3 hours of stroke onset but for whom IV thrombolysis was contraindicated.[40] The 8-hour time window was chosen based on the PROACT-II study, which suggested some benefit in recanalization after 8 hours despite an increase in sICH. However, for PROACT-II, the average time of onset of stroke symptoms to completion of treatment was 6 hours and 1 minute. Enrollment in the MERCI study was limited to patients with apparent large-vessel occlusions (MCA, intracranial internal carotid artery, vertebral artery, or basilar artery) who had moderate to severe strokes (NIHSS score $\geq$10). A total of 30 patients were enrolled, with 12 in the MERCI-only group and 18 in the MERCI plus IA tPA group. The study reported successful recanalization (TIMI 2–3) in 43% of the patients in the MERCI-only group, versus 64% when IA TPA was used in addition to the MERCI Retriever.[40] The study furthered showed a positive, although nonsignificant, 30-day outcome in 50% of the patients with successful recanalization (good outcome was defined as mRS score 0–2 in patients with baseline NIHSS of 10–20, and mRS score of 0–3 in patients with a baseline score of >20).

In 2005, a follow-up study showed an association between successful recanalization with the MERCI Retriever (up to 48% in all patients in whom retriever was used, $P<.0001$) and a better 90-day outcome (mRS $\leq$2) when compared with patients without successful recanalization (46% vs 10%; $P<.0001$).[41] The time window of enrollment was up to 8 hours, with the average symptom onset to groin puncture time of 4.3 hours. Results of this study also showed a similar mortality (32% vs 54%; $P = .01$) and an overall low incidence of sICH (7.8%) associated with recanalization. These findings were reproduced in the later Multi-MERCI trial, in which the L5 Retriever (a newer generation of the MERCI Retriever) was used in patients with persistent large-vessel occlusions after IV tPA treatment within the 8-hour window of stroke onset.[42] The Multi-MERCI investigators reported successful recanalization in 57.3% of patients treated with the retriever alone, and 69.5% when concomitant IA tPA was used. Like the earlier studies, the Multi-MERCI trial reported an association between successful recanalization and a good 90-day clinical outcome (36% of patients with mRS 0–2; 95% CI, 29–44) and lower mortality (34%; 95% CI, 26–41). The study also reported a low percentage of sICH (9.8%; 95% CI, 0.1–4.8). However, none of the MERCI trials was a randomized study, and the positive survival outcomes reported were not superior to the outcomes of the comparator historical controls of the PROACT-II study. Patient differences between the historical controls of the PROACT-II and the MERCI nonrandomized studies make any conclusions about the relative efficacy of this device problematic.[43]

In 2008, a small study[44] described outcomes with the Penumbra clot aspiration system. This study enrolled 23 patients who presented within 8 hours of stroke symptom onset (50% with stroke onset <3 hours) with intracranial vessel occlusions (TIMI 0–1) as verified by catheter cerebral angiography. There was successful recanalization in 100% of the patients, with a 45% positive 30-day outcome as defined by a 4-point improvement from baseline NIHSS or an mRS 0 to 2. The investigators reported an all-cause 30-day mortality of 45%, which they attributed to the high enrollment of patients (70%) with NIHSS greater than 20 or with basilar occlusions (BAO) in this pilot study. The larger prospective, multicenter nonrandomized Penumbra Pivotal Stroke Trial then enrolled 125 patients with an NIHSS of 8 or greater, with symptom onset of 8 hours or less, and who had a large intracranial vessel occlusion (TIMI 0 or 1) as determined by angiography.[45] Although 81.6% of patients treated with the Penumbra system had successful recanalizations (TIMI 2–3), these investigators were unable to show a positive association between vessel recanalization and a good 90-day clinical outcome (25% of overall patients with mRS 0–2, $P$ = .0596). Conducting a multivariate analysis on predictors that may have influenced this lower functional outcome, the investigators suggested that baseline NIHSS proved to be a significant factor in outcomes ($P$ value of 0.0005). Baseline NIHSS was also significant in predicting mortality (1.132; 95% CI, 1.035–1.239; $P$ = .0066) along with a history of previous stroke (OR, 3.498; 95% CI, 1.263–9.690; $P$ = .0160). Site of occlusion was also included in the multivariate analysis but was not shown to be significant in predicting mortality.

Most recently, the MR-RESCUE study failed to show benefit of mechanical embolectomy (n = 64) compared with standard of care (n = 54) in 118 fully eligible patients with large-vessel anterior circulation strokes randomized to treatment within 8 hours of symptom onset. The mean NIHSS score of the study population was 17 (range 6–29), and patients with a worse penumbral pattern, ascertained by CT or MRI, had higher NIHSS scores. The study was initiated in 2004 using any of the MERCI Retriever devices and, after 2009, the Penumbra system could also be used. In addition, IA tPA could be used as rescue therapy up to a maximum dose of 14 mg (the average dose used in the Multi-MERCI trial).[46] Of the 64 patients randomized to embolectomy, 3 had recanalization of the occluded target vessel by the time of angiography, 37 were treated with the MERCI retrievers, 14 with the Penumbra system, and 10 with both systems with mean time from symptom onset to groin puncture of 6 hours and 21 minutes (standard deviation, 1 hour and 14 minutes). Among all patients there was no difference at 90 days in the mRS scale between those who underwent embolectomy or standard of care (3.9 vs 3.9; $P$ = .99). This was the case regardless of stratification to either a favorable or unfavorable pattern for both treatments. Overall, IV tPA was given to 44 of 118 (37%) patients in the cohort. IV TPA was given to 27 of 34 (79%) patients with a favorable penumbral pattern who underwent embolectomy; 12 of 40 (30%) with an unfavorable pattern who underwent embolectomy; 16 of 34 (47%) patients who had a favorable penumbral pattern who underwent standard-of-care treatment; and 7 of 20 (35%) patients with an unfavorable pattern who underwent standard-of-care treatment ($P$ = .36). Across the cohort, the rate of all-cause mortality was 21%, the rate of sICH was 4%, and the rate of asymptomatic hemorrhage was 58%, with no difference between subgroups.

Among the currently approved FDA devices, the Solitaire intravascular stent retriever seems to be most promising, although it has not been compared with IV tPA therapy in a randomized fashion. In the SWIFT (SOLITAIRE FR With the Intention For Thrombectomy) study, the Solitaire device was compared in a randomized fashion with the MERCI Retriever in 3 separate areas: rate of vessel recanalization, 90-day neurologic outcome, and safety.[47] Revascularization to a TIMI score of 2 to 3 was more common in the Solitaire group than in the MERCI Retriever group (61% vs 24%; OR, 4.87; 95% CI, 2.14–11.10). Better 90-day neurologic outcomes (58% vs 33%; OR, 2.78; 95% CI, 1.25–6.22) and lower 90-day mortality (17% vs 38%; OR,

0.34; 95% CI, 0.14–0.81) were also seen with the Solitaire device compared with the MERCI Retriever. Whether this and other devices in development will justify routine use of mechanical thrombectomy for AIS remains to be elucidated.

### Sonothrombolysis

Sonothrombolysis is a promising adjunctive therapy to IV tPA. Mechanical pressure waves produced by ultrasonographic energy seem to help pharmacologic thrombolysis via nonthermal effects of ultrasound, possibly through creation of gas bubbles in liquid medium (acoustic cavitation).[48] In a human clinical trial, this benefit was seen using 2-MHz diagnostic TCD probes with ultrasonic energy applied for up to 2 hours after initiation of tPA.[49] In this CLOTBUST (Combined Lysis of Thrombus in Brain Ischemia using Transcranial Ultrasound and Systemic tPA) study, 126 patients were randomized to tPA alone or tPA plus sonothrombolysis. A good outcome, defined as complete recanalization (shown by ultrasonography) or clinic recovery (defined as a total NIHSS score $\leq$3 or improvement >10 within 2 hours of tPA administration), was observed in 49% of the sonothrombolysis group and 30% of the control group ($P$ = .03). The safety end point was sICH that led to a worsening greater than 4 points on the NIHSS; in the CLOTBUST study, there was no increase in sICH rates between the study and control groups. By contrast, the TRUMBI (Transcranial Low Frequency Ultrasound Mediated Thrombolysis in Brain Ischemia) trial was stopped because of a high rate of ICH (13 of 14 patients).[50] However, in the TRUMBI study, low-energy frequencies were used (300 $\pm$ 1.5 K HX pulsed ultrasound), and it has been suggested that low-frequency energy over a wider tissue footprint might predispose patients to a greater risk of brain hemorrhage.[48] Two systematic reviews of sonothrombolysis have been completed.[51,52] Both reviews noted that sample sizes in all studies were small, inclusion criteria were heterogeneous, and there was significant variation in ultrasonographic energies. Both reviews confirmed that there was no increase in hemorrhage with higher-frequency sonothrombolysis and suggested that statistically higher rates of recanalization might be associated with sonothrombolysis using the energies associated with routine TCD. Sonothrombolysis is an inexpensive therapeutic adjunct to IV tPA. Still, this approach remains unproved because of the availability of only a few small clinical trials. Furthermore, technical limits (operator-dependent variability in performing high-quality TCDs and limited ability to sonographically visualize arterial segments in many patients because of poor bony windows) and resource limits in providing sonothrombolysis acutely at most hospitals are such that widespread adoption of this approach remains questionable.

### CONCOMITANT THERAPIES

> **Unanswered question:**
> - What effects do AP and AC drugs have on thrombolysis?
> - Are these effects enough to maintain the current exclusion criteria for patients on AC/AP therapy?

In addition to sICH, early reocclusion after tPA thrombolysis is one of the major complications associated with thrombolytic therapy. Among the theories behind early reocclusion is that, after the initiation of cerebral ischemia, leukocyte and platelet activation remain high, causing platelet aggregation and microvascular occlusions, a concept referred as the no-reflow phenomenon.[8,53] Although concomitant thrombolysis with AP or AC therapy has been considered, the safety of concomitant therapy with thrombolytic agents is still unknown. The later discussion highlights the lack of data regarding the safety of thrombolysis in patients with acute stroke symptoms who were concurrently receiving AP or AC drugs. In addition to aspirin, the main AP and AC drugs in use for antithrombotic preventive therapy in cardiovascular disease include thienopyridines (eg, clopidogrel, prasugrel), nonthienopyridines/cyclopentyltriazolopyrimidines (eg, ticagrelor, cangrelor), dipyridamole (alone or in combination therapy with aspirin), warfarin, and new oral AC including factor Xa inhibitors (eg, rivaroxaban, apixaban) or direct thrombin inhibitors (eg, dabigatran).[54–57]

Considering the specific role of AP and AC drugs in the context of AIS, Ibrahim and colleagues[57] performed a retrospective review into the effects of aspirin, clopidogrel, extended-release dipyridamole plus aspirin, and warfarin, on functional outcomes and sICH risk compared with antithrombotic naive patients after being treated with IV TPA. The predictors for success included the presence of complete vessel recanalization (TIBI [Thrombolysis In Brain Ischemia]score of 4 or 5 after 2 hours of IV tPA), a positive 90-day outcome (mRS $\leq$2), and a low sICH risk. The study reported a significantly higher number of complete recanalization in patients taking clopidogrel (60%) or warfarin (55.6%) before IV tPA treatment, versus if they were AP naive (38.2%) or on aspirin alone (22.2%, $P$ = .017). Focusing on long-term outcomes and rates of sICH, this study showed that the clopidogrel group had a significantly lower frequency of patients with a good long-term outcome (38.5%, $P$ = .035), as well as a higher frequency of sICH (20%, $P$ = .029) compared with the other groups. By contrast, patients previously on warfarin before IV thrombolysis (even with a normal international normalized ratio [INR], as required before IV tPA) had the highest frequency of a good long-term outcome (55.6% vs 53.1% in the AP-naive group and 40.3% in the ASA group) as well as no recorded incidents of sICH (0% vs 5% in the AP naive group and 6.6% in the ASA group). However, only 9 patients on warfarin were included in this analysis, and all had a subtherapeutic INR before treatment. Furthermore, in the multiple regression analysis, previous antithrombotic use was not a predictor of recanalization rate ($P$ = .057) or of good outcome ($P$ = .27), although a significantly higher risk of sICH was present in patients on clopidogrel compared with antithrombotic naive patients (OR = 4.4; 95% CI, 1.03–21; $P$ = .04).

In addition, there are no current data about the risk of stroke thrombolysis complications in patients taking the newer AP drugs such as prasugrel. However, by extrapolation from the TIMI-38 study, it seems reasonable to be particularly cautious in considering stroke thrombolysis in a patient actively on prasugrel.[58–60] In TIMI-38, those patients treated for acute coronary syndromes (ACS) with prasugrel (as opposed to clopidogrel) were found to have greater risk of bleeding complications if they were older than 75 years, had a history of TIA/stroke, or had a body weight less than 60 kg.[60]

The risk of stroke thrombolysis might be theoretically safer in patients on concomitant ticagrelor or cangrelor, which had lesser bleeding complications when studied in patients with ACS. As with prasugrel, although there are ACS trials with ticagrelor or cangrelor, there are no data for their use in AIS, with or without thrombolytic therapy. The advantage of these 2 drugs is that they inhibit platelet aggregation with a shorter onset of action, higher potency, and have the added benefit of being reversible.[53,54] In the PLATO (Platelet Inhibition and Patient Outcomes) trial, ticagrelor was superior to clopidogrel in decreasing the incidence of vascular death, myocardial infarction, or stroke at 12 months (9.8% vs 11.7%; $P$<.001) without increasing the incidence of major bleeding (11.6% vs 11.2%; $P$ = .43) when given to ACS patients.[61]

As for concomitant oral AC therapy and the risk of complications with concomitant thrombolytic therapies, Vergouwen and colleagues[62] evaluated the association between immediate previous warfarin use (INR <1.7) and post-tPA hemorrhage and reported no significant association between preadmission warfarin use and sICH ($P = .29$) or gastrointestinal hemorrhage ($P = .57$). When analyzing the frequency of any ICH, a significant increase of ICH was present with preadmission warfarin use (16.8% vs 11.1%, respectively; $P = .054$), yet with no resultant differences in incidence of poor functional outcome ($P = .30$) or mortality ($P = .37$). Xian and colleagues[63] also reported that, although a higher unadjusted sICH rate was present in warfarin-treated patients than in those not taking warfarin (5.7% vs 4.6%; $P<.001$), warfarin use was not an independent predictor for sICH when the analysis was adjusted for the higher comorbid condition, older age, and increased severity of stroke present in the warfarin group (adjusted OR, 1.01; 95% CI, 0.82–1.25; $P = .94$). There were also no significant differences in sICH risk in patients on warfarin with an INR $\leq 1.7$ (adjusted OR, 1.10 per 0.1 unit increase in INR; 95% CI, 1.00–1.20; $P = .06$; adjusted RR, 1.09 per 0.1 unit increase; 95% CI, 1.00–1.20) or differences in in-hospital mortality (11.4% vs 7.9%; adjusted OR, 0.94; 95% CI, 0.79–1.13; $P<.001$). Furthermore, Kim and colleagues[64] analyzed the effects of warfarin discontinuation in patients with atrial fibrillation just before thrombolytic treatment. When comparing patients in whom warfarin had been discontinued versus those who remained on warfarin just before thrombolytic therapy, the investigators found an early neurologic deterioration (increase in NIHSS score within 7 days, 57.1% vs 26.9%; $P = .029$) and a poorer long-term functional outcome (mRS $\geq 3$; OR, 17.067; 95% CI, 2.703–107.748) in the group for whom warfarin had been discontinued previously.

Although some studies have argued that warfarin, even if subtherapeutic (INR $\leq 1.7$), increases the incidence of bleeding, most of these studies have enrolled only a few patients taking warfarin.[65–67] Those studies have fewer patients than the studies suggesting that previous warfarin use (even although subtherapeutic) is not harmful. Thus, the study by Vergouwen and colleagues[62] had 125 warfarin-treated patients compared with 1614 patients with no preadmission warfarin use; the study by Kim and colleagues[64] had 14 patients in their warfarin withdrawal group versus 134 patients in the no-withdrawal group; and the study by Xian and colleagues[63] compared 802 patients with previous warfarin use versus 21,635 with no preadmission warfarin use.

As for the newer factor Xa inhibitors and direct thrombin inhibitors, there are insufficient clinical data to determine what risk is associated with previous use of these agents in patients presenting with AIS for possible stroke thrombolysis. These drugs do have short half-lives.[56] Thus, it seems reasonable that if the patient had missed several doses before the stroke (approximately 24–48 hours depending on the agent), then the patient could safely be treated with IV or IA thrombolytic therapies. Otherwise, mechanical thrombectomy might be considered for these patients.

The risk of specific AP and AC drugs used for stroke prevention in the context of stroke thrombolytic therapy remains unclear, but IV thrombolysis might be contraindicated in the context of prasugrel and probably should be avoided in patients taking warfarin who have a therapeutic INR or who are actively taking one of the newer oral ACs.

## OUTCOME DETERMINANTS
### What Are the Determinants of Poor Outcome with Thrombolysis?

Unanswered question:

- Are there certain modalities or clinical characteristics that can be used to determine benefit and potential outcome with thrombolytic treatment beyond 3 hours?

One of the major concerns of thrombolytic therapy is posttreatment development of hemorrhagic transformation. Although studies such as the NINDS, ECASS, and ATLANTIS trials have shown an increased risk of sICH among treated groups, they have consistently shown that there is no increase in long-term mortality, and that the tPA-treated groups had better 90-day outcomes. Regardless, it remains a desirable goal to select patients who may respond favorably to thrombolytic treatment without bleeding. Use of imaging to screen for those at risk for ICH suggests that extent of CT hypoattenuation is the major determinant for bleeding risk.[12]

### Imaging modalities

Various studies within the last 2 decades have investigated the clinical benefit of using radiographic imaging to: (1) calculate the extent of ischemic damage, (2) determine the amount of salvageable tissue (called the penumbra), and (3) predict the likelihood of a favorable response to thrombolytic therapy. Common imaging modalities used include: MRI PWI-DWI mismatch, MRA-DWI mismatch, and CT perfusion hypoattenuation.[68–72]

The ASPECTS study investigators were among the first to suggest a benefit of using imaging modalities to predict the likelihood of a more favorable outcome.[68] Using noncontrast CT scans, Barber and colleagues created the ASPECTS 10-point scoring system, based on the presence of early ischemic changes (defined as focal swelling or parenchymal hypoattenuation) over 10 regions in the MCA territory. These investigators showed that individuals with an ASPECTS score of 7 or less had 14 times the risk for sICH compared with individuals with an ASPECTS score of greater than 7 (OR, 14; 95% CI, 1.8–117). Using logistic regression analysis, an ASPECTS score was also predictive of functional outcome after tPA thrombolysis (percent independent with ASPECTS $\leq$7 79.8% vs 4.6% with score >7; OR, 82; 95% CI, 23–290; sensitivity, 0.78; specificity, 0.96). Furthermore, although these results roughly correlated with those seen when patients were separated using the one-third MCA rule on NCCT, in terms of being a reliable imaging assessment modality, the ASPECTS score had consistently higher within-rater reliability compared with the one-third MCA rule (agreement range for ASPECTS scoring 0.67–0.82 vs one-third MCA rule 0.26–0.76).

Although it remains current practice to screen AIS thrombolytic-eligible patients with a baseline CT scan to rule out acute hemorrhage, identify other causes of stroke-like deficits, and identify previous infarcts or early acute infarct changes, MRI is an alternative imaging modality that can be used to screen thrombolytic-eligible patients. One study compared outcomes in 3 separate groups of patients (within 3 hours with CT, within 3 hours with MRI, and beyond 3 hours with MRI) to assess if there was a difference in outcomes of patients evaluated for thrombolytic treatment by MRI PWI-DWI mismatch versus by CT alone.[72] The investigators concluded that in patients who presented beyond the 3-hour time window (median time of onset 240 minutes; range, 181–1032 minutes), those who were treated with thrombolytic treatment based on an MRI PWI-DWI mismatch greater than 20% had better outcomes than those identified by CT alone (OR, 1.467; 95% CI, 1.017–2.117; $P$ = .040). Significant outcomes were not calculated when comparing the use of MRI versus CT within the 3-hour window; however, there was a nonsignificant trend for a better functional outcome in the MRI group versus the CT group (OR, 1.136; 95% CI, 0.841–1.534). Use of MRI, regardless of time window, was also associated with a significantly lower chance for sICH development (OR, 0.520; 95% CI, 0.270–0.999; $P$ = .05).

The concept of MRI PWI-DWI mismatch was used in the DEFUSE study and EPITHET studies to select patients who were likely to benefit from thrombolytic treatment within a 3-hour to 6-hour time of stroke onset (average onset in EPITHET, 4.2 hours; average onset in DEFUSE, approximately 5 hours).[18,70] The DEFUSE study showed a significant association in the mismatch group between early recanalization and the odds of a favorable clinical response (OR, 29; 95% CI, 1.01–397; $P$ = .047) and small infarct growth ($P$ = .024).[70] A smaller infarct growth was also associated with a favorable clinical response in the mismatch group ($P$ = .03).[70] These correlations were not present in the group without mismatch ($P$ = 1). In the assessment of patients with mismatch in the EPITHET study, reperfusion rates were higher after treatment with alteplase versus placebo (56% vs 26%, $P$ = .010).[18] Accurate assessment of reperfusion rates in patients without mismatch could not be completed because enrollment was small for those treated with alteplase (N = 3) versus placebo (N = 4).

MRI PWI-DWI mismatch might not only identify patients who would benefit from thrombolytic therapy but also might be a predictor of comparative benefit. Using the data from the DEFUSE study, Lansberg and colleagues[72] calculated a highly favorable response to tPA reperfusion in patients with MR-DWI mismatch (OR, 12.5; 95% CI, 1.8–83.9) compared with those without mismatch on MR imaging (OR, 0.2; 95% CI, 0.0–0.8). In the group without mismatch, patients initially seemed to do better if they were not reperfused (favorable outcomes in 3 of 14 patients with reperfusion vs 10 of 16 without reperfusion), yet this finding proved to be nonsignificant when adjusting for older age, higher baseline NIHSS score, and the larger PWI and DWI lesions that were more common in the no-mismatch group with reperfusion compared with the no-mismatch group without reperfusion ($P$ = .2).

Despite the inherent logic of using DWI-PWI mismatch to identify selected patients with greater potential for salvageable tissue, this strategy has not been supported by the clinical trial data of the MR-RESCUE study.[46] In the study, 55% of the 118 patients, with mean time to enrollment of 5.5 hours, had a favorable penumbral pattern assessed by either CT or MR perfusion imaging. Patients were randomized to either mechanical embolectomy or standard care (including in some cases IV tPA) and stratified by a favorable or nonfavorable ischemic penumbra. Yet, there were no clinical differences in outcome between the embolectomy and standard-of-care groups at 90 days, whether or not there was a favorable penumbral pattern.

The heterogeneity of the imaging approaches (CT vs MR) may have contributed, to some degree, to the failure of the study, because patients evaluated on CT apparently had larger predicted core volumes of infarction compared with MRI.[46] The MR-RESCUE investigators, in their discussion, also theorized that patients with a favorable penumbral window, especially those treated in a later time window (>3 hours) may have a good functional outcome regardless of treatment assessment, wherein a favorable penumbral pattern reflects the presence of good collateral flow. In a secondary prespecified analysis, patients with a favorable penumbral pattern had a better 90-day mRS than those with a poor penumbral pattern (3.6 mRS [95% CI, 3.3–4.0] vs 4.2 mRS [95% CI, 3.8–4.7] [$P$ = .047]).[46] Furthermore, a more favorable penumbral pattern, regardless of treatment assignment, was also associated with smaller infarct volumes. Nevertheless, the MR-RESCUE study failed to confirm the hypothesis that selecting patients for reperfusion, based on imaging characteristics, could identify a subgroup of patients that might derive greater benefit from intervention. Whether the failure of mechanical embolectomy in this study was related to the type of device used (associated with lower rats of revascularization) or the longer time to intervention in the study is unclear. Perhaps alternative imaging strategies other than measurement of perfusion mismatch might be necessary to identify patients with poor collateral flow who would then benefit from revascularization strategies with either IV or IA thrombolytic therapy.

## Presence of collaterals

Rapid restoration of adequate perfusion to tissue at risk for infarction increases a patient's chance for better outcomes. If perfusion could be maintained through vessels that could circumvent an arterial occlusion, it might be expected that the damaging effects of ischemia would be diminished, resulting in a better clinical outcome and potentially smaller infarct size. Might those patients with poor collateral flow then preferentially benefit from more aggressive attempts at flow restoration?[73–78] Early on, the NASCET investigators, in the context of internal carotid artery stenosis, explored the effects of a collateral system on stroke risk. They reported that patients with an angiographically visualized collateral system had a significantly decreased 2-year risk of suffering from a disabling or fatal stroke (6.3% vs 13.3%, $P = .11$) or any stroke (11.3% vs 27.8%, $P = .005$).[75] Christoforidis and colleagues[76] used a 5-point grading system to evaluate the effects of a good pial collateral system (score 1, full reconstitution up to site of occlusion vs score 5, little to no reconstitution) on clinical outcome and infarct volume of patients treated with IA tPA, urokinase, or r-proUK. These investigators reported a significant association between a poor collateral system (higher score) and a greater infarct volume irrespective of recanalization state after IA thrombolysis ($P = .003$ with complete recanalization; $P = .0067$ with partial and no recanalization). Bang and colleagues[77] similarly noted that patients with poor collaterals (American Society of Interventional and Therapeutic Neuroradiology [ASITN]/Society of Interventional Radiology [SIR] score 0–1) had a greater infarct growth after therapeutic revascularization compared with patients with good (ASITN/SIR score 2–3) or excellent (ASITN/SIR score 4) collaterals ($P = .012$). In addition to significantly decreased rates of complete revascularizations in the patients with poor collaterals (14.1% vs 25.2% with good collaterals and 41.5% with excellent collaterals; $P<.001$), higher rates of sICH were also noted in patients with poor collaterals ($P = .048$).[77,78]

## Stroke location

In 1988, Hacke and colleagues[29] published an observational study suggesting that patients with strokes caused by vertebrobasilar occlusive disease responded favorably to IA thrombolysis. In this analysis, these investigators reported a statistically significant better outcome in the subgroup of patients who had successful recanalization after IA thrombolysis (44% of all patients treated with thrombolysis) when compared with a control group treated only with AP and AC therapy ($P = .017$ for favorable/unfavorable outcome; $P = .0005$ for survival/death). A comparison of outcomes in all patients treated with thrombolysis versus control was not performed. Sairanen and colleagues[79] looked at predictors of BAO outcomes in 116 patients treated with mainly heparin or IV tPA and found that only 25.9% had good outcomes defined as mRS 0 to 1, with sICH rate of 15.7%. Partial or complete recanalization occurred in 64.8% of the patients with a posttreatment angiogram (59/91). Lower age and lower NIHSS score were associated with better outcome, and greater likelihood of recanalization was more likely associated with the top of the basilar syndrome. Despite the belief that posterior circulation strokes had a greater ischemic tolerance compared with anterior circulation strokes, leading to the suggestion that the time window for thrombolysis might be greater in patients with BAO, the main difference between the anterior circulation and posterior circulation stroke does not seem to be increased ischemic tolerance. Instead it seems that BAO are more resistant to hemorrhagic transformation.[80] Pagola and colleagues[80] described their cohort of 204 MCA strokes and 28 BAO strokes treated with IV tPA. These investigators noted that mean time to treatment was longer for patients with BAO ($P = .031$) and early recanalization was more frequent among MCA occlusions (41% vs 29%; $P = .039$)

but that the rate of persistent occlusion was equal in both groups, and furthermore, MCA strokes were more likely to be associated with hemorrhagic transformation than BAO strokes (OR, 8.2; $P = .043$).

Despite the widely held belief that posterior circulation strokes are best treated with endovascular thrombolysis, only 1 multicenter, randomized controlled trial has been conducted on IA thrombolysis in posterior circulation strokes.[81] Although patients in the treatment group had a better outcome compared with the control group (mRS 1 in survivors of treatment group vs mRS 3 in control), the enrollment rate was slow, resulting in an early termination of the study and an analysis of only a small study group of patients (n = 16). In a review of IA thrombolysis, Powers[82] noted that these results were not statistically significant as determined by a Fisher exact test ($P = .28$). Powers recommended that to justify acute interventions of BAO strokes, trials and observational data should be conducted to show that benefit significantly outweighs the risks and costs. However, because BAO strokes have an overall poor prognosis, Smith[83] argued that despite the lack of a randomized study, data had already been published showing a survival benefit in patients with acute BAO, if successful revascularization is achieved. Reviewing 10 studies published between 1988 and 2004 on recanalization rates and mortality in BAO patients, Smith calculated an overall recanalization rate of 64% and mortality of 56%.[83] Furthermore, when analyzing mortality with regards to recanalization status, 87% of patients with unsuccessful recanalizations had died versus only 37% for those in whom recanalization was successful ($P<.001$; Fisher exact test). Smith recommended that because there is a significant increase in the chance for survival after recanalization, IA thrombolysis should be considered.

Yet, although recanalization is associated with better outcome in posterior circulation strokes, it remains unclear as to whether all patients with BAO stroke should preferentially receive IA thrombolysis. Although a positive outcome with thrombolysis is possible in patients with BAO strokes, there is no good study that conclusively shows IA thrombolysis is the best treatment option. In a systematic analysis of 420 patients with BAO, comparing IA (n = 344) and IV (n = 76) thrombolysis for BAO, Lindsberg and Mattle[84] reported that death and dependency were equally common. Although recanalization was more common with IA thrombolysis versus IV thrombolysis (65% vs 53%; $P = .05$), survival rates were roughly equal (45% vs 50%; $P = .48$). These investigators noted that 24% of patients with IA thrombolysis and 22% of patients with IV thrombolysis had good outcomes ($P = .82$), albeit without recanalization the likelihood of good outcome was negligible (2%). Thus, there are no clear data that IA thrombolysis is superior to IV thrombolysis, but any aggressive strategy that results in successful recanalization may be preferable and the choice of intervention remains at the discretion of the clinician, the patient, or their family.

---

**Unanswered question:**

- What are the implications of these findings for patients with wake-up stroke?
- Is there evidence of benefit in treatment of patients older than 80 years with AIS?

---

*Wake-up strokes (unknown time window)*

Among the suggestions made by the DIAS study group was the notion of changing the management of stroke patients from a time clock to a tissue clock.[66] Schellinger and colleagues[72] showed that in patients presenting beyond the 3-hour window (median stroke onset 240 minutes), better outcomes were calculated with thrombolysis if a PWI-DWI mismatch greater than 20% was used to select for treatment compared with CT (OR, 1.467; 95% CI, 1.017–2.117; $P$ = .040). A year later, the DEFUSE study (average stroke onset ~5 hours) showed that with successful recanalization in patients with a PWI-DWI mismatch, odds for a favorable clinical response were high (OR, 29; 95% CI, 1.01–397; $P$ = .047) and infarct growth rates were small ($P$ = .024) when compared with patients without mismatch.[70] With regard to reperfusion rates, the EPITHET study showed high reperfusion rates in the mismatch group, when treated with alteplase versus placebo (56% vs 26%; $P$ = .010).[20]

The use of MRI to identify PWI-DWI mismatch, and thus patients who were likely to benefit from thrombolytic treatment, was one of the enrollment requirements of the DIAS and DEDAS studies.[24,25] Enrolling only patients with a PWI-DWI mismatch, both the DIAS and DEDAS trials showed a potential benefit of a novel thrombolytic, desmoteplase, which extended beyond the 3-hour window. The positive outcomes seen in these trials can give great insight into the management of a patient who presents with a wake-up stroke. From these studies, it might be inferred that patients with wake-up strokes who have a MRI PWI-DWI mismatch greater than 20% may have a better chance for a good outcome after thrombolytic therapy compared with someone who enters with a wake-up stroke without mismatch. However, this approach needs to be specifically validated in clinical trials, and the current accepted approach remains a time-based approach based on when the patient was last seen normal. Most wake-up patients with AIS remain ineligible for thrombolytic therapy.

### Older patients
The ECASS-II study is one of the few studies that included enrollment of patients older than 80 years; otherwise, most studies have made age older than 80 years an exclusion criterion for thrombolytic therapy.[4] With almost 30% of strokes occurring in the population older than 80 years, the degree of risk versus benefit of thrombolysis in patients older than 80 years had been unclear.[16] However, as noted earlier, IST-3 directly challenged this question, with a large subcohort of patients older than 80 years (n = 1617, 53%).[20] In the IST-3 analysis of the adjusted effect of treatment, there was a favorable odds ratio of 1.35 (0.97–1.88) when comparing the group older than 80 years with the group younger than 80 years ($P$ = .027). Thus, the results of the IST-3 trial can statistically justify extending IV tPA thrombolytic treatment in patients older than 80 years who present within 3 hours of stroke onset and possibly even up to 6 hours after stroke.[20]

### SUMMARY

In this review, various studies have been described that have taken into consideration factors such as the type of imaging modality used, whether the patient was on AP or AC therapy, age, location of stroke, and the particular type of intervention available (different types of IV thrombolytic drugs, IV or IA pharmacologic thrombolysis, and mechanical endovascular devices), in considering whether to treat a patient within or outside the preferred 3-hour time window. It is clear that early AIS treatment provides the best chance for a good outcome. Because many patients continue to present at less than optimal times immediately after stroke, extending the time window for treatment is critical. Although there remains a lack of clarity as to how to treat many of these patients with AIS, who would otherwise not fit the classic IV tPA paradigm, there are several evolving options. A strategy based on the available studies is summarized in **Fig. 3**. Better data to support an evidence-based approach to treatment of individual patients with AIS who do not meet the classic parameters for thrombolysis remain necessary.

## REFERENCES

1. Roger VL, Go AS, Lloyd-Jones DM, et al. Heart disease and stroke statistics–2012 update: a report from the American Heart Association. Circulation 2012; 125(1):e2–220.
2. The National Institute of Neurological Disorders and Stroke rt-PA Stroke Study group. Tissue plasminogen activator for acute ischemic stroke. N Engl J Med 1995;333:1581–7.
3. Hacke W, Donnan G, Fieschi C, et al. Association of outcome with early stroke treatment: pooled analysis of ATLANTIS, ECASS, and NINDS rt-PA stroke trials. Lancet 2004;363:768–74.
4. Hacke W, Kaste M, Bluhmki E, et al. Thrombolysis with alteplase 3 to 4.5 hours after acute ischemic stroke. N Engl J Med 2008;359:1317–29.
5. Lees KR, Bluhmki E, Von Kummer R, et al. Time to treatment with intravenous alteplase and outcome in stroke: an updated pooled analysis of ECASS, ATLANTIS, NINDS, and EPITHET trials. Lancet 2010;375:1695–703.
6. Clark WM, Wissman S, Albers GW, et al. Recombinant tissue-type plasminogen activator (alteplase) for ischemic stroke 3 to 5 hours after symptom onset: the ATLANTIS study–a randomized controlled trial. JAMA 1999;282:2019–26.
7. Del Zoppo GJ, Saver JL, Jauch EC, et al. Expansion of the time window for treatment of acute ischemic stroke with intravenous tissue plasminogen activator: a science advisory from the American Heart Association/American Stroke Association. Stroke 2009;40:2945–8.
8. Chavez JC, Hurko O, Barone FC, et al. Pharmacologic interventions for stroke: looking beyond the thrombolysis time window into the penumbra with biomarkers, not a stopwatch. Stroke 2009;40:e558–63.
9. Jung JE, Kim GS, Chen H, et al. Reperfusion and neurovascular dysfunction in stroke: from basic mechanisms to potential strategies for neuroprotection. Mol Neurobiol 2010;41:172–9.
10. Brott TG, Haley EC Jr, Levy DE, et al. Urgent therapy for stroke. I. Pilot study of tissue plasminogen activator administered within 90 minutes. Stroke 1992;23: 632–40.
11. Haley EC Jr, Levy DE, Brott TG, et al. Urgent therapy for stroke. II. Pilot study of tissue plasminogen activator administered 91–180 minutes from onset. Stroke 1992;23:641–5.
12. Larrue V, von Kummer R, Müller A, et al. Risk factors for severe hemorrhagic transformation in ischemic stroke patients treated with recombinant tissue plasminogen activator, a secondary analysis of the European-Australasian Acute Stroke Study (ECASS II). Stroke 2001;32:438–41.
13. Wahlgren N, Ahmed N, Davalos A, et al. Thrombolysis with alteplase for acute ischemic stroke in the Safe Implementation of Thrombolysis in Stroke-Monitoring Study (SITS-MOST): an observational study. Lancet 2007;369(9558):275–82.
14. Wahlgren N, Ahmed N, Dávalos A, et al. Thrombolysis with alteplase 3–4.5 hours after acute ischemic stroke (SITS-ISTR): an observational study. Lancet 2008; 372:1303–9.
15. Saver JL, Gornbein J, Grotta J, et al. Number needed to treat to benefit and to harm for intravenous tissue plasminogen activator therapy in the 3- to 4.5-hour window: joint outcome table analysis of the ECASS 3 trial. Stroke 2009;40: 2433–7.
16. Ford GA, Ahmed N, Azevedo E, et al. Intravenous alteplase for stroke in those older than 80 years old. Stroke 2010;41:2568–74.

17. Lansberg MG, Schrooten M, Bluhmki E, et al. Treatment time-specific number needed to treat estimates for tissue plasminogen activator therapy in acute stroke based on shifts over the entire range of the modified Rankin Scale. Stroke 2009;40(6):2079–84.
18. Davis SM, Donnan GA, Parsons MW, et al. Effects of alteplase beyond 3 h after stroke in the Echoplanar Imaging Thrombolytic Evaluation Trial (EPITHET): a placebo-controlled randomised trial. Lancet Neurol 2008;7:299–309.
19. Nagakane Y, Christensen S, Brekenfeld C, et al. EPITHET: positive result after reanalysis using baseline diffusion-weighted imaging/perfusion-weighted imaging co-registration. Stroke 2011;42(1):59–64.
20. The IST-3 Collaborative Group. The benefits and harms of intravenous thrombolysis with recombinant tissue plasminogen activator within 6 hours of acute ischaemic stroke (the third international stroke trial [IST-3]): a randomised controlled trial. Lancet 2012;6736(12):2352–63.
21. Wardlaw J, Murray V, Berge E, et al. Recombinant tissue plasminogen activator for acute ischaemic stroke: an updated systematic review and meta-analysis. Lancet 2012;6736(12):738.
22. Biller J, Dafer RM. Desmoteplase in the treatment of acute ischemic stroke. Expert Rev Neurother 2007;1:333.
23. Hacke W, Albers G, Al-Rawi Y, et al. The Desmoteplase in Acute Ischemic Stroke Trial (DIAS). A phase II MRI-based 9-hour window acute stroke thrombolysis trial with intravenous desmoteplase. Stroke 2005;36(6):6–73.
24. Furlan AJ, Eyding D, Albers GW, et al. Dose Escalation of Desmoteplase for Acute Ischemic Stroke (DEDAS) evidence of safety and efficacy 3 to 9 hours after stroke onset. Stroke 2006;37:1227–31.
25. Hacke W, Furlan AJ, Al-Rawi Y, et al. Intravenous desmoteplase in patients with acute ischaemic stroke selected by MRI perfusion-diffusion weighted imaging or perfusion CT (DIAS-2): a prospective, randomised, double-blind, placebo-controlled study. Lancet Neurol 2009;8(2):141–50.
26. Fiebach JB, Al-Rawi Y, Wintermark M, et al. Vascular occlusion enables selecting acute ischemic stroke patients for treatment with desmoteplase. Stroke 2012;4(3):1561–6.
27. Albers GW, von Kummer R; DIAS-3 and DIAS-4 Study Group. The Desmoteplase DIAS-3 and DIAS-4 clinical trials: an important milestone passed. Available at: http://kenes.com/stroke2012/abstractcd/pdf/1463.pdf. Accessed December 18, 2012.
28. Parsons M, Spratt N, Bivard A, et al. A randomized trial of tenecteplase versus alteplase for acute ischemic stroke. N Engl J Med 2012;366:1099–107.
29. Hacke W, Zeumer H, Ferbert A, et al. Intra-arterial thrombolytic therapy improves outcome in patients with acute vertebrobasilar occlusive disease. Stroke 1988;19:1216–22.
30. Mori E, Tabuchi M, Yoshida T, et al. Intracarotid urokinase with thromboembolic occlusion of the middle cerebral artery. Stroke 1988;19:802–12.
31. Furlan A, Higashida R, Wechsler L, et al. Intra-arterial prourokinase for acute ischemic stroke. The PROACT II study: a randomized controlled trial. PROlyse in Acute Cerebral Thromboembolism. JAMA 1999;282:2003–11.
32. Del Zoppo GJ, Higashida RT, Furlan AJ, et al. PROACT: a phase II randomized trial of recombinant pro-urokinase by direct arterial delivery in acute middle cerebral artery stroke. Stroke 1998;29:4–11.
33. Rubiera M, Ribo M, Pagola J, et al. Outcome in nonresponder intravenous tissue plasminogen activator-treated patients a case-control study. Stroke 2011;42:993–7.

34. The IMS Study Investigators. Combined intravenous and intraarterial recanalization for acute ischemic stroke: the interventional management of stroke study. Stroke 2004;35:904–11.
35. The IMS II Trial Investigators. The interventional management of stroke (IMS) II study. Stroke 2007;38:2127–35.
36. Khatri P, Hill MD, Palesch YY, et al. Methodology of the Interventional Management of Stroke (IMS) III trial. Int J Stroke 2008;3(2):130–7.
37. Broderick JP, Palesch YY, Demchuk AM, et al. Endovascular therapy after intravenous t-PA versus t-PA alone for stroke. N Engl J Med 2013. http://dx.doi.org/10.1056/NEJMoa1214300.
38. Chimowitz MI. Endovascular treatment for acute ischemic stroke–still unproven. N Engl J Med 2013. http://dx.doi.org/10.1056/NEJMe121573.
39. Ciccone A, Valvassori L, Nichelatti M, et al. Endovascular treatment for acute ischemic stroke. N Engl J Med 2013. http://dx.doi.org/10.1056/NEJMoa1213701.
40. Gobin YP, Starkman S, Duckwiler GR, et al. MERCI 1 a phase 1 study of mechanical embolus removal in cerebral ischemia. Stroke 2004;35:2848–54.
41. Smith WS, Sung G, Starkman S, et al. Safety and efficacy of mechanical embolectomy in acute ischemic stroke–results of the MERCI trial. Stroke 2005;36:1432–40.
42. Smith WS, Sung G, Saver J, et al. Mechanical thrombectomy for acute ischemic stroke–final results of the multi MERCI trial. Stroke 2008;39:1205–12.
43. Becker KJ, Brott TG. Approval of the MERCI clot retriever: a critical view. Stroke 2005;36:400–3.
44. Bose A, Henkes H, Alfke K, et al. The Penumbra System: a mechanical device for the treatment of acute stroke due to thromboembolism. AJNR Am J Neuroradiol 2008;29:1409–13.
45. The Penumbra Pivotal Stroke Trial Investigators. The penumbra pivotal stroke trial–safety and effectiveness of a new generation of mechanical devices for clot removal in intracranial large vessel occlusive disease. Stroke 2009;40:2761–8.
46. Kidwell CS, Jahan R, Jeffrey Gornbein J, et al. A trial of imaging selection and endovascular treatment for ischemic stroke. N Engl J Med 2013. http://dx.doi.org/10.1056/NEJMoa1212793.
47. Saver JL, Jahan R, Levy EI, et al. Solitaire flow restoration device versus the MERCI Retriever in patients with acute ischemic stroke (SWIFT): a randomised, parallel-group, non-inferiority trial. Lancet 2012;380(9849):1241–9.
48. Rubiera M, Alexandrov AV. Sonothrombolysis in the management of acute ischemic stroke. Am J Cardiovasc Drugs 2010;10(1):5–10.
49. Alexandrov AV, Molina CA, Grotta JC, et al. Ultrasound-enhanced systemic thrombolysis for acute ischemic stroke. N Engl J Med 2004;351:2170–8.
50. Daffertshofer M, Gass A, Ringleb P, et al. Transcranial low-frequency ultrasound-mediated thrombolysis in brain ischemia: increased risk of hemorrhage with combined ultrasound and tissue plasminogen activator: results of a phase II clinical trial. Stroke 2005;36:1441–6.
51. Ricci S, Dinia L, Del Sette M, et al. Sonothrombolysis for acute ischaemic stroke. Cochrane Database Syst Rev 2012;(10):CD008348.
52. Bor-Seng-Shu E, Nogueira Rde C, Figueiredo EG. Sonothrombolysis for acute ischemic stroke: a systematic review of randomized controlled trials. Neurosurg Focus 2012;32(1):E5.
53. Del Zoppo GJ. Virchow's triad: the vascular basis of cerebral injury. Rev Neurol Dis 2008;5(Suppl 1):S12–21.

54. Raju NC, Eikelboom JW, Hirsh J. Platelet ADP-receptor antagonists for cardiovascular disease: past, present and future. Nat Clin Pract Cardiovasc Med 2008;5(12):766–80.
55. Paikin JS, Eikelboom JW, Cairns JA, et al. New antithrombotic agents–insights from clinical trials. Nat Rev Cardiol 2010;7:498–509.
56. Morales-Vidal S, Schneck MJ, Flaster M, et al. Direct thrombin inhibitors and factor Xa inhibitors in patients with cerebrovascular disease. Expert Rev Neurother 2012;12(2):179–89.
57. Ibrahim MM, Sebastian J, Hussain M, et al. Does current oral antiplatelet agent or subtherapeutic anticoagulation use have an effect on tissue-plasminogen-activator-mediated recanalization rate in patients with acute ischemic stroke? Cerebrovasc Dis 2010;30:508–13.
58. Wiviott SD, Braunwald E, McCabe CH, et al. Prasugrel versus clopidogrel in patients with acute coronary syndromes. N Engl J Med 2007;357:2001–15.
59. Neumann F. Balancing efficacy and safety in the TRITON-TIMI 38 trial. Eur Heart J Suppl 2009;11(Suppl G):G14–7.
60. Serebruany VL, Alberts MJ, Hanley DF. Prasugrel in the poststroke cohort of the TRITON trial: the clear and present danger. Cerebrovasc Dis 2008;26:93–4.
61. Wallentin L, Becker RC, Budaj A, et al. Ticagrelor versus clopidogrel in patients with acute coronary syndromes. N Engl J Med 2009;361:1045–57.
62. Vergouwen MD, Casaubon LK, Swartz RH, et al. Subtherapeutic warfarin is not associated with increased hemorrhage rates in ischemic strokes treated with tissue plasminogen activator. Stroke 2011;42:1041–5.
63. Xian Y, Liang L, Smith EE, et al. Risks of intracranial hemorrhage among patients with acute ischemic stroke receiving warfarin and treated with intravenous tissue plasminogen activator. JAMA 2012;307(24):2600–8.
64. Kim YD, Lee H, Jung YH, et al. Effect of warfarin withdrawal on thrombolytic treatment in patients with ischaemic stroke. Eur J Neurol 2011;18:1165–70.
65. Prabhakaran S, Rivolta J, Vieira JR, et al. Symptomatic intracerebral hemorrhage among eligible warfarin-treated patients receiving intravenous tissue plasminogen activator for acute ischemic stroke. Arch Neurol 2010;67(5):559–63.
66. Seet RC, Zhang Y, Moore A, et al. Subtherapeutic international normalized ratio in warfarin-treated patients increases the risk for symptomatic intracerebral hemorrhage after intravenous thrombolysis. Stroke 2011;42:2333–5.
67. Ruecker M, Matosevic B, Willeit P, et al. Subtherapeutic warfarin therapy entails an increased bleeding risk after stroke thrombolysis. Neurology 2012;79:31–8.
68. Barber PA, Demchuk AM, Zhang J, et al. Validity and reliability of a quantitative computed tomography score in predicting outcome of hyperacute stroke before thrombolytic therapy. Lancet 2000;355:1670–4.
69. Kimura K, Sakamoto Y, Aoki J, et al. Clinical and MRI predictors of no early recanalization within 1 hour after tissue-type plasminogen activator administration. Stroke 2011;42:3150–5.
70. Olivot JM, Mlynash M, Thijs VN, et al. Relationships between infarct growth, clinical outcome, and early recanalization in Diffusion and Perfusion Imaging for Understanding Stroke Evolution (DEFUSE). Stroke 2008;39:2257–63.
71. Lansberg MG, Thijs VN, Bammer R, et al. The MRA-DWI mismatch identifies patients with stroke who are likely to benefit from reperfusion. Stroke 2008;39:2491–6.
72. Schellinger PD, Thomalla G, Fiehler J, et al. MRI-based and CT-based thrombolytic therapy in acute stroke within and beyond established time windows: an analysis of 1210 patients. Stroke 2007;38(10):2640–5.

73. Ribo M, Flores A, Rubiera M, et al. Extending the time window for endovascular procedures according to collateral pial circulation. Stroke 2011;42:3465–9.
74. Liebeskind DS, Kim D, Starkman S, et al. Collateral failure? Late mechanical thrombectomy after failed intravenous thrombolysis. J Neuroimaging 2010;20: 78–82.
75. Henderson RD, Eliasziw M, Fox AJ, et al. Angiographically defined collateral circulation and risk of stroke in patients with severe carotid artery stenosis. Stroke 2000;31:128–32.
76. Christoforidis GA, Mohammad Y, Kehagias D, et al. Angiographic assessment of pial collaterals as a prognostic indicator following intra-arterial thrombolysis for acute ischemic stroke. AJNR Am J Neuroradiol 2005;26:1789–97.
77. Bang OY, Saver JL, Kim SJ, et al. Collateral flow predicts response to endovascular therapy for acute ischemic stroke. Stroke 2011;42:693–9.
78. Bang OY, Saver JL, Kim SJ, et al. Collateral flow averts hemorrhagic transformation after endovascular therapy for acute ischemic stroke. Stroke 2011;42: 2235–9.
79. Sairanen T, Strbian D, Soinne L, et al. Intravenous thrombolysis of basilar artery occlusion: predictors of recanalization and outcome. Stroke 2011;42:2175–9.
80. Pagola J, Ribo M, Alvarez-Sabin J, et al. Thrombolysis in anterior versus posterior circulation strokes: timing of recanalization, ischemic tolerance, and other differences. J Neuroimaging 2011;21:108–12.
81. Macleod MR, Davis SM, Mitchell PJ, et al. Results of a multicentre, randomised controlled trial of intra-arterial urokinase in the treatment of acute posterior circulation ischaemic stroke. Cerebrovasc Dis 2005;20:12–7.
82. Powers WJ. Intra-arterial thrombolysis for basilar artery thrombosis: trial it. Stroke 2007;38(704):706.
83. Smith WS. Intra-arterial thrombolytic therapy for acute basilar occlusion: pro. Stroke 2007;38:701–3.
84. Lindsberg PJ, Mattle HP. Therapy of basilar artery occlusion a systematic analysis comparing intra-arterial and intravenous thrombolysis. Stroke 2006;37: 922–8.

# New Strategies for Endovascular Recanalization of Acute Ischemic Stroke

José E. Cohen, MD[a], Ronen R. Leker, MD[b],
Alejandro Rabinstein, MD[c],*

## KEYWORDS

- Acute ischemic stroke • Revascularization • Stent • Thrombolysis • Thrombectomy

## KEY POINTS

- Timely endovascular therapy can achieve reperfusion of brain tissue at risk of ischemic infarction (ischemic penumbra), thus providing the possibility of improving functional outcomes in patients with large intracranial artery occlusions and severe neurologic deficits.
- Acute endovascular therapy is safe when performed by experienced clinicians, and can be offered after failed intravenous thrombolysis as a rescue strategy or as primary therapy in patients with contraindications for intravenous thrombolysis.
- Mechanical thrombectomy devices have largely replaced intra-arterial thrombolysis as the preferred method of endovascular reperfusion therapy.
- Stent retrievers seem to be the most effective devices for acute interventional stroke therapy, based on early experience.
- Shortening the time to reperfusion and achieving complete or near-complete reperfusion are crucial to optimizing outcomes.
- More randomized trials are needed comparing intravenous thrombolysis versus primary endovascular thrombectomy and rescue thrombectomy versus placebo.

## INTRODUCTION

Early reperfusion is a strong predictor of good outcome in acute ischemic stroke (AIS).[1,2] This finding was the basis for the evaluation of intravenous (IV) recombinant tissue plasminogen activator (tPA), the first effective therapy for AIS, and the rationale for a change in the approach to this disease. IV tPA represents a first step beyond the

Disclosures: The authors did not receive funding in support of the preparation of this article, and have no conflicts of interest to disclose.

[a] Department of Neurosurgery, Hadassah-Hebrew University Medical Center, POB 12000, Jerusalem 91120, Israel; [b] Department of Neurology, Hadassah-Hebrew University Medical Center, POB 12000, Jerusalem 91120, Israel; [c] Department of Neurology, Mayo Clinic, 200 1st Street Southwest, Rochester, MN 55905, USA
* Corresponding author.
E-mail address: rabinstein.alejandro@mayo.edu

classic nihilism after failed neuroprotection and neurorestoration attempts with thousands of costly compounds and studies.[3]

However, soon after the general recommendation of its use gained acceptance, it become evident that the one-size-fits-all concept of IV tPA cannot be applied for all acute strokes, because not all strokes are the same. Patients with mild strokes, such as some with small vessel occlusions, may not require IV tPA because they can do well without it. On the other extreme of the spectrum, major strokes that are usually caused by either middle-size or large-size vessel occlusion represent the Achilles heel of IV thrombolysis.[4,5] The prognosis of patients with severe strokes (National Institutes of Health Stroke Score [NIHSS] ≥16) treated with IV tPA is poor. In landmark studies, one-third of these patients died, another one-third remained severely disabled (modified Rankin Scale [mRS] 4–5), and only one-fourth of patients were independent (mRS 0–2) at 3-month follow-up.[3–5] In internal carotid artery (ICA) occlusions, IV tPA therapy only allows a recanalization rate of close to 10% and, in occlusions of the proximal (M1 portion) middle cerebral artery (MCA), the recanalization rate is less than 30%.[1,2,6] Only one-third of patients with MCA occlusions who achieve recanalization after IV tPA have an excellent functional recovery (number needed to treat >10).[4,5,7] In these cases, the large clot burden responsible for the occlusion is often not effectively lysed by IV tPA during the brief therapeutic window allowed by the tissue at risk.

Limitations in achieving timely recanalization with IV tPA fueled the development of intra-arterial (IA) treatment strategies. These IA treatments for AIS are the focus of this article.

## IA THROMBOLYSIS: THERAPY, RATIONALE, AND RESULTS

IA administration of thrombolytics improves the efficiency of drug delivery into the clot, thus increasing the chances for recanalization and decreasing the dose of drug needed to achieve this goal. IA thrombolysis has been empirically used for the last 3 decades in patients with large intracranial vessel occlusions. IA thrombolysis is performed by selective placement of a microcatheter proximal to the occlusion and direct infusion of a high dose of fibrinolytic agent, with the aim of disintegrating the clot and recanalizing the artery. The intervention is considered technically simple, although it is frequently time consuming. Reported recanalization rates are usually modest in very proximal occlusions (less than 30% in carotid T occlusions), but better in more distal occlusions, such as in M2 branches. Complications, including hemorrhagic complications and distal emboli, are common.

Prolyse in Acute Cerebral Thromboembolism (PROACT) II was the main randomized trial to examine the safety and efficacy of IA thrombolysis in patients with AIS caused by angiographically proven occlusion of M1 or M2 branches of the MCA.[8] Outcomes in 121 patients treated with IA prourokinase plus heparin within 3 to 6 hours from stroke onset were compared with those in 59 patients treated with heparin alone. Patients in the two groups had similar risk factors and baseline criteria, and were randomized a mean of 4.7 hours from stroke onset in the treatment group and 5.1 hours in the control group. In the prourokinase plus heparin group, 40% of patients reached functional independence at 90 days, compared with only 25% of patients treated with heparin alone ($P = .04$). Recanalization was achieved within 2 hours of treatment in 66% of patients treated with prourokinase plus heparin compared with 18% of controls ($P < .001$). Complete recanalization, defined as Thrombolysis in Myocardial Infarction (TIMI) grade 3, was attained in 19% of treated patients and in only 4% of controls ($P = .003$). Symptomatic intracranial hemorrhage (sICH) was seen in 10% of treated patients compared with

2% of controls ($P = .06$), but the increase in sICH did not affect mortality rates, which were 25% and 27% respectively.

Despite these promising results, treatment with prourokinase plus heparin was not approved by the US Food and Drug Administration (FDA), which demanded a confirmatory study that was never performed. Nevertheless, IA thrombolysis with urokinase or tPA has continued to be used frequently in centers across the world for emergency treatment of patients presenting within 6 hours of onset with AIS caused by occlusion of large proximal vessels, such as the distal ICA, proximal MCA, or basilar artery.

PROACT II, a Japanese trial, and a meta-analysis have shown that IA fibrinolysis substantially increases recanalization rates and improves neurologic outcomes in patients with major vessel occlusions.[8–10] However, large thrombi are resistant to standard microcatheter-delivered thrombolysis and prolonged delivery is usually required to open these occlusions; thus IA fibrinolysis often fails to improve outcomes even after achieving recanalization.[11–13]

Several alternative strategies were not permitted and thus not evaluated in the context of PROACT II, including mechanical clot disruption with a microguidewire or repeatedly crossing the clot with the microcatheter with the goal of increasing clot surface exposure to the injected thrombolytic agent. Adjuvant clot angioplasty in refractory cases was also not included in the PROACT II design. Outside of the large formal studies, these alternatives were sometimes used in practice to increase the chances of recanalization and they were precursors to the development of novel endovascular therapies, including IA ultrasound, mechanical embolectomy, and acute stenting.

## COMBINED IV-IA TPA AND IA ULTRASOUND

The Interventional Management of Stroke (IMS) studies I (80 patients) and II (81 patients) examined the effects of initial lower dose of IV tPA (0.6 mg/kg) followed by IA tPA when recanalization was not achieved after the IV bolus.[14] Some patients were also treated with IA ultrasound administered with the EKOS EkoSonic Endovascular System after evidence showed that ultrasound energy could hasten clot breakdown.[15,16] Recanalization to TIMI 2 to 3 was achieved in 56% of patients in IMS-I, and 60% in IMS-II, with higher rates in patients who were also treated with the EKOS system. An mRS score of 0 to 2 was reached by 46% of IMS-II participants at 3 months after stroke. Mortality at 3 months was 16% in both IMS studies; sICH rates were 6.3% and 9.9%, respectively. The multicenter, randomized IMS-III trial was then designed to compare the standard IV tPA alone versus a combined IV/IA approach, with IV treatment initiated within 3 hours of AIS onset.[17] The recently published results of this trial are presented later.

The bridging concept tested in the IMS trials (ie, reduced-dose IV tPA followed if necessary by endovascular therapy) is no longer common in practice. Instead, most patients treated with combined therapy receive the full dose of IV tPA followed by endovascular intervention when this fails to achieve recanalization, a treatment paradigm known as rescue therapy. This practice has been supported by reports showing acceptable risks of sICH[18,19] and fueled by the development of neurothrombectomy devices that often allow recanalization without requiring IA administration of an additional thrombolytic dose.

## ENDOVASCULAR ANGIOPLASTY AND STENTING

Balloon angioplasty, with or without stent placement, is another technique that can be used to recanalize acute arterial occlusions. This strategy, which is similar to the approach commonly taken in patients with acute myocardial infarction, was hampered for a long time by the absence of dedicated catheters for the cerebral vasculature. The cerebral blood vessels are suspended in cerebrospinal fluid, without the firm muscular support of the myocardium, thus they are more prone to dissections and tears. Furthermore, the approach to intracranial arterial occlusions is often tortuous, making navigation more difficult. However, various catheters and other devices designed specifically for the cerebral vasculature have been developed in recent years, removing some of the obstacles to endovascular angioplasty and stenting in patients after acute stroke.

Levy and colleagues[20] proposed that stent-assisted recanalization may improve recanalization rates in patients with acute stroke and persistent intracranial vessel occlusions after thrombolysis. In their retrospective analysis of 19 patients, stenting afforded successful recanalization in 79% of cases. Lesions at the ICA terminus, older age, and higher baseline NIHSS score were identified as negative outcome predictors. There were no cases of sICH in this small series. From their preliminary experience, the investigators concluded that stent-assisted recanalization for acute stroke resulting from intracranial thrombotic occlusion is associated with a high recanalization rate and low rate of intracranial hemorrhage (ICH).

However, permanent stenting has the disadvantage of demanding the administration of dual antiplatelet therapy, including a loading dose of clopidogrel, which can increase the risk of symptomatic ICH from reperfusion injury. At present, the advent of embolectomy techniques has restricted the use of permanent stents to the treatment of patients with symptomatic subocclusive atherosclerotic stenoses, acute occlusions occurring on atherosclerotic stenosis, and, less frequently, those with embolic occlusions that are refractory to thrombolysis or thrombectomy.

## THE NEUROTHROMBECTOMY ERA

As it became increasingly clear that dissolving the clot with thrombolytic agents is not always possible, that dissolution may not be prompt enough to reduce the size of the infarction, and that thrombolysis carries a substantial risk of hemorrhage, new treatment approaches were sought. The advance of neuroendovascular techniques in parallel with the development of new devices has enabled mechanical removal of the occlusive clot from large intracranial vessels. Thrombectomy techniques have several potential advantages compared with pharmacologic thrombolysis, including higher rates of recanalization, lower risk of ICH, and a longer treatment window.[21–23] Several neurothrombectomy devices are now available, and they can be classified mechanistically into 4 groups (**Table 1**).

The Mechanical Embolus Removal in Cerebral Ischemia (MERCI) Retriever, the Penumbra System, and, more recently, the Solitaire FR Revascularization Device and TREVO Pro retriever have received 510(k) clearance from the FDA to treat patients with AIS. The other systems are approved for use in the European market. A summary of the main trials evaluating these devices is presented in **Table 2**.

### Clot Removal with MERCI or Aspiration with Penumbra

Several devices have been designed to retrieve or aspirate the occluding clot from large intracranial arteries. The snare and basket MERCI devices (Concentric Medical, Mountain View, CA) are deployed into the clot and work as a corkscrewlike retrieval tool.[26,27,33] The balloon of the guiding catheter is inflated proximally to the clot to achieve flow arrest and prevent distal embolization. The retrieval device is then pulled back into the catheter with the clot ensnared. Once the clot is removed, the procedure is completed by deflating the occluding proximal balloon and restoring circulation. This system received FDA approval in 2004.

**Table 1**
**Devices for thrombosis removal, aspiration, or fragmentation**

| Device | Supplier |
| --- | --- |
| Mechanical Thrombectomy | |
|   MERCI Retriever | Concentric Medical Systems, Mountain View, CA |
|   Phenox Clot Retriever | Phenox GmbH, Bochum, Germany |
|   Neuronet Device | Guidant Corp./Boston Scientific, Indianapolis, IN |
|   Amplatz Goosneneck Microsnare | Covidien/eV3, Plymouth, MN |
|   Alligator Retrieval Device | Covidien/eV3, Plymouth, MN |
|   Solitaire FR Revascularization Device | Covidien/eV3, Plymouth, MN |
|   TREVO Pro Retrieval System | Stryker Corp, Kalamazoo, MI |
|   ReVive SE Neurovascular Thrombectomy Device | Johnson & Johnson/Codman & Schurtleff, Raynham, MA |
| Thromboaspiration | |
|   Penumbra System | Penumbra, Alameda, CA |
|   AngioJet Ultra Thrombectomy System | MEDRAD, Warrendale, PA |
| Laser Thrombolysis and Mechanical Clot Fragmentation | |
|   Endovascular Photoacoustic Recanalization Laser | EndoVasix, Belmont, CA |
| Ultrasonification | |
|   EKOS Echosonic Endovascular System | EKOS Corp., Botell, WA |

Initial results published with the MERCI device explored its safety and efficacy in 151 patients with anterior or posterior circulation stroke secondary to large vessel occlusion who were treated within 8 hours of stroke onset.[26] Primary outcomes were recanalization at the end of the procedure, defined as TIMI 2 to 3, and safety. Secondary outcomes were mRS and NIHSS scores at 30 and 90 days, and death, myocardial infarction, or recurrent stroke within 30 days. A good neurologic outcome was defined as mRS less than or equal to 2 or NIHSS score improvement greater than or equal to 10 points. All patients included in the MERCI device study were ineligible for IV lysis. Mean age ($\pm$ standard deviation) was 67 $\pm$ 15.5 years and mean admission NIHSS score was 20.1 $\pm$ 6.6. Strokes in the anterior circulation were seen in 90% of participating patients; in 10%, strokes occurred in the posterior circulation. Mean onset time to treatment (OTT) was 4.3 $\pm$ 1.7 hours, and mean procedure duration was 2.1 hours, yielding a mean 5.5 hours from symptom onset to reperfusion.

Recanalization to TIMI 2 to 3 was achieved in 46% of treated patients, a significant improvement compared with 18% recanalization rates for historical controls treated with heparin alone in the PROACT II study ($P < .0001$). At 30 days after stroke, good outcomes were achieved by 22.6% of patients according to the mRS score and 34.1% as determined by improvement in the NIHSS score. At 90 days after stroke, these numbers improved to 27.7% and 32.4% respectively. Most importantly, the chance of attaining a good outcome was significantly greater in patients with vessel recanalization compared to those without. The chance for stroke, MI, or death at 30 days was 40%, and mortality was 43.5% at 90 days. Clinically significant procedural complications occurred in 10 of 141 patients (7.1%), and sICH was observed in 11 of 141 (7.8%). On multivariate analysis, recanalization was associated with good outcome, whereas increasing age and low admission NIHSS score were associated with higher mortality and poorer functional outcome.

**Table 2**
Leading studies of endovascular therapy for AIS

| | Number, Active Arm | NIHSS, Median | Successful Recanalization, TIMI 2–3/TICI 2b-3 (%) | Good Neurologic Outcome, mRS 0–2 90 d (%) | Mortality, 90 d (%) | sICH (%) |
|---|---|---|---|---|---|---|
| IA Thrombolysis | | | | | | |
| PROACT II[8] | 121 | 17 | 66 | 40 | 25 | 10 |
| Combined IV-IA Lysis | | | | | | |
| IMS-I[24] | 62 | 18 | 56 | 43 | 16 | 6 |
| IMS-II[14] | 55 | 19 | 60 | 46 | 16 | 10 |
| IMS-III[25] | 434 | 17 | 65–81[a] | 41 | 19 | 6 |
| Neurothrombectomy | | | | | | |
| MERCI[26] | 151 | 22 | 46 | 28 | 44 | 8 |
| Multi-MERCI[27] | 164 | 19 | 68 | 36 | 34 | 10 |
| Penumbra[28] | 125 | 18 | 82 | 25 | 33 | 11 |
| SWIFT (Solitaire)[29] | 58 | 17 | 83 | 37[b] | 17 | 2 |
| TREVO 2 (TREVO)[30] | 88 | 19 | 85 | 40 | 33 | 7 |
| MR-RESCUE[31,c] | 34;30 | 17;19 | 67;77 | 21;17 | 18;20 | 9;0 |
| Primary Modality | | | | | | |
| SYNTHESIS[32] | 181 | 13 | NA | 42 | 8 | 6 |

*Abbreviations:* NA, not available; NIHSS, National Institutes of Health Stroke Scale score; TICI, Thrombolysis in Cerebral Infarction; TIMI, Thrombolysis in Myocardial Infarction.
[a] Depending on the vessel treated.
[b] Fifty-eight percent when considering the definition of good functional outcome used in the trial: mRS 0 to 2, or mRS equal to the prestroke mRS if this was greater than 2, or NIHSS improvement greater than or equal to 10 points.
[c] Data presented for embolectomy in patients with favorable penumbral pattern on magnetic resonance imaging (MRI); embolectomy in patients without favorable penumbral pattern on MRI.

In the Multi-MERCI study, 160 patients were treated within 8 hours of stroke onset.[27] In this study, prior treatment with IV tPA, mechanical clot disruption, IA tPA, and other adjunctive therapies was allowed. Some of the patients were treated with the newer generation L5 device. Mean age was 68.1 ± 16.0 years and mean admission NIHSS score was 19 (range, 15–23). IV tPA had been administered to 29% of participants without recanalization before the procedure. The primary outcome measure was vessel recanalization; secondary outcomes were safety measures related to the device and the procedure. Mean OTT was 4.3 hours, and mean onset to recanalization was 5.9 hours. Overall, vessel recanalization was achieved in 55% of patients with the retriever alone, and in up to 68% when adjunctive therapies were used. Recanalization rates were higher in posterior circulation and M2-MCA occlusions (88% and 80% respectively) than in ICA and M1-MCA occlusions (59% and 48% respectively). mRS less than or equal to 2 was achieved in 36% of participants and NIHSS scores improved by more than 10 points in 26%. sICH occurred in 16 patients (9.8%); 4 patients (2.4%) had parenchymal hematoma type II. Clinically significant procedural complications occurred in 9 patients (5.5%). Treatment with IV tPA before MERCI device deployment did not increase the chance of sICH. Overall mortality at 90 days was 34%, with significantly improved outcomes in patients achieving revascularization.

Outcomes with the MERCI device now seem modest, but proximal intracranial vessel occlusion leading to stroke is associated with severe morbidity and mortality of about 80% without reperfusion;[34–36] thus, the results from the MERCI trials represented a significant leap forward in comparison with previous stroke outcomes.

The Penumbra Stroke System, which uses an aspiration catheter along with a separator to debulk and remove the thrombus, was approved by the FDA in 2007. A phase 1 prospective multicenter trial of the Penumbra System enrolled 125 patients presenting within 8 hours from symptom onset with NIHSS greater than 8 and complete occlusion of a large intracranial vessel.[28] The primary end points were vessel revascularization and device safety. Reperfusion rates were 81.6% and the serious adverse event rate was 3.2%, again a significant improvement compared with the outcomes in earlier trials with devices and thrombolytics. The analysis of the secondary end point showed that an NIHSS score improvement of greater than 4 points at discharge had been achieved in 57.8% of patients and 25% achieved mRS less than or equal to 2 at 90-day follow-up. Mortality in this study was 26.4% at 30 days and 32.8% at 90 days. Recent studies with the device corroborated these preliminary findings. In a series of patients with large arterial occlusions, Kulcsar and colleagues[37] reported TIMI 2 to 3 in 93% of patients with cerebral infarction, mRS less than or equal to 2 in 48% at 3 months, and all-cause mortality of 11% in cases treated with the Penumbra System. Menon and colleagues[38] also reported recanalization (TIMI 2–3) in 85% of patients with good clinical outcomes in nearly half of the patients treated with this system.

### Stent-based Thrombectomy

Stent-based mechanical thrombectomy is a new concept in interventional stroke treatment enabled by the introduction of stent retrievers. These self-expanding stents are partially deployed, the clot is captured, the stent is retrieved with the clot enmeshed, and the vessel is gently aspirated. All these steps are performed under proximal artery occlusion. Preliminary results with these devices have been encouraging, showing unprecedented recanalization rates and better functional outcomes than ever reported with other interventions. Stent-based thrombectomy has consequently gained rapid acceptance in the neurointerventional community.

The Solitaire FR Revascularization Device was the first to be released and remains the most tested of these stent retrievers. Castaño and colleagues[21,39] were among the first to evaluate the Solitaire AB stent for large artery occlusions of the anterior circulation in patients presenting within 8 hours from onset of AIS. Successful revascularization was achieved in 18 of 20 patients, and in 90% of vessels treated with this system; symptomatic ICH was found in 2 patients (10%), and 4 patients (20%) died during the 90-day follow-up period. Davalos and colleagues[40] reported their experience from 6 European centers using the Solitaire stent retriever to treat 141 patients with AIS from large intracranial artery occlusion. They achieved recanalization with complete or near-complete reperfusion (Thrombolysis in Cerebral Infarction [TICI] 2b–3) in 85% of cases. Good outcome (mRS 0–2) at day 90 was observed in 55% of patients despite a median baseline NIHSS of 18. Mortality at 90 days was 19% and the rate of sICH was 5%. Our initial experience has been consistent with these favorable results (**Fig. 1**).[41]

The Solitaire stent has been extensively used in Europe since 2010. In March 2012, Solitaire received FDA approval, based on results from the Solitaire With the Intention for Thrombectomy (SWIFT) trial.[29] This trial compared the performance of Solitaire (n = 58) versus MERCI (n = 55) in patients with AIS who received treatment within 8 hours of symptom onset. TIMI 2 to 3 recanalization rates were markedly superior with Solitaire (83% vs 48% when assessed by the local investigator and 69% vs 30%

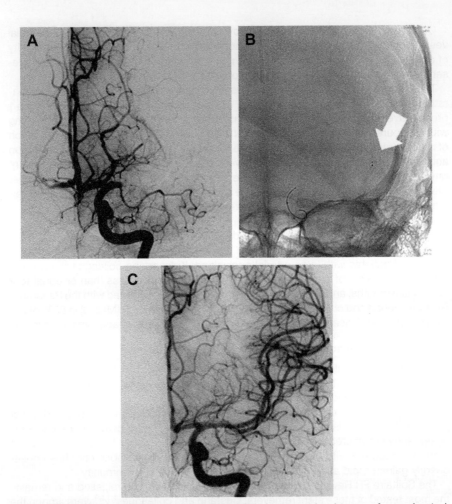

**Fig. 1.** Stent-based thrombectomy. This 50-year-old woman with a history of a mechanical prosthetic mitral valve, who was under oral anticoagulation with an International Normalization Ratio of 2.4, was transferred to our center for sudden-onset dysphasia and right hemiparesis that had begun 4 hours earlier (admission NIHSS 24). Head computed tomography was normal. The patient was urgently transferred to the interventional neuroradiology room for endovascular revascularization. (*A*) Selective angiogram of left ICA (anteroposterior view) shows the complete occlusion of the proximal left MCA. (*B*) The deployed stent across the occlusion. Note the distal markers of the stent (*arrow*) at the insular portion of the frontal MCA branch. (*C*) Complete vessel recanalization (TICI 3) was achieved in a single stent pass requiring only 37 minutes. The patient was discharged home after 7 days with no residual neurologic deficit.

when assessed by the core laboratory). Solitaire-treated patients also had significantly higher rates of favorable outcome at 90 days, defined as mRS 0 to 2, or equal to the pre-stroke mRS if the prestroke mRS was greater than 2, or NIHSS improvement of 10 points or more (58% vs 33%), as well as lower rates of 90-day mortality (17% vs 38%). The manufacturer of Solitaire has just released the results of the Solitaire FR Thrombectomy for Acute Revascularisation study, a prospective study conducted in

14 centers of Europe, Australia, and Canada that assessed the safety and efficacy of the device for patients with acute stroke symptoms for less than 8 hours and occlusion of a major intracranial vessel. Complete or near-complete reperfusion (TICI2b/3) was reportedly achieved in 160 of 190 patients (79.2%), 90-day mRS 0 to 2 was noted in 57.9% of patients, and the rate of sICH was 1.5%. These results remain unpublished at the time of writing this article.

More recently, we compared the efficacy of IV tPA with that of stent-based thrombectomy using the Solitaire device in patients with proximal MCA occlusions.[42] Although patients treated with the Solitaire device were treated at longer intervals from stroke onset, had higher NIHSS scores, and had higher probabilities of having an Alberta Stroke Program Early CT Study score lower than 7, which are all associated with poor outcome, they had significantly higher chances for good outcome (mRS$\leq$2 in 60% vs 37.5% of patients treated with tPA, $P = .001$) and larger improvements in NIHSS scores. No changes were noted in mortality or length of hospital admission.

The TREVO Pro Stent Retriever mechanical embolectomy device became the second device of this type to be approved by the FDA in August 2012. This approval was supported by results of the TREVO 2 trial, which compared the TREVO stent retriever (n = 88) with the MERCI device (n = 90) in patients with acute intracranial artery occlusions and stroke symptoms for less than 8 hours.[30] The primary efficacy end point, TICI 2 to 3 reperfusion assessed by a central laboratory, was achieved significantly more often in the TREVO-treated patients (86% vs 60%). The primary safety end point, a composite of procedure-related complications, was comparable for the two groups (15% vs 23%). Good functional outcome, defined as mRS 0 to 2, was also more common in patients treated with the stent retriever (40% vs 22%).

## TANDEM OCCLUSIONS: COMBINED INTERVENTIONS

AIS caused by tandem occlusions of the extracranial ICA and intracranial arteries have a poor natural history, and these cases are usually refractory to intravenous thrombolysis. In this setting, stenting of acute extracranial ICA occlusion followed by intracranial embolectomy or stent-based thrombectomy has been shown to be feasible and associated with high rates of recanalization and increased chances of good functional recovery.[43,44]

## ASSESSING THE RESULTS OF NEW TRIALS

Three important trials on acute endovascular stroke therapy were reported and published as we were completing this article. Although it is impossible for us to discuss them in detail here, because they will be debated in upcoming editorials, opinion pieces, and future reviews, it behooves us to present their main findings, limitations, and significance.

The largest and most anticipated of these trials was IMS-III.[25] This placebo-controlled trial evaluated endovascular intervention as a rescue therapy in patients who fail to improve after the administration of reduced-dose IV tPA (0.6 mg/kg) within 3 hours of stroke symptom onset. Confirmation of intracranial vessel occlusion by noninvasive angiography was not mandated before enrollment. The endovascular therapies used in the study included IA tPA, the EKOS catheter, the MERCI retriever, and the Penumbra System; almost no patients were treated with stent retrievers. Enrollment to the trial was prematurely halted because of futility after 656 patients had been enrolled (434 to endovascular therapy and 222 to IV tPA alone). This number, albeit large, is smaller than the planned population size of 900 subjects based on the power analysis of the research protocol. Despite better reperfusion rates (TICI 2–3) in the endovascular group, good functional outcome (mRS 0–2) at 90 days did not differ between the groups (40.8% with endovascular therapy vs 38.7% with IV tPA alone). Although there was a small trend toward better functional outcomes with endovascular therapy among patients with severe stroke (NIHSS 20 or higher), the difference (6.8%) was not statistically significant. A trend toward benefit with endovascular treatment was also noted for patients who received IV tPA within 120 minutes of symptom onset. Rates of mortality and sICH were similar between the groups.

The SYNTHESIS Expansion trial randomized patients with AIS symptoms for less than 4.5 hours to endovascular therapy (181 patients) or IV tPA (181 patients),[32] thus evaluating acute endovascular therapy as a primary modality. There was no minimal NIHSS score required for enrollment and no requirement for preenrollment demonstration of visible intracranial vessel occlusion. Median time to initiation of therapy was 1 hour longer in the endovascular arm (3.75 hours vs 2.75 hours in the IV tPA arm). Only a minority of patients (n = 56, including 18 patients treated with a stent retriever) were treated with a device. Recanalization/reperfusion rates were not reported. Good functional outcome rates were not different between the groups in the intention-to-treat analysis even after adjustment for age and stroke severity (90-day mRS 0–2 observed in 42.0% of patients in the endovascular therapy and 46.4% of patients in the IV tPA group). The results tended to favor IV tPA in older patients with milder deficits. Adverse events, including sICH, did not differ significantly between the groups.

Mechanical Retrieval and Recanalization of Stroke Clots Using Embolectomy (MR-RESCUE) was a trial assessing the value of embolectomy using the MERCI device or the Penumbra device and adjuvant IA tPA when deemed necessary within 8 hours of stroke onset in relation to whether patients had ischemic penumbra as defined by MR diffusion-perfusion mismatch. Overall, 58% of the 118 randomized patients had a favorable penumbral pattern on final review. Mean time to enrollment was 5.5 hours. Baseline NIHSS scores ranged between 6 and 29; they were greater in the nonpenumbral groups and well-balanced between the embolectomy and nonembolectomy groups. Embolectomy did not improve functional outcomes regardless of the presence of a favorable penumbra pattern on magnetic resonance imaging (MRI) despite the fact that more patients in the embolectomy groups initially receiving IV tPA (43.8% vs 29.6% in the nonembolectomy groups). The main finding that presence of penumbra did not predict better outcome after embolectomy could be interpreted to indicate that patients with persistent ischemic penumbra after several hours have enough collaterals to reduce the size of the infarction. However, although patients with penumbra had smaller final stroke volumes, the overall rates of good functional outcome were low even among patients with penumbra on MRI. Recanalization rates with embolectomy were good (67% among those with favorable penumbral pattern and 77% in those without penumbra), but they were unexpectedly better in patients not treated with embolectomy (93% and 78% in those with and without penumbra). Safety data were reassuring, confirming the findings of IMS-III and SYNTHESIS Expansion.

These three negative trials offer a wealth of information for critical analysis, but they do not preclude endovascular acute stroke therapy. Delayed time to endovascular treatment, inclusion of patients without intracranial vessel occlusion or with distal occlusions, use of devices that are less effective in achieving recanalization and reperfusion than the new stent retrievers, incomplete degrees of reperfusion considered as successful interventions, and better-than-expected recanalization rates and functional outcomes in the control groups may help explain the lack of benefit from embolectomy in these trials. There is still a lot to learn and additional research is more necessary than ever.

## LOOKING FORWARD

The history of major ischemic stroke is changing after constant advances in diagnosis and therapy. The prognosis for patients with major vessel occlusion can be significantly improved if timely reperfusion is achieved. Novel endovascular therapies, especially stent-based thrombectomy, can substantially increase reperfusion rates with acceptable risks. Stent-based thrombectomy has rapidly affected clinical practice and promises to revolutionize the endovascular management of major strokes. Among its most remarkable advantages are higher efficacy and shorter procedure times required to achieve arterial recanalization, with a reduced the rate of sICH.

The lack of evidence from randomized controlled trials to prove the clinical efficacy of endovascular therapy in improving functional outcomes is problematic,[45,46] but the strong association between early reperfusion and improved functional outcomes in patients with large intracranial artery occlusions and the increasing ability to achieve early reperfusion using modern devices are arguments that will continue to fuel the growth of acute interventional stroke therapy.

Despite the recent publication of controlled trials questioning the value of different strategies of endovascular stroke therapy (as a rescue in IMS-III, as primary modality in SYNTHESIS Expansion, and guided by advanced imaging in MR-RESCUE), many will continue offering the option of endovascular reperfusion therapy to select patients with disabling acute strokes from large artery occlusion who have either failed IV tPA or who have contraindications for this treatment and are not part of randomized trials. This is not mere obstinacy. We have seen too many patients who seemed destined to have major disability, but regained good and even full function after endovascular reperfusion therapy to proceed otherwise. We have also sometimes failed to intervene in the hope that IV tPA would be enough despite a persistent large intracranial vessel occlusion and then lamented the missed opportunity when seeing the patient remain incapacitated. As confirmed by the same trials questioning the efficacy of endovascular therapy, the intervention is safe when performed by qualified operators. Patients who, in our clinical judgment, deserve the chance of endovascular therapy should be offered that alternative. Our current practice is reflected in the algorithm illustrated in **Fig. 2**.

However, there is an urgent need for evidence from new trials to define how best to apply acute endovascular stroke therapy in practice. The stroke community must unite to ensure the prompt and successful conduction of these trials. To that purpose, when clinical equipoise is present, clinicians should try to randomize patients to a controlled trial. Completed trials can guide future research. They suggest that minimizing the time to recanalization and maximizing the degree of reperfusion are crucial. These principles apply to endovascular therapy when implemented as primary or rescue modality. Requiring a noninvasive angiogram (eg, computed tomography angiography) that shows a major intracranial vessel occlusion before enrollment should probably be mandatory. Refining the definition of clinical and angiographic end points is also essential. For instance, we are convinced that considering a TICI2a as successful reperfusion is inappropriate. Advanced imaging for patient selection also deserves another chance, especially considering that MR-RESCUE only included 34 patients with a favorable penumbral pattern who were treated with embolectomy.

We are confident that endovascular intervention will eventually become a fully accepted, evidence-based treatment of severe AIS. Trials that reflect current endovascular practices are in progress. Their results will clarify requirements for success, including emergency triaging, immediate availability of endovascular expertise, and optimal patient selection. Between now and then, acute stroke protocols will continue

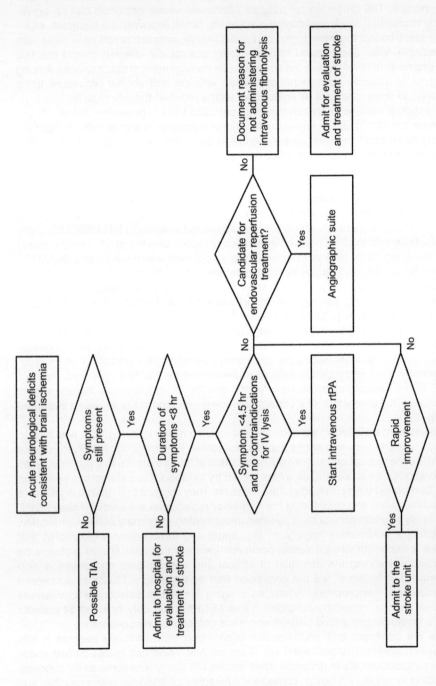

**Fig. 2.** Algorithm for the treatment of AIS. TIA, transient ischemic attack.

to vary across centers and clinical judgment should guide the best course of action for each patient, including the option of endovascular therapy if the expertise is available.

## ACKNOWLEDGMENTS

The authors wish to thank Shifra Fraifeld, a senior medical writer and research associate at the Hadassah-Hebrew University Medical Center, for her invaluable contribution to the preparation of this article.

## REFERENCES

1. Baird AE, Austin MC, McKay WJ, et al. Changes in cerebral tissue perfusion during the first 48 hours of ischaemic stroke: relation to clinical outcome. J Neurol Neurosurg Psychiatry 1996;61(1):26–9.
2. Barber PA, Davis SM, Infeld B, et al. Spontaneous reperfusion after ischemic stroke is associated with improved outcome. Stroke 1998;29(12):2522–8.
3. The National Institute of Neurological Disorders and Stroke rt-PA Stroke Study Group. Tissue plasminogen activator for acute ischemic stroke. The National Institute of Neurological Disorders and Stroke rt-PA Stroke Study Group. N Engl J Med 1995;333(24):1581–7.
4. Schellinger PD, Köhrmann M, Hacke W, et al. Chapter 57. Thrombolytic therapy for acute stroke. In: Fisher M, editor. Handbook of clinical neurology, stroke part III: investigation and management, vol. 94. Philadelphia: Elsevier; 2008. p. 1155–93.
5. European Stroke Organisation Executive, Committee, ESO Writing Committee. Guidelines for management of ischaemic stroke and transient ischaemic attack 2008. Cerebrovasc Dis 2008;25(5):457–507.
6. Saqqur M, Uchino K, Demchuk AM, et al. Site of arterial occlusion identified by transcranial Doppler predicts the response to intravenous thrombolysis for stroke. Stroke 2007;38(3):948–54.
7. Linfante I, Llinas RH, Selim M, et al. Clinical and vascular outcome in internal carotid artery versus middle cerebral artery occlusions after intravenous tissue plasminogen activator. Stroke 2002;33(8):2066–71.
8. Furlan A, Higashida R, Wechsler L, et al. Intra-arterial prourokinase for acute ischemic stroke. The PROACT II study: a randomized controlled trial. Prolyse in Acute Cerebral Thromboembolism. JAMA 1999;282(21):2003–11.
9. Lee M, Hong KS, Saver JL. Efficacy of intra-arterial fibrinolysis for acute ischemic stroke: meta-analysis of randomized controlled trials. Stroke 2010;41(5):932–7.
10. Ogawa A, Mori E, Minematsu K, et al. Randomized trial of intraarterial infusion of urokinase within 6 hours of middle cerebral artery stroke: the middle cerebral artery embolism local fibrinolytic intervention trial (MELT) Japan. Stroke 2007; 38(10):2633–9.
11. Arnold M, Nedeltchev K, Mattle HP, et al. Intra-arterial thrombolysis in 24 consecutive patients with internal carotid artery T occlusions. J Neurol Neurosurg Psychiatry 2003;74(6):739–42.
12. Eckert B, Kucinski T, Neumaier-Probst E, et al. Local intra-arterial fibrinolysis in acute hemispheric stroke: effect of occlusion type and fibrinolytic agent on recanalization success and neurological outcome. Cerebrovasc Dis 2003;15(4): 258–63.
13. Zaidat OO, Suarez JI, Santillan C, et al. Response to intra-arterial and combined intravenous and intra-arterial thrombolytic therapy in patients with distal internal carotid artery occlusion. Stroke 2002;33(7):1821–6.

14. IMS II Trial Investigators. The Interventional Management of Stroke (IMS) II Study. Stroke 2007;38(7):2127–35.
15. Mahon BR, Nesbit GM, Barnwell SL, et al. North American clinical experience with the EKOS MicroLysUS infusion catheter for the treatment of embolic stroke. AJNR Am J Neuroradiol 2003;24(3):534–8.
16. Tsivgoulis G, Alexandrov AV. Ultrasound-enhanced thrombolysis in acute ischemic stroke: potential, failures, and safety. Neurotherapeutics 2007;4(3):420–7.
17. Grunwald IQ, Wakhloo AK, Walter S, et al. Endovascular stroke treatment today. AJNR Am J Neuroradiol 2011;32(2):238–43.
18. Shaltoni HM, Albright KC, Gonzales NR, et al. Is intra-arterial thrombolysis safe after full-dose intravenous recombinant tissue plasminogen activator for acute ischemic stroke? Stroke 2007;38(1):80–4.
19. Shi ZS, Loh Y, Walker G, et al. Endovascular thrombectomy for acute ischemic stroke in failed intravenous tissue plasminogen activator versus non-intravenous tissue plasminogen activator patients: revascularization and outcomes stratified by the site of arterial occlusions. Stroke 2010;41(6):1185–92.
20. Levy EI, Ecker RD, Horowitz MB, et al. Stent-assisted intracranial recanalization for acute stroke: early results. Neurosurgery 2006;58(3):458–63 [discussion: 458–63].
21. Castaño C, Dorado L, Guerrero C, et al. Mechanical thrombectomy with the Solitaire AB device in large artery occlusions of the anterior circulation. A pilot study. Stroke 2010;41(8):1836–40.
22. Cohen JE, Gomori JM, Leker RR, et al. Preliminary experience with the use of self-expanding stent as a thrombectomy device in ischemic stroke. Neurol Res 2011; 33(2):214–9.
23. Baker WL, Colby JA, Tongbram V, et al. Neurothrombectomy devices for the treatment of acute ischemic stroke: state of the evidence. Ann Intern Med 2011; 154(4):243–52.
24. IMS Trial Investigators. Combined intravenous and intra-arterial recanalization for acute ischemic stroke: the Interventional Management of Stroke Study. Stroke 2004;35(4):904–11.
25. Broderick JP, Palesch YY, Demchuk AM, et al. Endovascular therapy after intravenous t-PA versus t-PA alone for stroke. N Engl J Med 2013;368:893–903.
26. Smith WS, Sung G, Starkman S, et al. Safety and efficacy of mechanical embolectomy in acute ischemic stroke: results of the MERCI trial. Stroke 2005;36(7):1432–8.
27. Smith WS, Sung G, Saver J, et al. Mechanical thrombectomy for acute ischemic stroke: final results of the Multi MERCI trial. Stroke 2008;39(4):1205–12.
28. Penumbra Pivotal Stroke Trial Investigators. The Penumbra Pivotal Stroke Trial: safety and effectiveness of a new generation of mechanical devices for clot removal in intracranial large vessel occlusive disease. Stroke 2009;40(8):2761–8.
29. Saver JL, Jahan R, Levy EI, et al. Solitaire flow restoration device versus the Merci Retriever in patients with acute ischaemic stroke (SWIFT): a randomised, parallel-group, non-inferiority trial. Lancet 2012;380(9849):1241–9.
30. Nogueira RG, Lutsep HL, Gupta R, et al. Trevo versus Merci retrievers for thrombectomy revascularisation of large vessel occlusions in acute ischaemic stroke (TREVO 2): a randomised trial. Lancet 2012;380(9849):1231–40.
31. Kidwell CS, Jahan R, Gornbein J, et al. A trial of imaging selection and endovascular treatment for ischemic stroke. N Engl J Med 2013;368:914–23.
32. Ciccone A, Valvassori L, Nichelatti M, et al. Endovascular treatment for acute ischemic stroke. N Engl J Med 2013;368:904–13.
33. Gonzalez A, Mayol A, Martinez E, et al. Mechanical thrombectomy with snare in patients with acute ischemic stroke. Neuroradiology 2007;49(4):365–72.

34. Brandt T, von Kummer R, Muller-Kuppers M, et al. Thrombolytic therapy of acute basilar artery occlusion. Variables affecting recanalization and outcome. Stroke 1996;27(5):875–81.
35. Hacke W, Schwab S, Horn M, et al. 'Malignant' middle cerebral artery territory infarction: clinical course and prognostic signs. Arch Neurol 1996;53(4):309–15.
36. Hacke W, Zeumer H, Ferbert A, et al. Intra-arterial thrombolytic therapy improves outcome in patients with acute vertebrobasilar occlusive disease. Stroke 1988; 19(10):1216–22.
37. Kulcsar Z, Bonvin C, Pereira VM, et al. Penumbra system: a novel mechanical thrombectomy device for large-vessel occlusions in acute stroke. AJNR Am J Neuroradiol 2010;31(4):628–33.
38. Menon BK, Hill MD, Eesa M, et al. Initial experience with the Penumbra Stroke System for recanalization of large vessel occlusions in acute ischemic stroke. Neuroradiology 2011;53(4):261–6.
39. Castaño C, Serena J, Davalos A. Use of the new Solitaire (TM) AB device for mechanical thrombectomy when Merci clot retriever has failed to remove the clot. A case report. Interv Neuroradiol 2009;15(2):209–14.
40. Davalos A, Pereira VM, Chapot R, et al. Retrospective multicenter study of Solitaire FR for revascularization in the treatment of acute ischemic stroke. Stroke 2012;43(10):2699–705.
41. Cohen JE, Gomori JM, Leker RR, et al. Stent for temporary endovascular bypass and thrombectomy in major ischemic stroke. J Clin Neurosci 2011;18(3):369–73.
42. Leker RR, Eichel R, Gomori JM, et al. Stent-based thrombectomy versus intravenous tissue plasminogen activator in patients with acute middle cerebral artery occlusion. Stroke 2012;43(12):3389–91.
43. Cohen JE, Gomori M, Rajz G, et al. Emergent stent-assisted angioplasty of extracranial internal carotid artery and intracranial stent-based thrombectomy in acute tandem occlusive disease: technical considerations. J Neurointerv Surg 2012. [Epub ahead of print]. http://dx.doi.org/10.1136/neurintsurg-2012-020340.
44. Malik AM, Vora NA, Lin R, et al. Endovascular treatment of tandem extracranial/intracranial anterior circulation occlusions: preliminary single-center experience. Stroke 2011;42(6):1653–7.
45. Broderick JP, Meyers PM. Acute stroke therapy at the crossroads. JAMA 2011; 306(18):2026–8.
46. Chimowitz MI. Endovascular treatment for acute ischemic stroke – still unproven. N Engl J Med 2013;368:952–5.

# New Developments in the Treatment of Intracerebral Hemorrhage

Joao A. Gomes, MD[a], Edward Manno, MD, FCCM[b],*

KEYWORDS

• Hemorrhage • Cerebrum • Edema • Blood pressure

KEY POINTS

• Understanding of intracerebral hemorrhage (ICH) pathophysiology and technological advances are now providing the opportunity to significantly reduce the morbidity and mortality associated with this debilitating type of stroke.
• This article reviews several ongoing clinical trials that may transform the way this patient population is treated within the next 5 years.
• Although more research is needed, a new era for ICH management is beginning.

## INTRODUCTION

Intracerebral hemorrhage (ICH) until recently was thought to be a monophasic event with secondary deterioration attributed to worsening cerebral edema. During the last several years, it has been discovered that ICH is a dynamic process evolving over the first few days. Better control of hypertension, the aging of the population, and increasing use of anticoagulation has changed the epidemiologic profile of patients experiencing cerebral hemorrhages. Surgical and medical options may expand as understanding of cerebral hematoma expansion, degradation, and pathophysiology develops.

This article explores the new developments in the past decade in the understanding of the best treatments for this disease, and potentially upcoming therapies are briefly discussed. Expert guidelines based on the best available scientific evidence have been published by the American Heart Association/American Stroke Association.[1] Challenges encountered in the management of this complex patient population are highlighted by the case report provided in **Box 1**.

---

[a] Neurointensive Care Fellowship program, Cerebrovascular Center, Cleveland Clinic Lerner School of Medicine at Case Western Reserve University, Cleveland Clinic, 9500 Euclid Avenue, Cleveland, OH 44195, USA; [b] Neurointensive Care Unit, Cerebrovascular Center, Cleveland Clinic, 9500 Euclid Avenue, Cleveland, OH 44195, USA
* Corresponding author.
E-mail address: mannoe@ccf.org

Neurol Clin 31 (2013) 721–735
http://dx.doi.org/10.1016/j.ncl.2013.03.002
0733-8619/13/$ – see front matter © 2013 Elsevier Inc. All rights reserved.

**Box 1**
**Case report**

A 62-year-old man with a history of hypertension, hyperlipidemia, and atrial fibrillation is admitted in transfer from an outside hospital for treatment of a warfarin-related ICH. On awakening, the patient had noted some left-sided paresthesias. His wife noted some slurred speech and he was taken to a local emergency room where head computed tomography (CT) revealed a small (10 cm³) right basal ganglia hemorrhage. His International Normalization Ratio (INR) was 6.2 and his blood pressure was 200/100 mm Hg. Ten milligrams of intravenous (IV) labetalol were administered, which lowered his blood pressure to 170/90 mm Hg. He was given 10 mg of IV vitamin K to treat his coagulopathy. While waiting for fresh frozen plasma to come from the blood bank, he abruptly deteriorated neurologically, requiring emergent endotracheal intubation. He was transferred to your hospital where a repeat head CT revealed expansion of the initial hemorrhage to 60 cm³. His blood pressure was lowered to 130/90 mm Hg with a continuous intravenous administration of nicardipine. He was given 50 IU/kg of an IV prothrombin complex concentrate formulation. Thirty minutes later his follow-up INR was 1.4. Neurosurgery was consulted for possible hematoma evacuation and decompressive hemicraniectomy. The family arrived 1 hour later and decided it was against the patient's wishes to proceed with aggressive medical or surgical management.

## MEDICAL MANAGEMENT
### Intensive Care Unit Management

Although the optimal blood pressure (BP) range following ICH has not been clearly established, both rapid reductions and marked increases in BP are associated with poor outcomes.[2,3] The Intensive Blood Pressure Reduction in Acute Cerebral Haemorrhage Trial (INTERACT) study assessed the safety and efficacy of BP reduction in the acute phase of ICH. Hypertensive patients were identified within 6 hours of stroke onset and were randomly assigned to either intensive BP control (target systolic BP [SBP] 140 mm Hg) or guideline-based management (target SBP 180 mm Hg). In this pilot trial, early intensive BP control was feasible, well tolerated, and associated with a trend toward decreased hematoma growth (6.2% vs 16.2%, $P = .06$). However, functional outcomes at 90 days were equal in both treatment groups.[4] A follow-up phase III trial (INTERACT2) finished recruiting more than 2800 patients in 140 sites worldwide in August 2012, although most of the patients were recruited in China and only 11 from US sites. Patient follow-up is still ongoing and final results have not been published. The primary end point of INTERACT2 was death or dependency as defined by modified Rankin scale (mRS) 3 to 5 at 90 days, and BP targets were similar to the ones used in the pilot study.[5]

The Antihypertensive Treatment of acute Cerebral Hemorrhage (ATACH) trial took a different approach to BP control. In this feasibility study, 3 different tiers of target SBP were chosen: 170 to 200 mm Hg, 140 to 170 mm Hg, and 110 to 140 mm Hg, and only 1 drug (nicardipine) was used as a continuous infusion to achieve the target BP. Three primary end points were assessed: feasibility of treatment, neurologic worsening within 24 hours, and any serious adverse events during the first 3 days. Patients assigned to the lowest tier of BP control were more likely to have treatment failure, neurologic deterioration, and serious adverse events; however, the rate of these events was less than the prespecified safety thresholds. Also, the 3-month mortality was lower than expected in all tiers of BP control.[6]

These preliminary data prompted the design of a phase III study (ATACH-II) that seeks to evaluate the effects of intensive BP reduction on mortality and disability at 3 months following treatment with nicardipine infusion. For this phase, only 2 BP tiers were chosen (<140 mm Hg and <180 mm Hg), and patients are required to start treatment within 4.5 hours after symptom onset. This trial is still ongoing and is expected to end in 2015.[5]

Evidence from animal experiments shows that increments in brain temperature have a major impact on histopathologic and functional consequences of various types of neuronal injuries. Clinical studies have also shown fever to be common following ICH and to be associated with poor clinical outcomes.[7,8] Moreover, in a cohort of patients with ICH, increased body temperature was associated with increased mortality and length of stay, and this relationship was proportional to the level of temperature increase.[9] Given the accumulating evidence on the detrimental effects of hyperthermia on morbidity and mortality following ICH, fever control may represent a major therapeutic intervention for the management of patients with severe ICH.

To date, only 1 clinical study has investigated the induction of forced normothermia in patients with severe cerebrovascular disease. By means of an endovascular catheter, body temperature was kept at 36.5°C in this trial, which included 41 patients with ICH. A significant reduction in fever burden compared with standard fever management was achieved in this mixed population that also included patients with subarachnoid hemorrhage and ischemic stroke. However, improved fever control did not translate into better clinical outcomes.[10] Lack of statistical power, the inclusion of different patient populations with severe disease status expected to carry a higher mortality, and increased incidence of infectious adverse events possibly related to the use of a cooling catheter likely contributed to the absence of improved outcomes. An ongoing trial, Targeted Temperature Management after ICH (TTM-ICH), seeks to establish the safety and tolerability of a protocol of ultraearly temperature management (normothermia vs mild induced hypothermia) and may represent the starting point for future trials of temperature modulation after ICH.[5]

The use of induced hypothermia in ICH has not been extensively studied. Although early hypothermia in a rodent model of ICH reduced perihematomal edema, blood-brain barrier disruption, and markers of inflammation, no evidence of improved functional outcomes was evident.[11] In 1956, Howell and colleagues[12] induced hypothermia in 8 patients with ICH and, although signs of herniation improved, 6 patients died of hypothermia-related complications. More recently, a randomized trial of selective brain cooling showed reduction in perihematomal edema volume, but clinical outcomes were not reported.[12] These results were replicated after induction of mild systemic hypothermia (35°C) for 10 days. Although a significant decrease in 90-day mortality and a trend toward improved functional outcomes were observed, almost all of the patients who underwent hypothermia developed pneumonia.[13,14] Metabolic stress related to shivering, immunosuppression and associated infections (particularly pneumonia), and cardiovascular complications (ie, hypotension, heart failure, arrhythmias) have been all postulated to potentially negate any beneficial effects derived from hypothermia induction. It is hoped that the ongoing CINCH (Cooling in Intracerebral Hemorrhage) trial, a randomized controlled study of hypothermia in ICH, will provide further data on the usefulness of prolonged hypothermia in patients with ICH.[15]

Following ICH, development of perihematomal edema (PHE) worsens mass effect, intracranial pressure (ICP), and brain tissue shifts, and contributes to neuronal cell injury. Furthermore, PHE is known to increase most rapidly in the first 2 or 3 days after ictus and peak toward the end of the second week.[16] Although osmotic diuresis for treatment of cerebral edema and increased ICP has traditionally been performed with the use of mannitol, more recent studies suggest equivalency, if not superiority, with hypertonic saline (HTS) use.[17,18] A recent meta-analysis of randomized clinical trials found that HTS was more effective than mannitol in controlling episodes of increased ICP in patients with cerebral edema.[17] Furthermore, a small clinical trial examined the effect of continuous 3% HTS infusion in 26 patients with ICH. In-hospital mortality, ICP crisis, and PHE volume were all improved with HTS treatment, and no significant increase in adverse events was documented.[19] Although encouraging, further randomized trials are needed to determine the role of osmotherapy with HTS in patients with ICH.

Multimodality monitoring of patients with acute brain injuries is becoming ubiquitous and provides brain-specific physiologic data obtained continuously or at frequent intervals, which in principle allows the implementation of interventions to minimize secondary brain injury.[20] The routine measurement of brain tissue oxygen tension in the setting of ICH has been limited. In a small series of 7 patients, brain desaturation episodes did not always correlate with instances of increased ICP or reductions in cerebral perfusion pressure, potentially adding another dimension to the acute phase management of this disease entity and another tool to help minimize secondary injury.[21] In another small pilot study, data derived from cerebral oximetry monitoring was used to characterize cerebral autoregulation.[22] Although provocative, more research is needed before this technique can be adopted in routine clinical practice.

The insertion of microdialysis (MD) probes into the brain parenchyma (ie, the perihematomal region) allows sampling of the interstitial fluid chemistry so that a metabolic signature of a particular brain region can be obtained. In principle, the measurement of certain compounds, such as lactate, pyruvate, glycerol, and glucose, can help determine early tissue ischemia, metabolic stress, and secondary brain damage. Only a few small studies have used MD to investigate the neurochemistry of the perihematomal region. Based on their findings, the concept of a metabolic penumbra has been proposed, referring to overactive glucose metabolism in the perihematomal region and likely reflecting ongoing neuronal injury.[22–24] In another series, lactate/pyruvate ratios correlated with patient outcomes and the investigators called for supranormal values of cerebral perfusion pressure to achieve this threshold.[25]

### Hemostatic Therapy

Because hematoma expansion has been documented in up to 70% of patients within 3 hours of symptom onset and because it has also been identified as an independent predictor of death and disability following ICH, strategies that could limit hematoma growth were considered to be an attractive therapeutic intervention. Activated recombinant factor VIIa (rFVIIa) acts locally at the site of tissue injury and results in accelerated thrombin generation and hemostasis. These characteristics made it a prime compound to be tested in patients with ICH.

A phase III trial (FAST) explored the safety and efficacy of rFVIIa in patients with spontaneous ICH. A total of 841 patients were randomly assigned to receive placebo, 20 μg/kg or 80 μg/kg of rFVIIa within 4 hours of stroke onset. Even though patients in the latter group had significant reduction in hematoma expansion, no significant difference in mortality or functional outcomes were identified. Furthermore, arterial thromboembolic adverse events were more frequent in the group receiving a higher dose of rFVIIa.[26]

Several explanations have been put forth to account for the negative results of the FAST trial, including a higher rate of intraventricular hemorrhage (IVH) present in patients treated with rFVIIa, the inclusion of octogenarians, inclusion of patients with large ICH (>60 cm³), and better-than-expected outcome in the placebo arm. Regardless, it has been postulated that patient selection (ie, those with higher risk of hematoma expansion) based on radiographic characteristics (the spot sign) or serum biomarkers may identify optimal candidates for hemostatic therapy.[27] This area of research remains active, but no further recommendations can be made at this point.

## Anticoagulant-related ICH

ICH related to oral anticoagulation therapy (OAT) is associated with substantially worse outcomes than spontaneous ICH. For instance, patients on OAT in the placebo arm of the CHANT (Cerebral Hemorrhagic and NXY-059 Treatment) trial had greater stroke severity, greater baseline median ICH volumes (30.6 vs 14.4 mL), were more likely to experience hematoma expansion, and had higher mortality (62% vs 17%) than patients with spontaneous ICH.[28]

It is thought that the higher propensity for hematoma expansion explains, at least in part, the worse prognosis associated with this condition, and therefore the rapid correction of the underlying coagulopathy should be the main goal of therapy. Fresh frozen plasma (FFP) and vitamin K administration have traditionally been used for the reversal of warfarin-related coagulopathy. However, significant delays in INR normalization have been documented with this approach and, in a recent retrospective study, the median time for door to INR normalization was 30 hours.[29] Significant complications (ie, pulmonary edema) and continued hematoma expansion after INR reversal were also documented in this series.

Another retrospective study of 69 patients with warfarin-related ICH showed that shorter time to FFP administration (median time 90 minutes) was the only intervention associated with successful INR reversal. Furthermore, every 30 minutes of delay in FFP administration was associated with a 20% decreased odds of INR normalization within the first 24 hours.[30]

Because of the shortcomings associated with FFP therapy, the use of alternative agents for warfarin reversal has been explored. For instance, rFVIIa has been shown to rapidly correct INR prolongation in patients treated with vitamin K antagonists.[31] In another small study, the coadministration of rFVIIa and FFP normalized INR faster (8.8 vs 32.2 hours) than the administration of FFP alone, but significant thromboembolic complications were observed in the former group.[32] Furthermore, using in vitro and in vivo models of warfarin anticoagulation, it has been shown that, although rapid normalization of PT/INR with rFVIIa use is almost universal, endogenous thrombin generation (and likely hemostasis) is not consistently restored.[33] Given all these issues and the lack of available clinical data, current guidelines advise against the use of rFVIIa as the sole agent for warfarin reversal in patients with ICH.[1,34]

Prothrombin complex concentrates (PCC) are plasma-derived factor concentrates that contain factors II, VII, IX, and X, have been used for acute warfarin reversal, and expert guidelines consider them a reasonable alternative to FFP for normalization of INR in patients with warfarin-related ICH.[1] Correction of INR in more than 70% of patients within 1 hour of administration can be achieved and a low thromboembolic event rate (2%–5%) was documented in a single-center registry.[35] Conflicting data exist as to their effect on hematoma enlargement and clinical outcomes, which may reflect the variability present between the different commercially available products (ie, 3-factor vs 4-factor PCC, activated vs nonactivated PCC), dosing, and population characteristics.[35,36] There is an ongoing multicenter, prospective, randomized clinical trial exploring the use of PCC and FFP in patients with warfarin-related ICH (the INCH trial).[37]

## Neuroprotective Strategies

To date, no neuroprotective therapy has been shown to improve either morbidity or mortality following ICH. Although several clinical trials have yielded negative results, a few promising agents are being actively investigated (**Fig. 1**).

Various agents have been tested in completed clinical trials, although only 1 phase III study has been conducted to date.[38] Gavestinel, an $N$-methyl-D-aspartate receptor

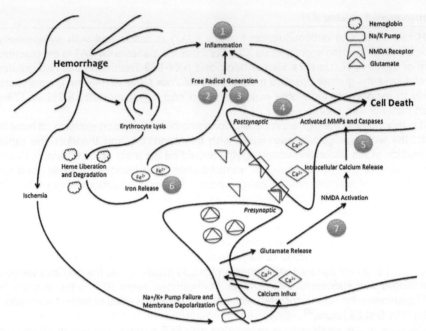

**Fig. 1.** Pathophysiology of ICH and targets in completed and ongoing clinical trials. (1) Celecoxib; (2) NXY-059; (3) rosuvastatin; (4) pioglitazone; (5) tauroursodeoxycholic acid; (6) deferoxamine; (7) gavestinel. NMDA, N-methyl-ᴅ-aspartate; MMP, matrix metalloproteinase. (*From* Ayer A, Hwang BY, Appleboom G, et al. Clinical trials for neuroprotective therapies in intracerebral hemorrhage: a new roadmap from bench to bedside. Transl Stroke Res 2012;3:411; with permission.)

antagonist, was the subject of the GAIN (Glycine Antagonist in Neuroprotection) Americas and GAIN International clinical trials.[39,40] A pooled analysis of the 571 patients with primary ICH enrolled in both studies showed no statistically significant difference in the distribution of trichotomized Barthel Index scores between gavestinel and placebo.[41] The free radical scavenger NXY-059 showed encouraging results in preliminary animal studies[42] and led to the CHANT trial in human subjects. In this randomized, placebo-controlled trial, 603 patients with ICH were enrolled within 6 hours of onset to test the clinical efficacy of NXY-059. Although the drug had a good safety and tolerability profile, the investigators found no evidence of clinical improvement.[43]

Inhibitors of HMG-COA reductase (ie, statins) through various pleiotropic effects may help reduce inflammation and superoxide free radicals, while increasing synaptogenesis and cellular survival. Animal models have shown significant decreases in hematoma volume and tissue loss as well as increases in neurogenesis and synaptic formation.[38] Preliminary clinical studies examining prior statin use have also suggested decreased perihematomal edema,[44] decreased mortality,[45] and even improvement in functional outcomes.[46] Two different statin agents have been tested in ICH to date. The effects of simvastatin were explored in a recent phase II randomized, placebo-controlled trial in which perihematomal edema, mortality, and the mRS were the main outcomes measured. However, the study was terminated because of poor enrollment.[38] Meanwhile, rosuvastatin was shown to improve mortality and functional outcomes in a small nonrandomized study conducted by a Mexican group.[46] Although encouraging, given the nonrandomized design and the small number of patients included in this study, further trials are needed to establish the efficacy of rosuvastatin in patients with ICH.

Citicoline, a compound needed for the synthesis of structural phospholipids, has also been tested as a neuroprotective agent in patients with ICH. Muscular strength was reportedly improved in 32 patients with ICH who participated in a small clinical study and received citicoline for 14 days. However, issues regarding validation of the scale used to measure strength made interpretation of these findings challenging.[38] In another randomized pilot study that included 38 patients, the safety and efficacy of citicoline in ICH was tested. Although a positive trend favoring citicoline was observed, insufficient data are available to recommend its routine use in patients with ICH.[27] The selective cyclooxygenase-2 inhibitor celecoxib has similarly been investigated in ICH therapy because of its antiinflammatory properties. A recent retrospective study suggested decreased perihematomal edema in patients treated with the drug.[47] This suggestion led to a randomized, open-label study sponsored by the Seoul National University Hospital. Forty patients were enrolled to receive either placebo or celecoxib 400 mg twice a day for 2 weeks, and the primary outcome assessed was the volume of perihematomal edema. Although the trial was completed in 2010, no results have been made available to date.[5]

Iron released from red blood cell hemolysis after ICH has been implicated in neurotoxicity via autophagy, exacerbation of excitotoxicity, hydroxyl radical formation, and oxidative stress.[48,49] Deferoxamine (DFO), an iron chelator, is a promising therapeutic intervention to help limit brain injury and improve outcomes following ICH. Besides its iron-chelating properties, DFO is thought to exert neuroprotective effects by inhibiting apoptosis, decreasing oxidative stress, and through antiinflammatory mechanisms.[50] Animal studies support this putative neuroprotective effect of DFO, and improved neurologic function has been shown in several species in experimental models of ICH.[51] A recent phase I, dose-finding study in humans established the safety, feasibility, and tolerability of DFO in patients with ICH. The maximum tolerated dose in this study was 62 mg/kg/d and the daily drug infusion was not associated with significant serious adverse events or increased mortality.[52] One of the few ongoing clinical trials in ICH (**Table 1**) is a prospective, randomized, placebo-armed, phase II futility study to determine whether it is futile to move DFO forward to phase III efficacy testing. Planned enrollment will include 324 patients who will be randomized to receive either placebo or a daily infusion of DFO for 5 days.[5]

Pioglitazone, an agonist of the peroxisome proliferator activated receptor gamma (a member of the nuclear receptor superfamily) is currently being investigated because

**Table 1**
**Ongoing neuroprotection trials in spontaneous ICH**

| Agent | Trial | Phase | # Patients | Outcomes | Completion Date |
|---|---|---|---|---|---|
| Deferoxamine | HI-DEF | II/III | 324 | Safety and efficacy (dichotomized mRS) | 2017 |
| Pioglitazone | SHRINC | II | 80 | Safety and mortality | September 2013 |
| Albumin | ACHIEVE | II | 40 | Safety and BBB disruption | September 2013 |
| Celecoxib | ACE-ICH | II | 40 | Safety and PHE | Completed in 2010 |

*Abbreviation:* ACHIEVE, albumin for intracerebral hemorrhage intervention; ACE-ICH, administration of celecoxib for treatment of intracerebral hemorrhage; BBB, blood-brain barrier; Hi-Def, high dose deferoxamine in intracerebral hemorrhage; SHRINC, safety of pioglitazone for hematoma resolution in intracerebral hemorrhage.

of the pathway's impact on pathogenic cascades triggered by hematoma formation.[38] The Safety of Pioglitazone for Hematoma Resolution in Intracerebral Hemorrhage (SHRINC) trial seeks to enroll 80 patients with spontaneous ICH and it aims to establish the safety and determine the duration of treatment of hematoma/edema resolution in ICH.[5] In addition, because of its putative neuroprotective effects, albumin is also being explored as a possible therapy for ICH. In the albumin for intracerebral hemorrhage intervention (ACHIEVE) trial, patients are being randomized to placebo or albumin infusion for 3 consecutive days and blood-brain barrier disruption is being assessed in serial MRIs using the hyperintense acute reperfusion marker on postcontrast fluid-attenuated inversion recovery sequences.[5]

## SURGICAL MANAGEMENT
### Open Craniotomy

Open craniotomy has been the most widely studied surgical modality for ICH treatment, and early attempts to establish its efficacy date back to the preimaging era.[53] Since then, several clinical studies have attempted to show a clinical benefit based on imaging, clinical, anatomic, or surgical timing characteristics, but with little success.[54]

In 2005, the results of a randomized study comparing early surgery (mean time from ictus onset 30 hours) versus initial conservative treatment in patients with spontaneous supratentorial ICH (STICH trial) were published. A total of 503 patients were allocated to the surgical arm, whereas 530 received medical therapy initially, and both groups seemed to be well matched at baseline. The primary outcome measure was mild or moderate disability as measured by the Glasgow Outcome Scale at 6 months. The participants were randomized into either group only after the investigators had determined that they were not candidates for urgent hematoma evacuation. No overall benefit from early surgery could be shown and a favorable outcome was observed in 26% of patients allocated to surgery compared with 24% in those allocated to initial conservative treatment.[55]

A preplanned subgroup analysis of the STICH trial showed a trend toward improved functional outcomes with early surgical therapy in patients with a hematoma within 1 cm of the cortical surface. Given this encouraging trend, 601 patients with lobar ICH have been enrolled in the follow-up STICH II trial. The investigators intend to address 2 of the common criticisms of the original study, namely surgery on deeply seated hematomas and late timing for surgery. The STICH II trial is currently closed to recruitment and is in the final stages of the follow-up period.[56]

The role of early decompressive craniectomy (DC) in patients with large areas of ischemia involving the territory of the middle cerebral artery was established in a pooled analysis of 3 European trials. Both mortality and functional outcomes were improved with surgery in this patient population.[57] Because mass effect secondary to hematoma volume and perihematomal edema are thought to contribute to poor outcome after ICH, DC has been explored in small studies as a therapeutic option for large ICH.

In a rodent model of ICH with autologous blood injection into the basal ganglia, DC improved mortality and behavioral scores when performed early (before 24 hours from onset). Postcraniectomy mortality was only 10% in the group randomized to DC within 6 hours.[58] Most of the few clinical series published to date on DC in ICH have focused on a combined treatment of hematoma evacuation and craniectomy. One such retrospective series included 12 patients with nondominant ICH who underwent DC and hematoma evacuation. Of these, 92% survived to discharge and 54.5% had a good outcome, as measured by an mRS score between 0 and 3.[59] The only report of DC without hematoma evacuation available included a small number of patients. Overall, it seemed to be feasible and safe and an improvement in mortality and functional outcome was suggested, although some concerns were raised about ultraearly DC and the risk of further hematoma expansion.[60] Future randomized trials are needed to properly evaluate the role, if any, of DC in ICH management and therefore a recommendation for routine DC cannot be made at this point.

### Minimally Invasive Strategies

In an effort to minimize surgical trauma associated with traditional hematoma evacuation, minimally invasive techniques have been refined over the years. They also offer the advantage of a shorter operative time, the potential for performing them at the bedside, and minimization of potential secondary brain injury associated with general anesthesia and brain manipulation and retraction. Furthermore, a consensus conference sponsored by the National Institutes of Health concluded that minimally invasive strategies to evacuate intraparenchymal clots were a promising area for future investigations.[61]

Backlund and von Host[62] (1978) first pioneered a CT-guided stereotactic system that allowed the aspiration of intracerebral hematomas using cannulas based on the water-screw principle of Archimedes. However, significant residual ICH was left behind because of the physical characteristics of the coagulated blood mass, and the use of urokinase infused through a stereotactically placed tube into the center of the hematoma resulted in removal of major parts of the clot without any significant side effects.[63] An ultrasonic surgical aspirator was subsequently developed to enhance aspiration of dense clots in the acute stage.[64]

The largest study to date of minimally invasive hematoma evacuation was conducted in China and reported in 2009. A total of 377 patients with basal ganglia ICH were randomized to either medical management or minimally invasive craniopuncture with clot aspiration and urokinase infusion. Overall, independent survival at 90 days was significantly better in the treatment group and the investigators reported that, in 50% of the treated cases, half of the hematoma was removed in the first aspiration attempt. There was a slightly higher rate of rebleeding (9.7% vs 5%) in the craniopuncture group, but the in-hospital case fatality rate was similar between the two groups.[65]

Neuroendoscopic aspiration of intraparenchymal clot through a burr hole has also been reported. In this technique, the hematoma cavity is accessed under direct visual control and artificial cerebrospinal fluid is infused under low pressure with subsequent drainage of blood clots through a separate channel on the endoscope. This endoscopic technique also allowed the coagulation of small oozing vessels in the hematoma bed. Although only 50 patients were included in the endoscopy group, functional outcomes were significantly better in those with a hematoma size of less than 50 cm$^3$ and age less than 60 years. In patients with hematomas larger than 50 cm$^3$, mortality was decreased, but functional outcomes remain unchanged.[66]

Urokinase and streptokinase were the initial thrombolytic agents used to facilitate hematoma aspiration, but more recently tissue plasminogen activator (t-PA) has become the agent of choice.[61] For instance, in a small series of 15 patients, frameless stereotactic clot aspiration-thrombolysis using 2 mg of t-PA every 12 hours resulted in a 17% decrease in hematoma volume and a trend toward improved 30-day survival. Even though ventriculitis and hematoma expansion were reported, the overall complications did not exceed the expected incidence rates.[67]

The MISTIE trial was a phase II proof-of-concept study that tested the safety, feasibility, and reproducibility of surgical performance combining minimally invasive stereotactic surgery with t-PA infusion for hematoma evacuation versus standard medical management. A total of 93 patients were enrolled (54 in the surgical arm) and this technique was safe and effective at decreasing ICH volume (on average 28 cm$^3$ by the third day of therapy). Standardization of the surgical procedure across different centers was shown to be feasible. Achieving an ICH volume of less than 15 cm$^3$ at the end of treatment (day 3) was associated with an odds ratio of 3.6 for benefit using dichotomized mRS ($P$ = .053), potentially establishing a surgical goal for future trials.[68] A larger, phase III study to confirm these preliminary findings is in the planning stages.

Sonothrombolysis is a new technology that relies on the delivery of ultrasound energy locally to the clot, which is thought to enhance t-PA penetration into the parenchymal hematoma thus facilitating thrombolysis (**Fig. 2**). When this novel drug delivery method of enhanced thrombolysis was tested in 9 patients, it resulted in a faster and greater reduction in hematoma volume compared with patients enrolled in the MISTIE trial who were treated with t-PA alone. Although promising, these results need confirmation in larger studies. Furthermore, catheters specifically designed for intracranial use are currently being developed.[69]

The infusion of thrombolytic agents to enhance clot drainage in patients with IVH, either primary or secondary to ICH, has also been tested. In the CLEAR (Clot Lysis: Evaluating Accelerated Resolution of ICH) study, the safety of intraventricular injections of 3 mg of t-PA every 12 hours was assessed. Mortality was 18% in the treated group (vs 23% in the placebo arm), whereas symptomatic bleeding occurred in 23% of patients who received t-PA. Clot resolution was highest in the t-PA group (18% vs 8%, $P$<.001) and patients were liberated from a ventriculostomy earlier than their untreated counterparts.[70] It has also been shown that t-PA leads to IVH resolution in a

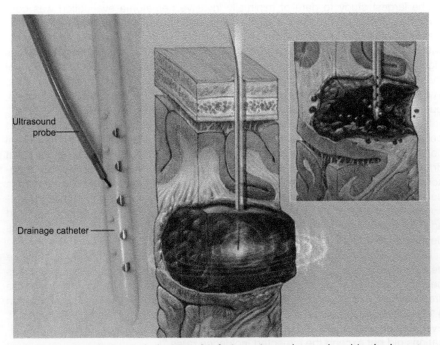

**Fig. 2.** Drainage catheter and ultrasound infusion microcatheter placed in the hematoma bed. Enhanced thrombolysis as a result of ultrasound energy and t-PA infusion. (*From* Newell DW, Shah MM, Wilcox R, et al. Minimally invasive evacuations of spontaneous intracerebral hemorrhage using sonothrombolysis. J Neurosurg 2011;115:594. *Courtesy of* David W. Newell, M.D, Seattle, WA; with permission.)

dose-dependent manner and that most of this effect is observed in the midline ventri-cles.[71] The CLEAR III trial is currently actively recruiting (planned recruitment of 500 patients) and it will assess functional outcomes at 90 and 180 days after IVH.[5]

## SUMMARY

Understanding of ICH pathophysiology and technological advances are now providing the opportunity to significantly reduce the morbidity and mortality associated with this debilitating type of stroke. As reviewed in this article, several ongoing clinical trials may transform the way this patient population is treated within the next 5 years. Although more research is needed, a new era for ICH management is beginning.

## REFERENCES

1. Morgenstern LB, Hemphil CJ, Anderson C, et al. Guidelines for the management of spontaneous intracerebral hemorrhage: a guideline for healthcare professionals from the American Heart Association/American Stroke Association. Stroke 2010;41:2108–29.
2. Vemmos KN, Tsivgoulis G, Spengos K, et al. U-shaped relationship between mortality and admission blood pressure in patients with acute stroke. J Intern Med 2004;255:257–65.
3. Qureshi AI, Bliwise DL, Bliwise NG, et al. Rate of 24-hour blood pressure decline and mortality after spontaneous intracerebral hemorrhage: a retrospective analysis with a random effects regression model. Crit Care Med 1999;27: 480–5.
4. Anderson CS, Huang Y, Wang JG, et al. Intensive Blood Pressure Reduction in Acute Cerebral Haemorrhage Trial (INTERACT): a randomised pilot trial. Lancet 2008;7:391–9.
5. Available at: http://clinicaltrials.gov/. Search: ongoing ICH trials. Accessed January 3, 2013.
6. ATACH investigators. Antihypertensive treatment of acute cerebral hemorrhage. Crit Care Med 2010;38:637–48.
7. Saini M, Saqqur M, Kamruzzaman A, et al. Effect of hyperthermia on prognosis after acute ischemic stroke. Stroke 2009;40:3051–9.
8. Leira R, Davalos A, Silva Y, et al. Early neurological deterioration in intracerebral hemorrhage: predictors and associated factors. Neurology 2004;63: 461–7.
9. Diringer MN, Reaven NL, Funk SE, et al. Elevated body temperature independently contributes to increased length of stay in neurologic intensive care unit patients. Crit Care Med 2004;32:1489–95.
10. Broessner G, Beer R, Lackner P, et al. Prophylactic, endovascularly based, long-term normothermia in ICU patients with severe cerebrovascular disease: bicenter prospective, randomized trial. Stroke 2009;40:e657–65.
11. MacLellan CL, Davies LM, Fingas MS, et al. The influence of hypothermia on outcome after intracerebral hemorrhage in rats. Stroke 2006;37:1266–70.
12. Feng H, Shi D, Wang D, et al. Effect of local mild hypothermia on treatment of acute intracerebral hemorrhage, a clinical study. Zhonghua Yi Xue Za Zhi 2002;10:1622–4.
13. Kollmar R, Staykov D, Dorfler A, et al. Hypothermia reduces perihemorrhagic edema after intracerebral hemorrhage. Stroke 2010;41:1684–9.

14. Satykov D, Wagner I, Volbers B, et al. Mild prolonged hypothermia for large intracerebral hemorrhage. Neurocrit Care 2013;18(2):178–83.

15. Kollmar R, Juetler E, Huttner HB, et al. Cooling in intracerebral hemorrhage (CINCH) trial: protocol of a randomized German-Austrian clinical trial. Int J Stroke 2012;7:168–72.

16. Venkatasubramanian C, Mlynash M, Finley-Caufield A, et al. Natural history of perihematomal edema after intracerebral hemorrhage measured by serial magnetic resonance imaging. Stroke 2011;42:73–80.

17. Kamel H, Navi B, Nakagawa K, et al. Hypertonic saline versus mannitol for the treatment of elevated intracranial pressure. Crit Care Med 2011;39:554–9.

18. da Silva JC, de Lima Fde M, Valenca MM, et al. Hypertonic saline more efficacious than mannitol in lethal intracranial hypertension model. Neurol Res 2010; 32:139–43.

19. Wagner I, Hauer EM, Staykov D, et al. Effects of continuous hypertonic saline infusion on perihemorrhagic edema evolution. Stroke 2011;42:1540–5.

20. Wartenberg KE, Schmidt JM, Mayer SA. Multimodality monitoring in neurocritical care. Crit Care Clin 2007;23:507–38.

21. Hemphill JC III, Morabito D, Farrant M, et al. Brain tissue oxygen monitoring in intracerebral hemorrhage. Neurocrit Care 2005;03:260–70.

22. Diedler J, Karpel-Massler G, Sykora M, et al. Autoregulation and brain metabolism in the perihematomal region of spontaneous intracerebral hemorrhage: an observational pilot study. J Neurol Sci 2010;295:16–22.

23. Vespa PM. Metabolic penumbra in intracerebral hemorrhage. Stroke 2009;40: 1547–8.

24. Zazulia AR, Videen TO, Powers WJ. Transient focal increase in perihematomal glucose metabolism after acute human intracerebral hemorrhage. Stroke 2009;40:1638–43.

25. Nikaina I, Paterakis K, Paraforos G, et al. Cerebral perfusion pressure, microdialysis biochemistry, and clinical outcome in patients with spontaneous intracerebral hematomas. J Crit Care 2012;27:83–8.

26. Mayer SA, Brun NC, Begtrup K, et al. Efficacy and safety of recombinant activated factor VII for acute intracerebral hemorrhage. N Engl J Med 2008;358:2127–37.

27. Adeoye O, Broderick JP. Advances in the management of intracerebral hemorrhage. Nat Rev Neurol 2010;6:593–601.

28. Cucchiara B, Messe S, Sansing L, et al. Hematoma growth in oral anticoagulation related intracerebral hemorrhage. Stroke 2008;39:2993–6.

29. Lee SB, Manno EM, Layton KF, et al. Progression of warfarin-associated intracerebral hemorrhage after INR normalization with FFP. Neurology 2006;67: 1272–4.

30. Goldstein JN, Thomas SH, Frontiero V, et al. Timing of fresh frozen plasma administration and rapid correction of coagulopathy in warfarin-related intracerebral hemorrhage. Stroke 2006;37:151–5.

31. Freeman WD, Brott TG, Barret KM, et al. Recombinant factor VIIa for rapid reversal of warfarin anticoagulation in acute intracranial hemorrhage. Mayo Clin Proc 2004;79:1495–500.

32. Brody DL, Aiyagari V, Shackelfor AM, et al. Use of recombinant factor VIIa in patients with warfarin-associated intracranial hemorrhage. Neurocrit Care 2005;2: 263–7.

33. Tanaka AK, Szlam F, Dickneite G, et al. Effects of prothrombin complex concentrate and recombinant activated factor VII on vitamin K antagonist induced anticoagulation. Thromb Res 2008;122:117–23.

34. Rosovsky RP, Crowther MA. What is the evidence for the off-label use of recombinant factor VIIa (rFVIIa) in the acute reversal of warfarin. Hematology Am Soc Hematol Educ Program 2008;1:36–8.

35. Dowlatshahi D, Butcher KS, Asdaghi N, et al. Poor prognosis in warfarin-associated intracranial hemorrhage despite anticoagulation reversal. Stroke 2012;43:1812–7.

36. Kuwashiro T, Yasaka M, Itabashi R, et al. Effect of prothrombin complex concentrate on hematoma enlargement and clinical outcomes in patients with anticoagulant-associated intracerebral hemorrhage. Cerebrovasc Dis 2011; 31:170–6.

37. Steiner T, Freiberger A, Husing J, et al. International normalized ratio normalisation in patients with coumarin-related intracranial hemorrhages – the INCH trial: a randomised, controlled, multicenter trial to compare safety and preliminary efficacy of fresh frozen plasma and prothrombin complex. Study design and protocol. Int J Stroke 2011;6:271–7.

38. Ayer A, Hwang BY, Appleboom G, et al. Clinical trials for neuroprotective therapies in intracerebral hemorrhage: a new roadmap from bench to bedside. Transl Stroke Res 2012;3:409–17.

39. Lees KR, Asplund K, Carolei A, et al. Glycine antagonist (gavestinel) in neuroprotection (GAIN International) in patients with acute stroke: a randomised controlled trial. Lancet 2000;355:1949–54.

40. Sacco RL, DeRosa JT, Haley EC, et al. Glycine antagonist in neuroprotection for patients with acute stroke. GAIN Americas: a randomized controlled trial. JAMA 2001;285:1719–28.

41. Haley EC, Thompson JL, Levin B, et al. Gavestinel does not improve outcome after acute intracerebral hemorrhage: an analysis from GAIN international and GAIN Americas studies. Stroke 2005;36:1006–10.

42. Lapchak PA, Araujo DM, Song D, et al. Effects of the spin trap agent disodium-[(tert-butylimino)methyl] benzene-1,3-disulfonate N-oxide (generic nxy-059) on intracerebral hemorrhage in a rabbit large clot embolic stroke model: combination studies with tissue plasminogen activator. Stroke 2002; 33:1665–70.

43. Lyden PD, Shuaib A, Lees KR, et al. Safety and tolerability of nxy-059 for acute intracerebral hemorrhage: the CHANT trial. Stroke 2007;38:2262–9.

44. Naval N, Abdelhak TA, Urrunaga N, et al. An association of prior statin use with decreased perihematomal edema. Neurocrit Care 2008;8:13–8.

45. Naval N, Abdelhak TA, Zeballos P, et al. Prior statin use reduces mortality in intracerebral hemorrhage. Neurocrit Care 2008;8:6–12.

46. Tapia-Perez H, Sanches-Aguilar M, Torres-Corzo JG, et al. Use of statins for the treatment of spontaneous intracerebral hemorrhage: results of a pilot study. Cent Eur Neurosurg 2009;70:15–20.

47. Park HK, Lee SH, Chu K, et al. Effects of celecoxib on volumes of hematoma and edema in patients with primary intracerebral hemorrhage. J Neurol Sci 2009;279:43–6.

48. Nakamura T, Keep RF, Hua Y, et al. Oxidative DNA injury after experimental intracerebral hemorrhage. Brain Res 2005;1039:30–6.

49. Chen M, Olatilewa O, Chen J, et al. Iron regulatory protein-2 knockout increases perihematomal ferritin expression and cell viability after intracerebral hemorrhage. Brain Res 2010;1337:95–103.

50. Selim M. Deferoxamine mesylate: a new hope for intracerebral hemorrhage: from bench to clinical trials. Stroke 2009;40:S90–1.

51. Gu Y, Hua Y, Keep RF, et al. Deferoxamine reduces intracerebral hematoma-induced iron accumulation and neuronal death in piglets. Stroke 2009;40: 2241–3.
52. Selim M, Yeatts S, Goldstein JN, et al. Safety and tolerability of deferoxamine mesylate in patients with acute intracerebral hemorrhage. Stroke 2011;42: 3067–74.
53. McKissock W, Richardson A, Taylor J. Primary intracerebral hemorrhage: a controlled trial of surgical and conservative treatment in 180 unselected cases. Lancet 1961;278:221–6.
54. Gomes JA, Kase CS, Caplan LR. Therapy of intracerebral hemorrhage. In: Brandt T, Caplan LR, Dichgans J, et al, editors. Neurological disorders: course and treatment. San Diego (CA): Academic Press; 2003. p. 403–20.
55. Mendelow AD, Gregson BA, Fernandes HM, et al. Early surgery versus initial conservative treatment in patients with spontaneous supratentorial intracerebral haematomas in the international Surgical Trial in Intracerebral Haemorrhage (STICH): a randomised trial. Lancet 2005;365:387–97.
56. Available at: http://research.ncl.ac.uk/stich/. Accessed December 26, 2013.
57. Vahedi K, Hofmeijer J, Juettler E, et al. Early decompressive surgery in malignant infarction of the middle cerebral artery: a pooled analysis of three randomised controlled trials. Lancet 2007;6:215–22.
58. Marinkovic I, Strbian D, Pedrono E, et al. Decompressive craniectomy for intracerebral hemorrhage. Neurosurgery 2009;65:780–6.
59. Murthy JM, Chowdary GV, Murthy TV, et al. Decompressive craniectomy with clot evacuation in large hemispheric hypertensive intracerebral hemorrhage. Neurocrit Care 2005;2:258–62.
60. Fung C, Murek M, Z'Graggen WJ, et al. Decompressive hemicraniectomy in patients with supratentorial intracerebral hemorrhage. Stroke 2012;43:3207–11.
61. Abdu E, Hanley DF, Newell DW. Minimally invasive treatment for intracerebral hemorrhage. Neurosurg Focus 2012;32:1–7.
62. Backlund EO, von Holst H. Controlled subtotal evacuation of intracerebral hematomas by stereotactic technique. Surg Neurol 1978;9:99–101.
63. Matsumoto K, Hondo H. CT-guided stereotaxic evacuation of hypertensive intracerebral hematomas. J Neurosurg 1984;61:440–8.
64. Hondo H, Uno M, Sasaki K, et al. Computed tomography controlled aspiration surgery for hypertensive intracerebral hemorrhage. Stereotact Funct Neurosurg 1990;54:432–7.
65. Wang WZ, Jiang B, Liu HM, et al. Minimally invasive craniopuncture therapy vs. conservative treatment for spontaneous intracerebral hemorrhage: results from a randomized clinical trial in China. Int J Stroke 2009;4:11–6.
66. Auer LM, Deinsberger W, Neiderkorn K, et al. Endoscopic surgery versus medical treatment for spontaneous intracerebral hematoma: a randomized study. J Neurosurg 1989;70:530–5.
67. Barret RJ, Hussain R, Coplin WM, et al. Frameless stereotactic aspiration and thrombolysis of spontaneous intracerebral hemorrhage. Neurocrit Care 2005; 03:237–45.
68. Hanley DF. MISTIE phase II results. Safety, efficacy and surgical performance. Presented at the 2012 International Stroke Conference (late-breaking science oral abstracts). New Orleans, February 2, 2012.
69. Newell DW, Shah MM, Wilcox R, et al. Minimally invasive evacuations of spontaneous intracerebral hemorrhage using sonothrombolysis. J Neurosurg 2011; 115:592–601.

70. Naff N, Milliams MA, Keyl PM, et al. Low-dose recombinant tissue-type plasminogen activator enhances clot resolution in brain hemorrhage: the Intraventricular Hemorrhage Thrombolysis Trial. Stroke 2011;42:3009–16.
71. Webb AJ, Ullman NL, Mann S, et al. Resolution of intraventricular hemorrhage varies by ventricular region and dose of intraventricular thrombolytic: the Clot Lysis: Evaluating Accelerated Resolution of ICH (CLEAR IVH) program. Stroke 2012;43:1666–8.

# New Therapies for Unruptured Intracranial Aneurysms

Philipp Taussky, MD[a,b], Rabih G. Tawk, MD[c],
David A. Miller, MD[c,d], William D. Freeman, MD[e],
Ricardo A. Hanel, MD, PhD[c],*

## KEYWORDS

- Aneurysm • Treatment • Endovascular • Flow diverter

## KEY POINTS

- The concept of flow diversion is based on placing a stent across the neck of an intracranial aneurysm, which then results in flow away from the aneurysm, inducing thrombosis and occlusion of the aneurysm over time.
- The stent itself experiences neointimal coverage, thus resulting in a remodeling of the parent vessel.
- As the use and application of flow diverters becomes more widespread, some important questions remain relating to the effective treatment of dual antiplatelet therapy, the occurrence of delayed aneurysm ruptures and intraparenchymal hemorrhages, and long-term patency rates.
- Novel flow diverters are currently being investigated for approval of the Food and Drug Administration in a large prospective multicentric trial, which may offer different treatment options and benefits, but whose safety and efficacy are currently under investigation.
- Intrasaccular devices lead to immediate aneurysm occlusion by deployment of a self-expanding ovoid-shaped metal mesh into the aneurysm sac, thus providing an intraluminal flow diversion, also indicated in acutely ruptured aneurysms.

## INTRODUCTION

The use of flow diverters introduced an exciting new concept in the current treatment of intracranial aneurysm. Standard endovascular treatment of aneurysms included

Disclosures: Covidien Proctor (R.A. Hanel).
[a] Department of Neurosurgery, Clinical Neurosciences Center, University of Utah, 175 North Medical Drive East Salt Lake City, UT 84132, USA; [b] Department of Radiology, University of Utah, 100 North Medical Drive Salt Lake City, UT 84132, USA; [c] Department of Neurosurgery, Mayo Clinic College of Medicine, 4500 San Pablo Road, Jacksonville, FL 32224, USA; [d] Department of Radiology, Mayo Clinic College of Medicine, 4500 San Pablo Road, Jacksonville, FL 32224, USA; [e] Department of Neurology, Mayo Clinic College of Medicine, 4500 San Pablo Road, Jacksonville, FL 32224, USA
* Corresponding author. Department of Neurosurgery, Mayo Clinic, 4500 San Pablo Road, Jacksonville, FL 32224.
E-mail address: hanel.ricardo@mayo.edu

packing the aneurysm with platinum coils, thus preventing inflow into the aneurysm, occlusion of the aneurysmal sac by the coil mass, and subsequent thrombosis. Flow diverters, which are essentially self-expanding, cylindrical meshed stents, cover the neck of the aneurysm and function by 2 distinct modes: The flow-diversion aspect diverts blood flow away from the aneurysm sac, thus promoting intra-aneurysmal stasis and subsequent thrombosis. In addition, the flow diverter induces neointimal growth along its mesh, resulting in neoendothelialization and remodeling of the parent artery, with occlusion of the neck of the aneurysm as the neointima covers the ostium of the aneurysm. The only flow diverter currently approved in the United States is the Pipeline embolization device (PED) (Covidien, Irvine, CA), which consists of 48 interwoven strands of 25% platinum tungsten and 75% cobalt chromium. It features diameters from 2.5 to 5 mm, with 0.025-mm increments, and lengths from 10 to 35 mm.

## CURRENT FLOW-DIVERSION INDICATIONS AND CONTRAINDICATIONS

Current indications for the use of Pipeline flow diverters include large and giant unruptured intracranial aneurysms ($\geq$10 mm) of the anterior circulation from the petrous segment to the superior hypophyseal segment. Aneurysms may be saccular or fusiform (**Box 1**). Patients need to be pretreated with dual antiplatelet therapy (aspirin and clopidogrel). Different loading algorithms exist; the authors' includes pretreatment for 7 days, after which the response to aspirin (325 mg) and clopidogrel (75 mg) is tested (aspirin function testing, P2Y12 testing [Accumetrics, San Diego, CA]) (**Box 2**). Aspirin and clopidogrel therapy is continued postprocedure for a duration of 3 to 6 months, again with different algorithms in place. Most centers will discontinue clopidogrel after 3 to 6 months and keep the patient on life-long daily aspirin therapy (81–325 mg).

Strict contraindications are ruptured aneurysms, prior stented aneurysms, patients with acute infection, and patients unable to remain on dual antiplatelet therapy for at least 3 to 6 months. As the use of flow diverters becomes more widespread, current treatment indications may expand, most notably with respect to aneurysm size and location, with the possibility of including smaller aneurysms, aneurysms to the carotid terminus, and posterior circulation aneurysms. Although many such as aneurysms are currently treated using Pipeline flow diverters, use of the device for such aneurysms is considered to be off-label.[1–4]

## INITIAL EXPERIENCE WITH FLOW DIVERTERS

In the United States, the PUFS trial (Pipeline for Uncoilable or Failed Aneurysms) led to approval by the Food and Drug Administration (FDA) in April 2011. The trial was a multicenter, prospective, interventional, single-arm trial of the PED for the treatment of uncoilable or failed aneurysms of the internal carotid artery, enrolling patients from November 2008 to July 2009. A total of 108 patients were enrolled.[5] The primary effectiveness end point was angiographic evaluation that demonstrated complete

---

**Box 1**
**Current indications for Pipeline flow diverter**

- Unruptured intracranial aneurysms
- Large or giant intracranial aneurysms with a diameter of 10 mm or greater
- Internal carotid artery from the petrous to the superior hypophyseal artery segments

---

**Box 2**
**Recommended loading and treatment schemes for dual antiplatelet therapy for Pipeline flow diverters**

- Aspirin 325 mg for 7 days
- Clopidogrel 75 mg for 7 days

Followed by aspirin function testing (aspirin reaction unit) with a goal of less than 550 aspirin reaction units

Followed by P2Y12 testing with a goal of 100 to 150 P2Y12 reaction units.

---

aneurysm occlusion and absence of major stenosis at 180 days. The primary safety end point was occurrence of major ipsilateral stroke or neurologic death at 180 days.[5] Placement was technically successful in 107 of 108 patients (99.1%). Mean aneurysm size was 18.2 mm; 22 aneurysms (20.4%) were giant (>25 mm). Of the 106 aneurysms in the effectiveness cohort, 78 met the study's primary effectiveness end point (73.6%; 95% posterior probability interval: 64.4%–81.0%). Six of the 107 patients in the safety cohort experienced a major ipsilateral stroke or neurologic death (5.6%; 95% posterior probability interval: 2.6%–11.7%).

An earlier study in 2007, the PITA trial (Pipeline Embolization Device for the Intracranial Treatment of Aneurysms), was a multicenter, single-arm clinical trial of the Pipeline device conducted at 3 medical centers in Europe and 1 center in Argentina.[6] Subjects were included if they had wide-necked intracranial aneurysms (neck of >4 mm or dome/neck ratio of <1.5) or intracranial aneurysms that had failed previous attempts at endovascular treatment. Patients were excluded if they had subarachnoid hemorrhage within 60 days, an unstable neurologic deficit, or greater than 50% stenosis of the parent artery. Thirty-one patients with 31 intracranial aneurysms with an average age of 54.6 years were treated during the study period. Twenty-eight aneurysms arose from the intracerebral artery (5 cavernous, 15 paraophthalmic, 4 superior hypophyseal, and 4 posterior communicating segments), 1 from the middle cerebral artery, 1 from the vertebral artery, and 1 from the vertebrobasilar junction. Mean aneurysm size was 11.5 mm and mean neck size was 5.8 mm. Twelve (38.7%) aneurysms had failed (or recurred after) a previous endovascular treatment. PED placement was technically successful in 30 of 31 patients (96.8%). Most aneurysms were treated with either 1 (n = 18) or 2 (n = 11) PEDs. Fifteen aneurysms (48.4%) were treated with a PED alone while 16 were treated with both PED and embolization coils. Two patients experienced major periprocedural stroke. Follow-up angiography demonstrated complete aneurysm occlusion in 28 (93.3%) of the 30 patients who underwent angiographic follow-up. No significant in-construct stenosis (≥50%) was identified at follow-up angiography.

Since then several real-life clinical experiences have been published, of both a retrospective and prospective nature. Yu and colleagues[7] reported their results in a prospective study of 143 patients with 178 aneurysms. In one of the largest reported series, Saatci and colleagues[4] reported their experience with 251 aneurysms in 191 patients. Indications were side-wall aneurysms with a wide neck (≥4 mm) or unfavorable dome-neck ratio (≤1.5); large/giant, fusiform, dissecting, blister-like, and recurrent side-wall aneurysms; aneurysms at difficult angles; and aneurysms in which a branch was originating directly from the sac. Clinical and angiographic follow-up information for up to 2 years were included. Ninety-six aneurysms (38.3%) were large or giant (≥10 mm). In 34 of 251 (13.5%), the Pipeline device was used for retreatment.

Adjunctive coiling was performed in 11 aneurysms (2.1%). The mean number of devices per aneurysm was 1.3. One aneurysm ruptured in the fourth month after treatment (0.5%), and symptomatic in-construct stenosis was detected in 1 patient (0.5%) treated with percutaneous transarterial angioplasty. Any-event rate was 27 of 191 (14.1%), with a permanent morbidity of 1% and mortality of 0.5%. Control angiography was available in 182 (95.3%) patients with 239 (95.2%) aneurysms. In 121 aneurysms (48.2%), 1- to 2-year control angiography was available. The aneurysm occlusion rate was 91.2% in 6 months, increasing to 94.6%.[4]

## CONTROVERSIES IN THE USE OF FLOW DIVERTERS: LIMITATIONS AND AREAS OF INVESTIGATION

Although flow diversion offers to be a promising endovascular tool to treat challenging intracranial aneurysms, real-life experience with the device and its properties is only beginning. One of the most concerning aspects in the use of flow diverters is the occurrence of delayed aneurysm rupture after flow diversion, which seems to occur after all types of flow diversion.[4,7–9] Although there was no delayed aneurysm rupture in the PUFS trial, there was one cavernous carotid artery aneurysm that on follow-up showed features of a carotid-cavernous fistula, which may imply a delayed rupture of the treated cavernous aneurysm.[5] Numerous retrospective and prospective studies have reported about the occurrence of delayed aneurysm rupture after flow diversion, with the RADAR study (rupture after flow diversion), a multicentric retrospective study, finding a 1% delayed rupture risk after flow diversion in 1421 studied aneurysms.[10]

The cause of delayed rupture is poorly understood, and 2 main hypotheses are put forward. The first hypothesis stresses the association with aggressive and rapid thrombus formation in the aneurysm sac, possibly triggering increased autolysis, which may overload the biological defense mechanisms of the vessel wall and result in aneurysm rupture.[8–10] Similar biological processes have been noted in abdominal aortic aneurysms, where mural thrombi within aortic aneurysms are characterized by an absence of organization and cell colonization and are associated with a thinner arterial wall and more extensive elastolysis. The mural thrombus acts as a source of secreted proteases within the aneurysm, leading to further chemical degradation and weakening of the aneurysm wall.[11–13] Alternatively, delayed aneurysm rupture may be caused by the flow-diversion device causing an inflow jet into the aneurysm wall with minimal outflow from the aneurysmal sac, thus causing a rupture of the vessel wall by force of the inflow jet.[14,15] This theory stresses the importance of an increase in the intra-aneurysmal pressure, which can potentially cause the rupture of the aneurysm, especially giant aneurysms that may have very weak walls.[14]

Although the exact pathologic mechanisms leading to delayed aneurysm rupture after flow diversion remain unclear at this point, some common characteristics that may predispose an aneurysm to rupture after flow diversion have been identified. These characteristics, elucidated by Kulcsar and colleagues,[9] include: large and giant aneurysms; symptomatic aneurysms suggesting recent growth and wall instability; saccular aneurysms with an aspect ratio of greater than 1.6; and morphologic characteristics predisposing to an inertia-driven inflow at baseline.

The occurrence of delayed aneurysm rupture may be the most concerning aspect of flow diversion, and unanswered questions remain with respect to the use of flow diversion. Such aspects include the optimal use of antiplatelet therapy, including platelet inhibition testing; the length of antiplatelet therapy; the occurrence of intraparenchymal hemorrhages or subarachnoid hemorrhages not associated with aneurysm rupture; and technical aspects, including optimal sizing and placement of the device.

Finally, although early long-term results appear to be very promising, reported outcomes beyond a few years are missing at this point.

## ONGOING STUDIES AND OUTLOOK FOR THE FUTURE

Several studies are currently investigating real-life experiences with the Pipeline flow diverter (**Box 3**). The ASPIRE study (Aneurysm Study of Pipeline in an Observational Registry) is an observational, case-only prospective registry analyzing the incidence of neurologic adverse events following the use of the Pipeline device until last follow-up, for an average of 3 years of follow-up for each subject enrolled. The primary end point will consist of a composite of any/all of the events including: incidence of spontaneous rupture of Pipeline-treated aneurysm; other (nonaneurysmal) intracranial hemorrhage, ipsilateral and contralateral; ischemic stroke; symptomatic and asymptomatic parent artery stenosis; permanent cranial neuropathy; and change in baseline neurologic signs/symptoms related to Pipeline-treated internal carotid arteries at last assessment.

At present, the Pipeline device is the only FDA-approved flow diverter in the United States. The Surpass NeuroEndograft (Stryker Neurovascular, Fremont, CA) is a

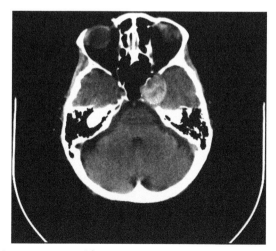

**Fig. 1.** Giant right cavernous carotid aneurysm as seen on noncontrast computed tomography of the head.

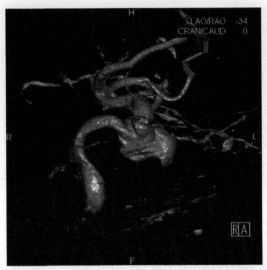

**Fig. 2.** Three-dimensional conventional angiogram showing partially thrombosed right cavernous segment aneurysm.

next-generation flow diverter currently being tested in the United States as part of the ongoing surpass intracranial aneurysm embolization system pivotal (SCENT) trial. This trial is a multicenter, prospective, interventional, single-arm trial of the Surpass Neuro-Endograft device aimed at obtaining FDA approval. The Surpass device consists of a chromium cobalt mesh with 12 platinum markers for visibility and is preloaded onto its own microcatheter delivered using an over-the-wire technique.

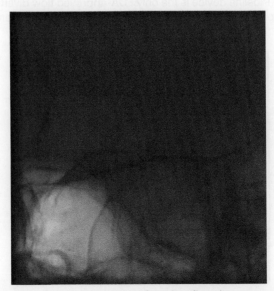

**Fig. 3.** Native angiogram showing placement of Pipeline flow diverter across the neck of the aneurysm with the device extending into the petrous portion.

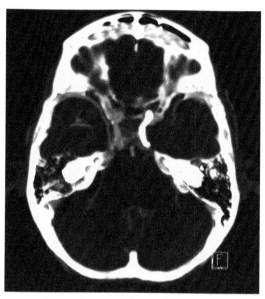

**Fig. 4.** Computed tomographic angiogram at 3 months, showing near complete occlusion of the aneurysm with minimal neck residual.

Other companies are currently in the process of developing flow diverters for intracranial aneurysms, which will be tested over the coming years. With new flow diverters being developed, questions arise as to whether the current indication for flow diverters will be expanded and may possibly include smaller aneurysms and aneurysms of the posterior circulation. Finally, questions remain as regards whether flow diversion manifests a true paradigm shift and performs more favorably in terms of safety and efficacy

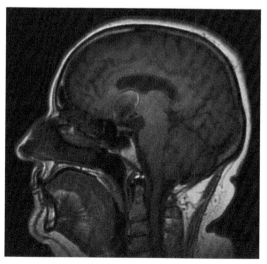

**Fig. 5.** Magnetic resonance image showing a giant partially thrombosed supraclinoidal aneurysm.

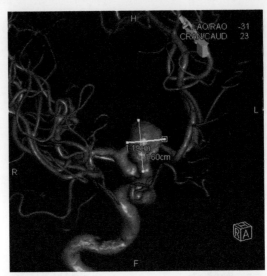

**Fig. 6.** Three-dimensional conventional angiogram showing 16-mm residual filling of this supraclinoidal aneurysm.

when compared with other treatment options. Critics of flow diverters have noted the absence of any randomized controlled trials comparing flow diverters with other conventional endovascular aneurysm treatments, such as balloon-assisted or stent-assisted coiling. In Canada, the FIAT trial (Flow Diversion of Intracranial Aneurysms) aims at comparing flow diversion with best standard treatment in the context

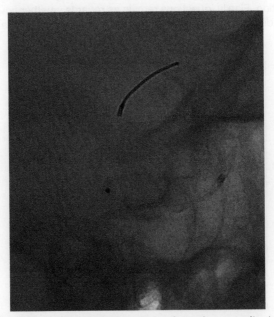

**Fig. 7.** Native view of the deployed Pipeline device from the supraclinoidal portion across the neck of the aneurysm into the cavernous segment.

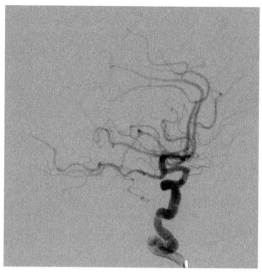

**Fig. 8.** Follow-up at 6 months, showing complete aneurysm occlusion and remodeling of the dysplastic supraclinoidal segment.

of a randomized controlled trial. In the study protocol, best standard treatment is left to the physician's discretion and may include conservative management, coiling with or without high-porosity stenting, parent vessel occlusion with or without bypass, or surgical clipping.

## INTRASACCULAR FLOW DIVERSION

One of the main limitations of flow diversion is its application only for unruptured aneurysm and the strict adherence to dual antiplatelet therapy. Because the treated aneurysm will only thrombose and occlude over weeks and months, flow diversion is not indicated in the acute phase of ruptured aneurysm. New devices, so-called intrasaccular occlusion devices, consist of different shapes of self-expanding mesh deployed into the aneurysm, thus attaining immediate aneurysm occlusion by intraluminal flow diversion.[16,17] Such devices as the Woven Endobridge (WEB) device (Sequent Medical, Inc, Aliso Viejo, CA) and the Luna device (NFocus Neuromedical, Palo Alto, CA) have currently achieved a CE Mark in Europe and are being used for ruptured aneurysms as well as bifurcation and trifurcation aneurysms. Because these devices are intrasaccular (ie, placed inside the sac of the aneurysm covering the neck) there seems to be no need for dual antiplatelet therapy, which is clinically significant in the context of a subarachnoid hemorrhage. Although these devices are not currently

---

**Case study 1**

A 78-year-old woman presented acutely with new-onset headaches and complete ophthalmoplegia. A computed tomography (CT) scan of her head showed a giant, partially thrombosed, cavernous carotid aneurysm. The patient was loaded on dual antiplatelet therapy and treated with placement of a Pipeline flow diverter across the neck of the aneurysm. A CT angiogram at 3 months showed near complete occlusion of the aneurysm with a minimal 4-mm neck residual and clinical improvement of her ophthalmoplegia (**Figs. 1–4**).

---

**Case study 2**

A 76-year-old woman presented with progressive visual loss. A magnetic resonance image showed a giant supraclinoidal aneurysm with partial thrombosis. The aneurysm was treated using a Pipeline flow diverter deployed across the neck of the aneurysm. A follow-up at 6 months showed complete occlusion of the aneurysm and remodeling of this dysplastic segment (**Figs. 5–8**).

---

available in the United States, it is anticipated that they will undergo testing and seek FDA approval in the near future, adding further tools to the treatment armamentarium for intracranial aneurysms.[16,17]

## REFERENCES

1. Piano M, Valvassori L, Quilici L, et al. Midterm and long-term follow-up of cerebral aneurysms treated with flow diverter devices: a single-center experience. J Neurosurg 2013;118:408–16.
2. Consoli A, Renieri L, Nappini S, et al. Endovascular treatment with 'kissing' flow diverter stents of two unruptured aneurysms at a fenestrated vertebrobasilar junction. J Neurointerv Surg 2013;5:e9.
3. Burrows AM, Zipfel G, Lanzino G. Treatment of a pediatric recurrent fusiform middle cerebral artery (MCA) aneurysm with a flow diverter. J Neurointerv Surg 2012. [Epub ahead of print].
4. Saatci I, Yavuz K, Ozer C, et al. Treatment of intracranial aneurysms using the pipeline flow-diverter embolization device: a single-center experience with long-term followup results. AJNR Am. J Neuroradiol 2012;33:1436–46.
5. Becske T, Kallmes OF, Saatci I, et al. Pipeline for Uncoilable or Failed Aneurysms: Results from a Multicenter Clinical Trial. Radiology 2013. [Epub ahead of print].
6. Nelson PK, Lylyk P, Szikora I, et al. The pipeline embolization device for the intracranial treatment of aneurysms trial. AJNR Am. J Neuroradiol 2011;32: 34–40.
7. Yu SC, Kwok CK, Cheng PW, et al. Intracranial aneurysms: midterm outcome of pipeline embolization device–a prospective study in 143 patients with 178 aneurysms. Radiology 2012;265:893–901.
8. Turowski B, Macht S, Kulcsar Z, et al. Early fatal hemorrhage after endovascular cerebral aneurysm treatment with a flow diverter (SILK-Stent): do we need to rethink our concepts? Neuroradiology 2011;53:37–41.
9. Kulcsar Z, Houdart E, Bonafe A, et al. Intra-aneurysmal thrombosis as a possible cause of delayed aneurysm rupture after flow-diversion treatment. AJNR Am J Neuroradiol 2011;32:20–5.
10. Kulcsár Z, Szikora I. The ESMINTRetrospective Analysis of Delayed Aneurysm Ruptures after flow diversion (RADAR)study. EJ Minim Invas Neurol Ther 2012; 2012:1244000088.
11. Touat Z, Ollivier V, Dai I, et al. Renewal of mural thrombus releases plasma markers and is involved in aortic abdominal aneurysm evolution. Am J Pathol 2006;168:1022–30.
12. Fontaine V, Jacob MP, Houard X, et al. Involvement of the mural thrombus as a site of protease release and activation in human aortic aneurysms. Am J Pathol 2002;161:1701–10.
13. Coutard M, Touat Z, Houard X, et al. Thrombus versus wall biological activities in experimental aortic aneurysms. J Vasc Res 2010;47:355–66.

14. Cebral JR, Mut F, Raschi M, et al. Aneurysm rupture following treatment with flow-diverting stents: computational hemodynamics analysis of treatment. AJNR Am J Neuroradiol 2011;32:27–33.
15. Fiorella O, Sadasivan C, Woo HH, et al. Regarding "Aneurysm rupture following treatment with flow-diverting stents: computational hemodynamics analysis of treatment". AJNR Am J Neuroradiol 2011;32:E95–97. [author reply E98–100].
16. Kwon SC, Ding YH, Dai O, et al. Preliminary results of the luna aneurysm embolization system in a rabbit model: a new intrasaccular aneurysm occlusion device. AINR Am J Neuroradiol 2011;32:602–6.
17. Klisch J, Sychra V, Strasilla C, et al. The Woven EndoBridge cerebral aneurysm embolization device (WEB II): initial clinical experience. Neuroradiology 2011; 53:599–607.

# The Diagnosis and Management of Brain Arteriovenous Malformations

Roberta L. Novakovic, MD[a,b], Marc A. Lazzaro, MD[b],
Alicia C. Castonguay, PhD[b], Osama O. Zaidat, MD, MS[a,b,c],*

## KEYWORDS

- Arteriovenous malformations • AVM treatment • Embolization • Radiosurgery
- Surgical resection

## KEY POINTS

- The natural history of asymptomatic brain cerebral arteriovenous malformations (AVMs) remains poorly understood.
- Hemorrhagic presentation of a brain AVM is a significant independent predictor of future hemorrhage.
- For diagnosis and visualization of AVMs, cerebral angiography is considered the gold standard in the evaluation of AVM architecture.
- Advances in noninvasive imaging have led to an increase in the identification of unruptured AVMs, which presents new challenges in their management and treatment.
- Management of cerebral AVMs includes observation with medical management, endovascular embolization, surgical resection, stereotactic radiotherapy, and multimodal approaches.

## AVM BIOLOGY/PATHOPHYSIOLOGY

AVMs are an abnormal connection between arteries and veins via a network of vessels, called the nidus, that lack an intervening capillary bed. AVMs are considered congenital vascular lesions; however, the precise pathogenetic mechanisms leading to the lack of capillaries in the AVM nidus remain unclear. Although it is assumed that AVMs appear during fetal development, they are rarely detected in utero or found in infants.[1–3] Distal arterial branches are commonly involved in brain AVMs.

Funding Sources: None.
Conflict of Interest: None.

[a] Neuroradiology Division, Department of Radiology, UT Southwestern Medical Center, 5323 Harry Hines Boulevard, Dallas, TX 75390-9178, USA; [b] Department of Neurology, UT Southwestern Medical Center, 5323 Harry Hines Boulevard, Dallas, TX 75390-9178, USA; [c] Division of Neurointervention, Department of Neurology, Neurosurgery and Radiology, Froedtert Hospital and Medical College of Wisconsin, 9200 West Wisconsin Avenue, Milwaukee, WI 53226, USA
* Corresponding author.
*E-mail address:* szaidat@mcw.edu

Neurol Clin 31 (2013) 749–763
http://dx.doi.org/10.1016/j.ncl.2013.03.003
0733-8619/13/$ – see front matter © 2013 Published by Elsevier Inc.

**neurologic.theclinics.com**

Approximately half of AVMs are situated at the border-zone watershed area between the distal anterior, middle, and posterior cerebral arteries.[4] This distal watershed territory represents anatomic remnants to the manifold artery-to-artery connections that cover the brain surface during the lissencephalic state. During the 29th gestational week, the cortical gyration starts and the original arterial mesh regresses, eventually giving rise to the leptomeningeal arteries. This vascular topographic finding suggests that AVMs potentially arise within or after the formation of the arterial border zones.[5]

Different theories propose that AVMs represent persistence of direct connections between arteries and veins within the primitive vascular plexus; result from a derangement in vessel growth proliferative capillaropathy[6]; result from the dysfunction of the remodeling process at the junction between capillaries and veins[7]; or represent fistualized cerebral venous angiomas.[8] Most theories about the embryogenesis of AVMs suggest a congenital nature to these lesions and attribute them to either a persistence of a primitive arteriovenous connection or development of such after the initial closure of the primitive connection.

Brain AVMs are frequently pyramid-shaped, with the base parallel to the cortical surface and the apex directed toward the ventricle. Functionally important brain tissue may be displaced and thus absent within a compact AVM, or intervening normal brain tissue may be found within a loose nidus. A commonly used grading scale for brain AVMS is the Spetzler-Martin grading scale. A composite score is derived from the nidus size, eloquence of adjacent brain, and presence of deep venous drainage.[9] The Spetzler-Martin score can correlate with the expected incidence of postoperative neurologic complications (discussed later).

The nidus is composed of coiled and tortuous vessels that connect the feeding arteries to the draining veins. It is the absence of the capillary network that allows for high-flow AV shunting. The permanent intraluminal stress arising from abnormal flow and pressure may lead to some of the secondary angiopathy within the AVM and neighboring vessels.[10] As such, the feeding arteries are typically dilated, with regions of subendothelial thickening and abnormal or absent media and elastic lamina.[11] The degenerative changes are presumably due to the shear stress on the vessel wall caused by the high flow state of the arterial to venous shunting. Meanwhile, the nidal vessels may contain a hypertrophic media, which can blur the distinction between artery and vein. Aneurysms may be found on either nidal or feeding vessels to the AVM. The veins that accommodate the outflow of the AVM may exhibit thickening of the wall due to cellular proliferation,[12] with poorly developed muscular and elastic components. If hemorrhage has occurred, the surrounding parenchyma show evidence of gliosis and hemosiderin staining.

## NATURAL HISTORY

AVMs of the brain account for approximately 1.4% to 2% of hemorrhagic strokes.[13,14] The estimated prevalence of AVM varies from less than 10 to 18 per 100,000.[15,16] Meanwhile, the New York Islands AVM Study,[17] a prospective population-based incidence and case-control study, found an annual brain AVM detection rate of 1.34 per 100,000 person-years (95% CI, 1.18–1.49). In general, AVMs are thought to be congenital lesions that occur sporadically. The familial incidence of brain AVMs seems rare, with only a few reported cases in the literature, although there is an association with other abnormalities (Osler-Weber-Rendu disease and Sturge-Weber syndrome).[18,19]

Advanced imaging has led to a better identification of AVMs, including asymptomatic lesions. Brain AVMs are found incidentally on 0.05% of brain MRI screens.[20] The natural history of asymptomatic brain AVMs remains poorly understood and conflicting information can be found on symptomatic lesions in the literature. The ongoing ARUBA (A Randomized trial of Unruptured Brain Arteriovenous Malformations) will hopefully further understanding of the natural history of brain AVMs and whether treatment improves morbidity and mortality for unruptured brain AVMs.[21]

Spontaneous obliteration of pial brain AVMs has been reported, with an incidence of 0.8% to 1.3% of cases; however, selection bias inherent to the databases may influence these reported rates.[22,23] Although investigators have not been able to reliably identify anatomic predictors, spontaneous obliteration may be more likely to occur in small AVMs (less than 2.5 cm) that present with hemorrhage and have fewer arterial feeders.[23] One publication suggests a predisposition to this phenomenon, with AVMs drained by a single draining vein, and confirmed the association with smaller AVMs and a hemorrhagic presentation.[22]

## CLINICAL PRESENTATION

Brain AVMs can lead to intracranial hemorrhage, seizures, headaches, and long-term disability. When symptomatic, the most common presenting symptoms are hemorrhage and seizures.[24]

### Hemorrhage

Based on current literature, the annual incidence of hemorrhage of previously unruptured and untreated brain AVMs lies approximately in the range of 2% to 4%.[24–28] Population-based studies show that approximately 38% to 71% of patients with brain AVMs present with intracranial hemorrhage,[24,25,27,29–32] with a crude incidence of first-ever hemorrhage of 0.51 per 100,000 (95% CI, 0.41–0.61) person-years in the New York Islands AVM Study[17] and Scottish Intracranial Vascular Malformation Study.[33] The initial presentation of hemorrhage most commonly occurs in patients between 20 and 40 years of age[28,29,34,35]; however, there are conflicting data in regards to association of age and risk of hemorrhage.[25,27,31,34] Although data seem conflicted in regards to the effect of gender,[26] evidence seems to support no effect of gender on the risk of hemorrhage.[14,31]

Hemorrhagic presentation is a significant independent predictor of future hemorrhage.[24,26,27,31,35,36] Ondra and colleagues[25] published the results of approximately 24 years of follow-up in a prospectively followed cohort of unoperated symptomatic patients with brain AVMs and found a mean time interval of 7.7 years between initial presentation and subsequent hemorrhage. Mast and colleagues[26] found that among patients with hemorrhage as the initial presentation, the risk of subsequent hemorrhage fell from 32.9% during the first year to 11.3% per year in subsequent years. Meanwhile, the study from Toronto found an annual risk of hemorrhage of 9.65% during the first year and 3.67% after 5 years from a hemorrhagic presentation.[24] After an initial presentation of hemorrhage, the potential for declining risk of subsequent hemorrhage overtime was supported in other studies as well.[28,32,35,37]

Several factors are mentioned in the literature as other potential risk factors for hemorrhage, including AVM with deep location, infratentorial location, size, male gender, venous outlet restriction, mean pressure, and type of feeding vessels.[26,28,31,32,34,35,37,38] Although the literature is divergent in regards to these factors, there is some agreement for a higher association of subsequent hemorrhage when (1) AVM has exclusively deep venous drainage (typically defined as drainage through the periventricular, galenic, or cerebellar pathways),[24,31] (2) AVM has associated aneurysms,[24,39–41] (3) AVM is deep in location,[31,35] or (4) AVM is infratentorial in location.[41] In a prospective study of 678 patients, brain AVMs with associated aneurysms had an overall hemorrhage rate of 6.93% per year compared with 3.99% per year for patients without associated aneurysms.[24] This increased annual risk of hemorrhage remained elevated at 2 to 5 years as well as beyond 5 years of follow up (5.41% and 6.01%, respectively). The annual risk of hemorrhage was elevated in the first year after a presentation of hemorrhage (9.65%) but dropped to 6.3% at 2 to 5 years and returned to 3.67% beyond 5 years.

It is evident from the literature that brain AVMs are heterogeneous, with different clinical outcomes inherent to each AVM's specific features of anatomy and angio-architecture. The risk of hemorrhage can be as low as 0.9% per year in patients without factors like hemorrhagic presentation, deep AVM location, or deep venous drainage,[31,36] and may be as high as 34.4% in patients with these features.[31] The risk of hemorrhage does not seem to be altered by partially treated AVMs and remains present until complete AVM obliteration.[24,42] In the Toronto study, the elevated risk of hemorrhage was not significantly altered even when the partial treatment targeted endovascular occlusion of an associated aneurysm.[24]

Clinical outcomes from the initial hemorrhagic presentation of a brain AVM can be favorable. Each hemorrhage from a brain AVM has an associated neurologic morbidity of 20% to 30% and mortality of 10% to 40%.[25,27,28,30,32,43] Choi and colleagues[44] found that 14% of patients had a modified Rankin score (mRS) of 4 to 5, and 11% had a National Institutes of Health Stroke Scale score of greater than 13 at a median of 11 days from AVM rupture. In this study, multivariate testing showed age, gender, race, and AVM size had no significant effect on clinical outcome. At a mean follow-up of 16.2 months, Hartmann and colleagues[45] showed 47% (95% CI, 0.38–0.56) had no neurologic deficit after the incident hemorrhage; 37% (95% CI, 0.28–0.46) were independent in their daily activities (mRS 1); 13% (95% CI, 0.07–0.19) were moderately disabled (mRS 2 or 3); and 3% (95% CI, 0–0.06) were severely disabled (mRS $\geq$4). In this study, 74% of patients with recurrent hemorrhage were normal or independent (mRS 0 or 1). Similarly, in the Toronto study, only 35% of patients had a significant functional impairment (Glasgow Outcome Scale score 2 or 3).[24]

In a Finnish study by Ondra and colleagues,[25] the mean age at death from an AVM hemorrhage was 44.4 years, which was significantly lower than that of patients dying from other causes in the study (59.4 years). The yearly mortality rate was 1% per year in this study and the rate of both hemorrhage and death remained constant over the entire length of the study.

### Seizures

Approximately 18% to 40% of brain AVMs present with seizures[24,25,27,29] and response to treatment with antiepileptic drugs seems favorable.[46] A study of 1289 patients with brain AVMs found that of those with seizures, 30% were generalized and 10% were focal seizures.[29] In the Toronto-based prospective study of 678 patients, the hemorrhage rate for patients presenting with seizure was 4.16% per year, which remained close to the rate for the entire cohort (4.61%).[24] Likewise, other population-based studies have shown patients presenting with seizure were not more likely to suffer a rupture during follow-up.[24,30] In another study of 131 patients followed for an average of 8 years, there was a 26.9% incidence of hemorrhage in those who presented with seizure.[32] Additionally, Mast and colleagues[26] confirmed no significant association of hemorrhage with initial presentation with seizure, FNDs, or headaches.

### Headaches

Approximately 5% to 14% of patients with brain AVMs present with headaches.[25,29] Headaches associated with AVMs are not distinctive,[47] can be unilateral or bilateral, and can have the character of a migraine even with the classic associated aura.[48] The rates of response to pharmacologic treatment and AVM obliteration have not been studied.

### Neurologic Deficits

Focal neurologic deficits (FNDs) at presentation unrelated to hemorrhage or seizure are uncommon. Approximately 5% to 15% of patients with brain AVMs present with persistent or progressive neurologic deficits.[25,29,32,44] The underlying pathophysiology of this phenomenon remains unclear. Although an unlikely mechanism of FNDs, evidence suggests perinidal arterial steal, which is presumed to result from the high-flow shunting through the AVM and leads to low blood pressure in the feeding arteries and surrounding brain tissue.[49–51] Another study suggests that mass effect, possibly related to the compressive effect of venous dilatation and white matter pathway vulnerability, could be associated with the occurrence of FND.[44] The Columbia AVM Databank (n = 735), using a multivariate logistic regression model, found an independent association of FND with increasing age, female gender, deep brain location, and venous ectasia. Meanwhile, no association was found for lobar location, size, arterial supply, or venous drainage pattern and two-thirds of patients did not have progression of symptoms.[44]

## DIAGNOSIS

For diagnosis and visualization of AVMs, cerebral angiography is considered the gold standard in the evaluation of AVM architecture, including morphology, location of nidus, presence and location of associated aneurysms, and venous drainage pattern, and is commonly used for treatment planning.[52–54] Other techniques, such as CT, CT angiography, MRI, and magnetic resonance angiography, may be used to visualize AVMs; however, they are limited in their sensitivity and ability to provide detailed imaging of AVM architecture.[53,54] Initial imaging is often done using CT and MRI, because these modalities are able to readily identify large AVMs and are used to evaluate symptoms that are not specific to AVMs, such as seizure, headache, and hemorrhage.[55,56] Although CT angiography provides better vascular detail of AVMs, MRI and magnetic resonance angiography provide greater visualization of surrounding structures adjacent to the nidus. (**Fig. 1** shows the MRI findings in an AVM patient

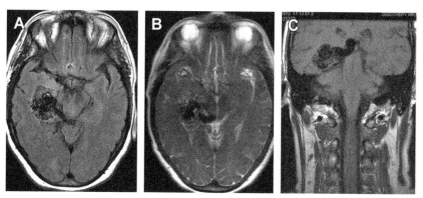

**Fig. 1.** MRI showing multiple flow void signals with large venous varix draining into the straight sinus in axial fluid-attenuated inversion recovery (*A*) and T2 (*B*) and coronal T1 (*C*) images sequences.

presenting with seizure, showing flow void and draining into the deep venous system.[54]) Functional MRI may provide guidance and information that can be helpful in treatment planning. As imaging techniques become more sophisticated, noninvasive neuroimaging modalities will continue to play a significant role in the management and treatment of AVMs.

## CEREBRAL ARTERIOVENOUS MALFORMATION MANAGEMENT

Management of cerebral AVMs includes observation with medical management, endovascular embolization, surgical resection, and stereotactic radiotherapy. The high rate of morbidity and mortality from ruptured brain AVMs presents compelling justification for invasive treatments. AVMs that have not bled, however, present a more challenging decision in the setting of a poorly defined natural history and the seemingly low annual hemorrhage rates. The clinical equipoise in the broad management of brain AVMs has driven the development of ARUBA, which aims to compare the natural history with modern multimodal therapy over 5 years.[21] Among the various therapies available, reported outcomes vary, and no rigorous randomized study has compared treatments. A large meta-analysis identified 137 observational studies, including 142 cohorts and 13,698 patients undergoing treatment for brain AVMs.[57] The cohorts were composed of microsurgery, 41 (29%); embolization, 14 (10%); stereotactic radiosurgery, 69 (48%); fractionated radiotherapy, 7 (5%); and multimodal therapies, 11 (8%). Severe complications were observed in a median of 5.1% to 7.4% patients and median obliteration rate was from 13% to 96%. Case fatality after treatments decreased over time as did complication rates after radiosurgery and embolization, likely attributed to recent technical advances and experience. Direct comparison between treatment modalities cannot be made; however, notable treatment risks and incomplete obliteration warrant randomized comparison study of treatment modalities.

### Observation

Observation is considered for management of asymptomatic AVMs; however, it is rarely considered for those patients who have presented with hemorrhage. Conservative management may include management of associated symptoms, general medical care, and surveillance imaging of an AVM. Presentation can include seizures, which may be related to hemorrhage, hemosiderin deposition from recurrent microhemorrhages, venous hypertension, and ischemia from high-flow shunting. Anticonvulsant therapy is appropriate for those patients presenting with seizures. Similar outcomes in seizure frequency have been reported in an observational study comparing conservative management and AVM treatment.[58] General medical care includes management of hypertension and conventional regimens for headaches. Time intervals for surveillance imaging are not well defined and may include noninvasive MRI brain imaging annually or biennially.

### Treatment

Treatment may include single or multimodal therapy with the goal of eradication, which may be dictated by various factors, including operator skill, and AVM characteristics, including size, location, surgical or endovascular accessibility, venous drainage, and presence of high-risk features, such as a feeding artery aneurysm. Technological advancements continue to shape treatment modalities, and multimodal therapy is increasingly used for brain AVM treatment due to the potential benefits of combination therapy (**Table 1**).

**Table 1**
Treatment modalities for brain arteriovenous malformations

| Modality | Approach | Benefits | Limitations |
|---|---|---|---|
| Endovascular embolization | Catheter delivery of <br> • Liquid embolics (glue) <br> • Coils <br> • Particles | • Minimally invasive <br> • Concomitant angiography | • Lower rate of obliteration <br> • Decreased durability |
| Surgical resection | • Microsurgical excision | • Higher rate of obliteration | • Invasive |
| Radiotherapy | • Gamma Knife | • Noninvasive | • 1–2 y latency for obliteration <br> • Parenchymal radiation injury <br> • Limited to smaller lesions |

## Endovascular Treatment

Endovascular treatment of brain AVMs has become an increasingly popular method of therapy, partly because of advances in endovascular technologies, including microcatheter design, and the development of liquid embolics with unique properties.

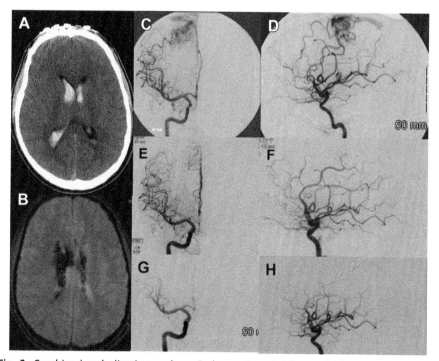

**Fig. 2.** Combined embolization and surgical resection. A 16-year-old boy presented with sudden onset of headache and mental status change. CT scan and MRI gradient echo showed acute intraventricular blood (*A, B*). Angiogram showing the right frontal AVM, pre-embolization (*C, D*) and postembolization (*E, F*), combined with surgical resection (*G, H*) with complete AVM removal.

Superselective catheterization with microcatheters and flow-guided ultrathin micro-catheters has overcome barriers to delivery beyond tortuous anatomy. Common approaches include delivery of liquid embolics, such as n-butyl cyanoacrylate and ethylene vinyl alcohol copolymer (Onyx), and platinum embolic coils.

Endovascular therapy is often performed as preoperative embolization to surgical resection or in conjunction with stereotactic radiotherapy. Small malformations can be obliterated and larger malformations can be reduced in size for excision (**Fig. 2**) or radiosurgery (**Fig. 3**). In some cases, curative embolization can be achieved (**Fig. 4**), whereas palliative embolization can be used in selected cases to attempt seizure control or stabilize progression of neurologic deficits when they are not amenable to radiosurgery or microsurgical excision. Preoperative embolization has

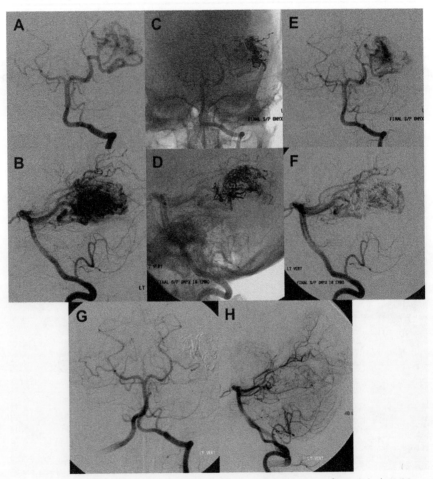

**Fig. 3.** Combined embolization and Gamma Knife radiosurgery. Left occipital AVM: pre-embolization angiogram—(*A*) anteroposterior (AP) and (*B*) lateral—and postembolization using Onyx material (AP and lateral unsubtracted [*C, D*] and subtracted [*E, F*]), showing reduction in the AVM nidus size with complete obliteration after Gamma Knife radiosurgery on 3-year angiogram (*G, H*).

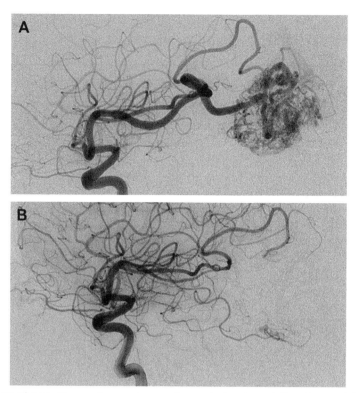

**Fig. 4.** Lateral projection angiogram images demonstrate a large left parieto-occipital AVM (*A*) with near-complete obliteration after liquid embolization (*B*).

been reported with acceptable rates of clinically significant complications (up to 6.5%).[59]

The benefits of endovascular therapy include a minimally invasive approach, immediate occlusion, and intraprocedure angiographic evaluation. Challenges of endovascular therapy include incomplete embolization, intracranial hemorrhage, unintended vessel embolization, and normal perfusion pressure breakthrough, leading to swelling or hemorrhage.[60]

### Surgical Resection

Microsurgical excision of the AVM involves a careful dural opening with circumferential nidus dissection until complete AVM resection is achieved. Postoperative angiography is performed to document complete excision.

A decision tool for the microsurgical approach is the Spetzler-Martin grading system, which is used to estimate the risk of surgical resection of an AVM (**Table 2**). The 3 elements are size, venous drainage, and location. Higher grades are associated with greater surgical morbidity and mortality.[9]

The benefits of microsurgical excision include high rates of complete obliteration. The limitations of this approach include intraoperative rupture, anatomic accessibility, edema from retraction, resection of normal brain tissue, feeding vessel thrombosis, and normal perfusion pressure breakthrough. Despite these adverse events, early reports showed high rates of favorable outcomes.[9] A meta-analysis comprising

**Table 2**
**Spetzler-Martin grading scale for arteriovenous malformations**

| Characteristic | Points |
| --- | --- |
| Size | |
| Small (<3 cm) | 1 |
| Medium (3–6 cm) | 2 |
| Large (>6 cm) | 3 |
| Location | |
| Noneloquent site | 0 |
| Eloquent site[a] | 1 |
| Pattern of venous drainage | |
| Superficial only | 0 |
| Deep component | 1 |

[a] Eloquent site includes sensorimotor, language, visual cortex, hypothalamus, thalamus, internal capsule, brainstem, cerebellar peduncles, and cerebellar nuclei.

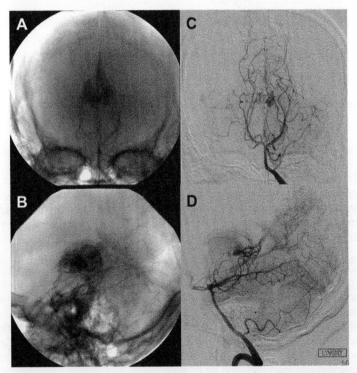

**Fig. 5.** A young woman who presented with headaches was found on noninvasive imaging to have a large vein in the region of the thalamus. A catheter cerebral angiogram demonstrated a brain AVM involving the area of the bilateral thalami—unsubtracted anteroposterior (*A*) and lateral (*B*) projections. After stereotactic radiosurgery, marked reduction in AVM size was noted on 3-year follow-up catheter angiogram—anteroposterior (*C*) and lateral projections (*D*).

2425 patients treated between 1990 and 2000 showed a surgical mortality of 3.3% and a permanent postoperative morbidity of 8.6%, with an increasing morbidity-mortality rate associated with an increasing Spetzler-Martin grade.[61]

### Radiosurgery

Radiosurgery can be an effective therapy for properly selected patients with brain AVMs. Sharply localized high-dose radiation is delivered to the AVM to produce a vascular injury response. Gradual sclerosis of the blood vessels ensues with eventual obliteration over a period of 1 to 2 years (**Fig. 5**). Focused radiation is ideally delivered to the abnormal vessels; however, neighboring and interspace parenchymal tissue exposure necessarily poses a challenge in cases of diffuse nidus. AVMs smaller than 3.5 cm are considered more favorable for treatment.

A multicenter analysis of 1255 patients receiving radiotherapy reported 102 (8%) patients who developed a neurologic deficit after the radiation.[62] Successful treatment with radiosurgery depends on various factors, including AVM volume; angioarchitecture, including the density of the nidus; AVM location; and radiation dosage.

The benefits of radiotherapy include a noninvasive therapy and reasonable obliteration rates. The challenges for this treatment modality include risk of bleeding during the latency of 1 to 2 years, individual sensitivity to radiation and unknown long-term outcome, and neurologic deficits from edema and necrosis of normal brain tissue (**Fig. 6**).

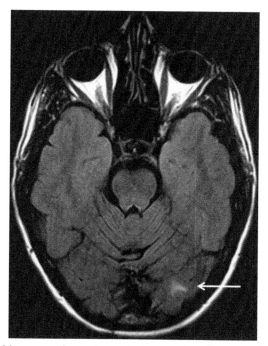

**Fig. 6.** A 41-year-old woman who underwent stereotactic radiosurgery for a left transverse sinus dural arteriovenous fistula noted visual disturbances. Axial T2-weighted fluid-attenuated inversion recovery images demonstrate a region of subcortical signal abnormality in the left occipital lobe (*arrow*) in the region of irradiated brain and consistent with radiation leukoencephalitis.

## FUTURE DIRECTIONS AND CONCLUSIONS

Cerebral AVMs remain a considerable cause of morbidity and mortality and the expanded use of noninvasive brain imaging has led to an increase in identification of these lesions. Challenges remain in management decisions for asymptomatic AVMs, given the poorly defined natural history, and also in selecting optimal treatment in symptomatic AVMs, using single or multimodal therapy. Variations in practice exist due to limited available skill for therapies and lack of rigorous data. Advancements in technologies to treat AVMs and experience will continue to shape management, and continued support and development of randomized controlled trials to elucidate the natural history and compare available treatments is needed.

## REFERENCES

1. Mullan S, Mojtahedi S, Johnson DL, et al. Embryological basis of some aspects of cerebral vascular fistulas and malformations. J Neurosurg 1996; 85(1):1–8.
2. Suh DC, Alvarez H, Bhattacharya JJ, et al. Intracranial hemorrhage within the first two years of life. Acta Neurochir (Wien) 2001;143(10):997–1004.
3. Baird WF, Stitt DG. Arteriovenous aneurysm of the cerebellum in a premature infant. Pediatrics 1959;24:455–7.
4. Stapf C, Mohr JP, Sciacca RR, et al. Incident hemorrhage risk of brain arteriovenous malformations located in the arterial border-zones. Stroke 2000;31: 2365–8.
5. Van der Eecken HM, Fisher CM, Adams RD. The anatomy and functional significance of the meningeal arterial anastomoses of the human brain. J Neuropathol Exp Neurol 1953;12:132–57.
6. Yasargil MG. AVM of the brain, history, embryology, pathological considerations, hemodynamics, diagnostic studies, microsurgical anatomy. Stuttgart (Germany): George Thieme Verlag; 1987.
7. Lasjaunias P. A revised concept of the congenital nature of cerebral arteriovenous malformations. Interv Neuroradiol 1997;3:275–81.
8. Mullan S, Mojtahedi S, Johnson DL, et al. Cerebral venous malformation-arteriovenous malformation transition forms. J Neurosurg 1996;85(1):9–13.
9. Spetzler RF, Martin NA. A proposed grading system for arteriovenous malformations. J Neurosurg 1986;65(4):476–83.
10. Lasjaunias P. Vascular diseases in neonates, infants and children: interventional neuroradiology management. Berlin: Springer-Verlag; 1997.
11. Mandybur TI, Nazek M. Cerebral arteriovenous malformation. A detailed morphological and immunohistochemical study using actin. Arch Pathol Lab Med 1990;114(9):970–3.
12. Challa VR, Moody DM, Brown WR. Vascular malformations of the central nervous system. J Neuropathol Exp Neurol 1995;54(5):609–21.
13. Stapf C, Labovitz DL, Sciacca RR, et al. Incidence of adult brain arteriovenous malformation hemorrhage in a prospective population-based stroke survey. Cerebrovasc Dis 2002;13(1):43–6.
14. Perret G, Nishioka H. Report on the cooperative study of intracranial aneurysms and subarachnoid hemorrhage. Section VI. Arteriovenous malformations: an analysis of 545 cases of cranio-cerebral arteriovenous malformations and fistulae reported to the cooperative study. J Neurosurg 1966;25:467–90.
15. Berman MF, Sciacca RR, Pile-Spellmann J, et al. The epidemiology of brain arteriovenous malformations. Neurosurgery 2000;47:389–96.

16. Al-Shahi R, Fang JS, Lewis SC, et al. Prevalence of adults with brain arteriovenous malformations: a community based study in Scotland using capture-recapture analysis. J Neurol Neurosurg Psychiatry 2002;73(5):547–51.
17. Stapf C, Mast H, Sciacca RR, et al. The New York Islands AVM study design, study progress, and initial results. Stroke 2003;34:e29–33.
18. Kikuchi K, Kowada M, Sasajima H. Vascular malformations of the brain in hereditary hemorrhagic telangiectasia (Rendu-Osler-Weber disease). Surg Neurol 1994;41:374–80.
19. Laufer L, Cohen A. Sturge-Weber syndrome associated with a large left hemispheric arteriovenous malformation. Pediatr Radiol 1994;24:272–3.
20. Morris Z, Whiteley WN, Longstreth WT Jr, et al. Incidental findings on brain magnetic resonance imaging: systematic review and meta-analysis. BMJ 2009;339: b3016.
21. Mohr JP, Moskowitz AJ, Stapf C, et al. The ARUBA Trial: current status, future hopes. Stroke 2010;41:e537–40.
22. Abdulrauf SI, Malik GM, Awad IA. Spontaneous angiographic obliteration of cerebral arteriovenous malformations. Neurosurgery 1999;44(2):280–7.
23. Patel MC, Hodgson TJ, Kemeny AA, et al. Spontaneous obliteration of pial arteriovenous malformations: a review of 27 cases. AJNR Am J Neuroradiol 2001;22: 531–6.
24. da Costa L, Wallace MC, Ter Brugge KG, et al. The natural history and predictive features of hemorrhage from brain arteriovenous malformations. Stroke 2009;40: 100–5.
25. Ondra SL, Troupp H, George ED, et al. The natural history of symptomatic arteriovenous malformations of the brain: a 24-year follow-up assessment. J Neurosurg 1990;73:387–91.
26. Mast H, Young WL, Koennecke HC, et al. Risk of spontaneous haemorrhage after diagnosis of cerebral arteriovenous malformation. Lancet 1997;350: 1065–8.
27. Crawford PM, West CR, Chadwick DW, et al. Arteriovenous malformations of the brain: natural history in unoperated patients. J Neurol Neurosurg Psychiatry 1986;49:1–10.
28. Graf CJ, Perret GE, Torner JC. Bleeding from cerebral arteriovenous malformations as part of their natural history. J Neurosurg 1983;58:331–7.
29. Hofmeister C, Stapf C, Hartmann A, et al. Demographic, morphological, and clinical characteristics of 1289 patients with brain arteriovenous malformation. Stroke 2000;31:1307–10.
30. Brown RD Jr, Wiebers DO, Torner JC, et al. Frequency of intracranial hemorrhage as a presenting symptom and subtype analysis: a population-based study of intracranial vascular malformations in Olmsted County, Minnesota. J Neurosurg 1996;85:29–32.
31. Stapf C, Mast H, Sciacca RR, et al. Predictors of hemorrhage in patients with untreated brain arteriovenous malformation. Neurology 2006;66(9):1350–5.
32. Fults D, Kelly DL. Natural history of arteriovenous malformations of the brain: a clinical study. Neurosurgery 1984;15:658–62.
33. Al-Shahi R, Bhattacharya JJ, Currie DG, et al. Prospective, Population-based detection of intracranial vascular malformations in adults: The Scottish Intracranial Vascular Malformation Study (SIVMS). Stroke 2003;34:1163–9.
34. Stapf C, Khaw AV, Sciacca RR, et al. Effect of age on clinical and morphological characteristics in patients with brain arteriovenous malformation. Stroke 2003; 34:2664–70.

35. Hernesniemi JA, Dashti R, Juvela S, et al. Natural history of brain arteriovenous malformations: a long-term follow-up study of risk of hemorrhage in 238 patients. Neurosurgery 2008;63(5):823–9.

36. Pollock BE, Flickinger JC, Lunsford LD, et al. Factors that predict the bleeding risk of cerebral arteriovenous malformations. Stroke 1996;27:1–16.

37. Itoyama Y, Uemura S, Ushio Y, et al. Natural course of unoperated arteriovenous malformations: study of 50 cases. J Neurosurg 1989;71:805–9.

38. Duong DH, Young WL, Vang MC, et al. Feeding artery pressure and venous drainage pattern are primary determinants of hemorrhage from cerebral arteriovenous malformations. Stroke 1998;29:1167–76.

39. Marks MP, Lane B, Steinberg GK, et al. Hemorrhage in intracerebral arteriovenous malformations: angiographic determinants. Radiology 1990;176:807–13.

40. Meisel HJ, Mansmann U, Alvarez H, et al. Cerebral arteriovenous malformations and associated aneurysms: analysis of 305 cases from a series of 662 patients. Neurosurgery 2000;46(4):793–802.

41. Khaw AV, Mohr JP, Sciacca RR, et al. Association of infratentorial brain arteriovenous malformations with hemorrhage at initial presentation. Stroke 2004;35: 660–3.

42. Miyamoto S, Hashimoto N, Nagata I, et al. Posttreatment sequelae of palliatively treated cerebral arteriovenous malformations. Neurosurgery 2000;46:589–94 [discussion: 594–5].

43. Wilkins R. Natural history of intracranial vascular malformations of the brain: a review. Neurosurgery 1985;16:421–30.

44. Choi JH, Mast H, Sciacca RR, et al. Clinical outcome after first and recurrent hemorrhage in patients with untreated brain arteriovenous malformation. Stroke 2006;37:1243–7.

45. Hartmann A, Mast H, Mohr JP, et al. Morbidity of intracranial hemorrhage in patients with cerebral arteriovenous malformations. Stroke 1998;29:931–4.

46. Osipov A, Koennecke HC, Hartmann A, et al. Seizures in cerebral arteriovenous malformations: type, clinical course, and medical management. Interv Neuroradiol 1997;3:37–41.

47. Ghossoub M, Nataf F, Merienne L, et al. Characteristics of headache associated with cerebral arteriovenous malformations. Neurochirurgie 2001;47:177–83.

48. Lees F. The migrainous symptoms of cerebral angiomata. J Neurol Neurosurg Psychiatry 1962;25:45.

49. Mast H, Mohr JP, Osipov A, et al. "Steal" is an unestablished mechanism for the clinical presentation of cerebral arteriovenous malformations. Stroke 1995;26: 1215–20.

50. Meyer B, Schaller C, Frenkel C, et al. Physiological steal around AVMs of the brain in not equivalent to cortical ischemia. Neurol Res 1998;20(Suppl 1): S13–7.

51. Meyer B, Schaller C, Frenkel C, et al. Distribution of local oxygen saturation and its response to changes of mean arterial blood pressure in the cerebral cortex adjacent to arteriovenous malformation. Stroke 1999;30:2623–30.

52. Turjman F, Massoud TF, Vinuela F, et al. Aneurysms related to cerebral arteriovenous malformations: superselective angiographic assessment in 58 patients. AJNR Am J Neuroradiol 1994;15:1601–5.

53. Mossa-Basha M, Chen J, Gandhi D. Imaging of cerebral arteriovenous malformations and dural arteriovenous fistulas. Neurosurg Clin N Am 2012;23:27–42.

54. Friedlander B. Arteriovenous malformations of the brain. N Engl J Med 2007; 356:2704–12.

55. Brown RD Jr, Flemming KD, Meyer FB, et al. Natural history, evaluation, and management of intracranial vascular malformations. Mayo Clin Proc 2005;80: 269–81.
56. Choi JH, Mohr JP. Brain arteriovenous malformations in adults. Lancet Neurol 2005;4:299–308.
57. van Beijnum J, van der Worp B, Buis DR. Treatment of brain arteriovenous malformations a systematic review and analysis. JAMA 2011;306(18):2011–9.
58. Josephson CB, Bhattacharya JJ, Cousell CE. Seizure risk with AVM treatment or conservative management: prospective, population-based study. Neurology 2012;79:500–7.
59. Ledezma CJ, Hoh BL, Carter BS. Complications of cerebral arteriovenous malformation embolization: multivariate analysis of predictive factors. Neurosurgery 2006;58:602–11.
60. Spetzler RF, Wilson CB, Weinstein P. Normal perfusion breakthrough theory. Clin Neurosurg 1978;25:651–72.
61. Castel JP, Kantor G. Postoperative morbidity and mortality after microsurgical exclusion of cerebral arteriovenous malformations. Current data and analysis of recent literature. Neurochirurgie 2001;47:369–83.
62. Flickinger JC, Kondziolka D, Lunsford LD. A multi-institutional analysis of complication outcomes after arteriovenous malformation radiosurgery. Int J Radiat Oncol Biol Phys 1999;44:67–74.

# Advances and Controversies in the Management of Cerebral Venous Thrombosis

Michael Star, MD, Murray Flaster, MD, PhD*

## KEYWORDS

- Cerebral venous thrombosis • Anticoagulation • Venous infarction • Cerebral edema
- Hemicraniectomy • Thrombectomy

## KEY POINTS

- CVT should be considered in any young patient who presents with an unexplained headache in combination with known hypercoagulable state, focal neurologic deficits, seizure, or lobar hemorrhage. In addition, MRI brain and MRV head should be done in any patient suspected of idiopathic intracranial hypertension (pseudotumor cerebri) to rule out CVT.
- Diagnosis of CVT has been made significantly easier since the advent of MRV, which together with MRI is now the gold standard for quick and noninvasive diagnosis.
- Early anticoagulation with either unfractionated heparin or low-molecular-weight heparin for patients presenting with CVT, even in patients who present initially with intracranial hemorrhage, prevents propagation of the thrombus and has been demonstrated to improve long-term outcomes.
- Endovascular thrombolysis or mechanical thrombectomy is a reasonable intervention in patients with CVT without intracranial hemorrhage who are clinically deteriorating despite anticoagulation.
- Emergent craniotomy can be effective in cases of threatened cerebral herniation.
- Pediatric patients with CVT have similar presentations to adults, aside from neonates, who often present with seizures.
- Older children with CVT should be treated with anticoagulation. However, treatment of neonates with anticoagulation is more controversial, and more conservative treatment is often pursued.

## INTRODUCTION

Cerebral venous thrombosis (CVT) is an uncommon, serious, and treatable cause of vascular insult to the brain. Usually the result of a combination of thrombosed venous sinuses and cerebral veins, CVT incidence is about five cases per 1 million population and accounts for about 0.5% to 1% of all strokes.[1] Because of its low incidence, large

Department of Neurology, Loyola University Chicago Stritch School of Medicine, 2160 South 1st Avenue, Maywood, IL 60153, USA
* Corresponding author.
*E-mail address:* mflaster@lumc.edu

Neurol Clin 31 (2013) 765–783
http://dx.doi.org/10.1016/j.ncl.2013.03.013
0733-8619/13/$ – see front matter © 2013 Elsevier Inc. All rights reserved.

double-blinded studies promising statistically significant results are difficult to arrange. There are few randomized studies and consequently recommendations for diagnosis and management are based mostly on case series.[2] Unlike ischemic stroke, CVT most often affects patients 50 year old and younger, making poor outcomes even more costly and tragic. As opposed to arterial strokes, CVT has a significantly higher incidence in women, with a 3:1 female/male ratio.[3] This gender imbalance is prominent during the female reproductive years, reaching a female preponderance of five-fold to sevenfold. Before pubescence and in senescence gender mismatch is not present.

CVT can be especially difficult to diagnose because of the variability of its clinical manifestations and its ability to mimic other diseases. Still, in large part because of less invasive and more definitive diagnostic techniques and larger and better documented clinical series, significant progress has been made in recent years in terms of diagnosis, treatment, and probably outcome.

CVT can be divided into two subtypes based on location and mechanism. The first, occurring when the cerebral venous sinuses are primarily involved, leads to impaired cerebrospinal fluid (CSF) resorption and secondarily, intracranial hypertension. The second mechanism, occurring when smaller cerebral veins, often contiguous superficial cortical veins or the paired internal cerebral veins are involved, results in focal edema and venous infarction. Neither process is mutually exclusive.[4] Where the first mechanism predominates, raised intracranial pressure and its clinical consequences, typically headache, impaired visual acuity, and papilledema, become manifest. When the second mechanism predominates, focal venous ischemia leads to focal neurologic deficits and then to secondary venous hemorrhage, which together drive clinical manifestations (**Fig. 1**).

## CLINICAL FINDINGS

The diagnosis of CVT is largely made based on clinical suspicion and imaging. The clinical presentation of CVT is protean, and often missed. Common presenting

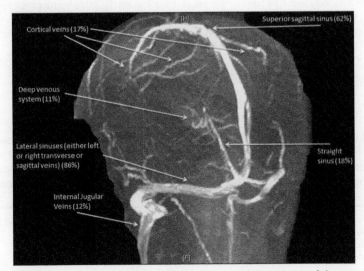

**Fig. 1.** Magnetic resonance venography with frequencies of thrombosis of the noted sinuses based on the International Study on Cerebral Venous and Dural Sinuses Thrombosis.[3] Most patients have thrombosis in more than one location.

symptoms in the International Study on Cerebral Venous and Dural Sinuses Thrombosis (ISCVT) were headache (89%); seizures (39.3%); unilateral or bilateral weakness (37.2%); papilledema (28.3%); and mental status changes (22%).[3]

The most common presenting symptom of CVT is headache, which occurred in 89% of patients.[3] The headaches can be diverse and misleading, with little association between the location of the thrombus and the location and quality of the headache. An exception to this includes patients with thrombosis of the sigmoid sinus who often present with occipital headache.[5] Case studies have demonstrated patients with CVT presenting initially with thunderclap headache,[6] migrainous headache,[7] postural headache,[8] and cluster-like headache.[9] One retrospective study analyzed the quality of headaches in 200 patients with CVT, finding that 20% were described as "band like"; 9% throbbing; 5% thunderclap; and 20% as other, which included stabbing, pounding, and exploding. The study also found that 37% were unilateral, 19% localized, and 20% were diffuse headaches.[5] Because the quality of the headache is not particularly informative, the wary clinician must look for new headache or progressive headache as a significant symptom. Headache is far more common in CVT than in arterial ischemic syndromes, where overall headache frequencies are 25% or less.[10]

In the ISCVT trial, 243 patients (39.3%) presented with seizures, of which about a quarter were focal seizures, a quarter began as focal seizures and then generalized, and half were generalized seizures.[11] Only three patients, slightly more than 1%, presented in status epilepticus. CVT stands apart from other causes of ischemic stroke in having such a high incidence of secondary seizures. A reasonable estimate of seizure frequency during the acute phase is 4% in arterial ischemic stroke and 10% in intracerebral hemorrhage (ICH).[12] A definitive explanation for the high seizure frequency observed in CVT is not available; however, seizures are associated with cortical parenchymal abnormalities and focal neurologic deficits.[11] The presence of intracerebral blood products may also be important because an association between seizure and ICH has also been observed.[13]

Other common presenting symptoms in the ISCVT were unilateral or bilateral weakness (37.2%), papilledema (28.3%), and mental status changes (22%), including delirium, amnesia, and mutism in patients with thrombosis of the deep venous system and coma or death in patients with larger infarcts and hemorrhages.[3,4] It should be remembered that bilateral motor deficits or preferential involvement of the lower extremities suggest parasagittal involvement as may be seen in thrombosis involving the superior sagittal sinus and neighboring superficial cortical veins. Patients with headache and no other findings make up 32% of patients eventually diagnosed with CVT[5] and pose a difficult diagnostic challenge. This, along with other diagnostic dilemmas, is discussed later.

## NEUROIMAGING

A crucial component of diagnosing CVT is by neuroimaging. Rapid progress in the last two decades has made multiple noninvasive and invasive imaging modalities available to help make this diagnosis.

Noncontrast computed tomography (CT) head may show a thrombus as a hyperintense signal in one of the large sinuses, also known as the "cord sign."[4] Currently, the gold standard for the diagnosis of CVT is magnetic resonance venography (MRV) together with magnetic resonance imaging (MRI), including T2* (gradient recalled echo [GRE]) weighted imaging. The major pitfall of MRV is the difficulty in differentiating between a thrombosed sinus vein and a hypoplastic one,[2] particularly the transverse sinuses where asymmetry is common and the left transverse sinus is more frequently hypoplastic. In some instances, a thrombosed sigmoid sinus can be differentiated from a hypoplastic sinus by scrutinizing the outline of the sinus on the bone window of a noncontrast CT. If any ambiguity remains, then a contrast-enhanced MRV or a CT venography (CTV) should directly demonstrate thrombus or define the vessel. Echoplanar susceptibility-weighted images, also known as T2* and GRE, can also help make this distinction. One study demonstrated 97% detection of CVT with T2* sequences, compared with 78% with T1 and less than 40% with FLAIR.[1,14] If MRI is not obtainable, CTV has been shown to be just as effective as MRV in the diagnosis of CVT,[2] although it requires the addition of radiation exposure, the potential for iodine contrast allergy, and problems with contrast exposure in patients with poor renal function.[2] MR contrast studies also carry the risk of nephrogenic systemic fibrosis in patients with poor renal function.[15]

Imaging findings in brain parenchyma in CVT have many interesting and important features. First, the pattern of brain edema, infarction, or hemorrhage is not typically easily accounted for by an arterial ischemic distribution. Second, the mixed features of edema, blood products, and diffusion restriction are also fairly distinct. The frequency of hemorrhagic transformation in venous ischemia is remarkably high, involving one-third of cases.[16]

Invasive techniques, such as catheter cerebral angiography and direct cerebral venography, are less commonly performed, usually reserved for situations in which there are equivocal results from noninvasive imaging techniques or in special circumstances, in preparation for invasive treatment, or where real-time imaging of clot burden is needed. Thrombosis of the vein of Labbe can be difficult to confirm without catheter angiography (see case report in **Fig. 2**).

In neonates suspected of CVT, power Doppler ultrasonography can be used in lieu of MRV and CTV. One series found that power Doppler ultrasonography detected CVT in 10 of 12 neonates undergoing both MRI and ultrasound.[17]

## RISK FACTORS

The ISCVT found that 87.5% of patients with CVT had a demonstrable predisposing condition for CVT.[3] The most common conditions were either a genetic or acquired thrombophilia or oral contraceptive (OCP) use.[2,3] A total of 34% of patients had a genetic or acquired prothrombotic condition, such as antithrombin III deficiency, protein C deficiency, protein S deficiency, factor V Leiden, resistance to activated protein C, mutation G20210 A of factor II, hyperhomocysteinemia, and the antiphospholipid antibody syndromes.[3] OCP use was found in 54.3% of female patients younger than age 50, 33% of all patients.[2,3] A total of 21% of patients with CVT were associated with pregnancy and puerperium. Most of these cases occur late in pregnancy or during the puerperium; however, a few cases do occur earlier and are sometimes associated with hyperemesis gravidarum.[18] Other causes include parameningeal infections (12.3%), either otitis, mastoiditis, or sinusitis; and hematologic disorders (12%), such as polycythemia vera or essential thrombocytosis and iron deficiency anemia. Malignancies were found in 7.5% of cases, whereas systemic disease, such as hyperthyroidism and inflammatory bowel disease, explained 7.2% of cases.[3]

CVT often seems multifactorial with a proximate cause (closed head injury or dehydration) readily obtained from patient history and examination and an underlying cause elucidated later.[3] In the ISCVT nearly 44% of patients had more than one risk factor (**Box 1**).

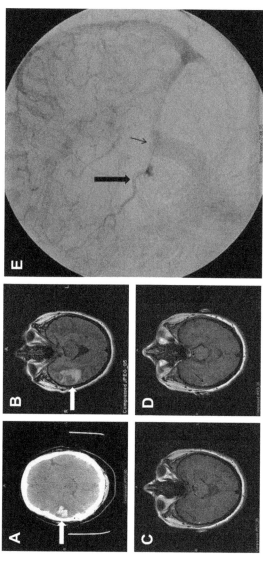

**Fig. 2.** A 34-year-old woman presented with 24 hours of nausea, vomiting, and confusion preceded by 1 week of progressive headache. (A) CT scan of the head revealed a small right temporal hemorrhage (*arrow*). Past medical history included four pregnancies, two normal deliveries, one set of twins delivered by cesarean section, and a stillbirth at 5 months gestational age 15 months before presentation. Her examination was remarkable for persistent inattentiveness and intermittent right-sided neglect. (B) T2 Weighted FLAIR MRI demonstrated a mixture of acute blood products and edema suggestive of venous infarction (*arrow*). (C, D) MRV (not shown) was normal; however, high-resolution T1 imaging demonstrated a linear T1 bright lesion suggestive of a thrombosed vein (*arrows*). (E) Catheter angiography demonstrated a slightly late draining vein of Labbe (*thick arrow*) with a poorly resolved termination into the turn from the right transverse to the sigmoid sinus (*thin arrow*) suggesting partial thrombosis. An electroencephalogram showed mild generalized slowing, focal slowing in the right temporal region, but no epileptiform activity. Intravenous unfractionated heparin was begun along with oral levetiracetam and a brief course of dexamethasone. The patient's headache and inattentiveness began to improve within 48 hours. Conversion to oral anticoagulation with warfarin was begun 4 days after treatment was initiated. Search for a prothrombotic state yielded a positive antinuclear antibody titer, weakly positive lupus anticoagulant, elevated anticardiolipin IgG, and elevated β₂ glycoprotein-1 and the patient was diagnosed with lupus-associated antiphospholipid antibody syndrome. She proved to be poorly compliant with medications and suffered a spontaneous abortion 2 years later followed by a right lower extremity deep vein thrombosis that was successfully treated.

**Box 1**
**Causes of and risk factors associated with cerebral venous sinus thrombosis**

*Genetic prothrombotic conditions*
- Antithrombin deficiency
- Protein C and protein S deficiency
- Factor V Leiden mutation
- Prothrombin gene mutation
- Methyltetrahydrofolate reductase (MTHFR) mutation

*Acquired prothrombotic states*
- Nephroptic syndrome
- Antiphospholipid antibody syndrome
- Hyperhomocysteinemia
- Pregnancy or puerperium

*Infections*
- Otitis, mastoiditis, sinusitis
- Meningitis
- Systemic infectious disease

*Inflammatory disease*
- Systemic lupus erythematosus
- Wegener granulomatosis
- Sarcoidosis
- Inflammatory bowel disease
- Behçet syndrome

*Hematologic conditions*
- Polycythemia, primary and secondary
- Thrombocythemia
- Leukemia
- Anemia
- Paroxysmal nocturnal hemoglobinuria
- Elevated factor VIII

*Drugs*
- Oral contraceptives
- L-Asparaginase

*Mechanical causes, trauma*
- Head injury
- Injury to sinuses or jugular vein, jugular catheterization
- Neurosurgic procedures
- Lumbar puncture

*Miscellaneous*
- Dehydration
- Cancer

*Data from* Stam J. Thrombosis of the cerebral veins and sinuses. N Engl J Med 2005;352:1791–8.

## DIAGNOSTIC DILEMMAS

As suggested by the multitude of different clinical presentations, the diagnosis of CVT can be elusive and often goes undiagnosed for long periods of time. In the ISCVT the delay from symptom onset to diagnosis of CVT was 7 days but the interquartile range was 3 to 16 days.[19] Although there are many disorders that mimic CVT (**Box 2**), certain diagnoses of exclusion, including idiopathic intracranial hypertension (IIH) (pseudotumor cerebri), necessitate patients' undergoing MRV to exclude CVT. This is because of the high likelihood of incorrect diagnosis, illustrated by a study in which nine consecutive patients previously diagnosed with IIH underwent direct retrograde cerebral venography and manometry and five demonstrated CVT,[20] and another study in which 10% of 131 patients presenting with symptoms suggesting IIH, such as papilledema, were found to have CVT on MRV.[21]

Even more vexing to the clinician is the multitude of instances where the only presenting clinical finding in patients eventually diagnosed with CVT was an isolated headache.[1] Although it is economically unfeasible to order an MRV for every patient who presents with a headache, a good rule of thumb is that CVT should be considered in any young patient who presents with an unexplained headache in combination with either known hypercoagulable state, focal neurologic deficits, seizure, or lobar hemorrhage. The work-up for IIH should include an MRV to rule out CVT.

Multiple studies have evaluated the usefulness of measuring D dimer levels to help diagnose or exclude CVT. In a study of 73 patients diagnosed with CVT, 10% were found to have originally presented with a negative D dimer[22] indicating insufficient sensitivity. Specificity of D dimer is also lacking.[2] Still, it must be remembered that primary headache disorders are always a diagnosis of exclusion and patients with subtle presentations must be considered thoughtfully and followed appropriately. It is vital to evaluate patients with unexplained headache for papilledema at each visit.

---

**Box 2**
**Possible CVT mimics**

- Arterial ischemic stroke
- Thunderclap headache
- Postepidural headache
- Migraine
- Orthostatic headache
- Cluster headache
- Intracranial hypertension (pseudotumor cerebri)
- Tension headache
- Transient ischemic attacks
- Isolated psychiatric disturbances
- Tinnitus
- Isolated or multiple cranial nerve palsies, especially sixth nerve palsy
- Subarachnoid hemorrhage

*Data from* Bousser MG, Ferro JM. Cerebral venous thrombosis: an update. Lancet Neurol 2007;6(2):162–70; and Wasay M, Kojan S, Dai AI, et al. Headache in cerebral venous thrombosis: incidence, pattern and location in 200 consecutive patients. J Headache Pain 2010;11(2):137–9.

## MANAGEMENT OF CVT

After a patient has been diagnosed with CVT, there are multiple issues that must be considered. Where should the patient be moved for optimal treatment? What pharmacologic or nonpharmacologic interventions should be considered acutely? What symptomatic treatment should be initiated? What is the length of treatment? What long-term treatments should be considered to avoid recurrence? How should long-term complications be managed?

### Setting

It has been well established in the stroke literature that early assessment by a stroke neurologist, admission to a stroke unit, physiotherapy, and occupational therapy are among the most important factors in reducing morbidity and mortality after acute stroke.[22,23] Because CVT is a type of stroke, it is recommended that patients be treated in a qualified stroke unit.[2]

### Acute Treatment

Although it was initially controversial when introduced by the British gynecologist Stansfield in 1941, it has become the standard of care to treat patients with CVT acutely with anticoagulation. The rationale behind anticoagulation is to prevent propagation of the thrombus, aid in spontaneous thrombus resolution, and to prevent systemic deep vein thrombosis and pulmonary embolism. Not surprisingly, controversy regarding anticoagulation arose because of the possibility of hastening or worsening hemorrhagic conversion. Anticoagulation has since become accepted as the gold standard of acute pharmacologic treatment.

There have been two controlled trials that compared anticoagulation with placebo, one of which was stopped early because of benefit of treatment with heparin. The initial trial of anticoagulation versus placebo used intravenous unfractionated heparin (UFH), titrating to a therapeutic activated partial thromboplastin time.[24] This trial was stopped early after 20 of the planned 60 patients were recruited when investigators found what was believed to be a benefit of treatment; all 10 patients treated with heparin had either completely resolved or had only mild deficits, whereas 3 of the 10 control patients had died.[24] Because of the small study size, the significance of these results was disputed and a second controlled study was launched. The second study enrolled 59 patients who received either the low-molecular-weight heparin (LMWH) nadroparin or placebo.[25] At a follow-up of 3 months, 13% of the group receiving anticoagulation and 21% of the placebo group suffered death or dependence, a trend favoring treatment that was not found to be statistically significant. Combining the two studies did not help demonstrate a statistically significant improvement in outcome with anticoagulation.[26] Still, based on trends in these studies and on results of observational studies, it is widely accepted at this time that anticoagulation is the appropriate initial treatment of acute CVT.[2]

Many clinicians favor using UFH over LMWH acutely in potentially unstable cases because the activated partial thromboplastin time normalizes within 1 to 2 hours after UFH is stopped if protamine is used. This may be advantageous when compared with LMWH, which can take 12 to 24 hours to wear off. Multiple studies comparing the efficacy of UFH against LMWH have been published, none achieving any statistical significance until 2010, when researchers with the ISCVT noted a statistically significant superiority in functional independence at 6 months, defined as a modified Rankin scale (mRS) from 0 to 2, in the patients receiving LMWH (91%) compared with UFH (78%).[26] One flaw of this analysis was that patients who started off on UFH and were switched to LMWH for any reason were not included in the analysis, and putting those patients back into the analysis would make the two treatments seem nearly identical.[26] Although one could argue that the reasons for switching were diverse enough to justify safely eliminating them from the study, one could alternatively argue that a large portion of those patients were the most successfully treated patients with UFH who were then being switched to LMWH for bridging to therapeutic Coumadin as an outpatient. The superiority of LMWH over UFH is in agreement with the conclusions of many large studies of noncerebral venous embolism. This was most robustly demonstrated in a major meta-analysis of venous thromboembolism (VTE) in which LMWH caused fewer recurrences, higher recanalization rates, and lower mortality than UFH.[27]

Anticoagulation is also advocated for in the setting of CVT presenting with ICH.[2] One of the randomized, controlled trials with anticoagulation demonstrated 15% mortality in patients with CVT presenting with ICH receiving UFH versus 69% mortality in those not receiving anticoagulation.[24] There is no sufficiently large trial supporting anticoagulation in patients presenting with ICH, and likely never will be, because of the wide acceptance of its safety and efficacy.[2] The one exception to treating CVT with anticoagulation acutely is in patients who have developed severe intracranial hypertension and require serial lumbar punctures (LP) to remove cerebrospinal fluid to preserve the patient's vision.[28] Anticoagulation must be discontinued temporarily but may be reinstituted with care after each LP.

### Thrombolysis and Mechanical Thrombectomy

Although most patients presenting with CVT have a good prognosis when treated with anticoagulation, 9% to 13% of patients deteriorate despite this treatment.[2] In this setting, many clinicians seek alternative interventions including systemic thrombolysis, direct catheter thrombolysis, and direct mechanical thrombectomy. None of these treatments for CVT, however, have been studied in randomized clinical trials. A recent meta-analysis of retrospective and prospective studies in which patients with CVT were treated with thrombolysis with urokinase or alteplase concluded that a not negligible number of patients subsequently had extracranial and intracranial bleeding or died.[29] It is not clear how useful this information is, because one can assume that most of the patients in these studies had significant clot burden and were likely to have a higher incidence of ICH and death compared with patients treated with standard anticoagulation.

In light of this dilemma, the Thrombolysis or Anticoagulation for Cerebral Venous Thrombosis Trial (TO-ACT) is currently underway. TO-ACT will recruit and randomize patients with CVT who have a poorer prognosis (defined by the presence of one or more of the following risk factors: mental status disorder, coma, intracranial hemorrhagic lesion, or thrombosis of the deep cerebral venous system) to treatment with either endovascular thrombolysis or standard anticoagulation.[26]

Mechanical thrombectomy using a variety of different devices is a potential alternative or supplement to thrombolysis. Thus far, studies are limited to observation but this avenue of treatment should be considered as potentially safer and more effective than thrombolysis alone. Further study is warranted.

It is the authors' opinion that it is currently reasonable to treat patients with CVT who have no ICH and are demonstrating signs of clinical deterioration despite treatment with anticoagulation with endovascular thrombolysis. Mechanical thrombectomy may prove to be safer in the presence of hemorrhagic conversion.

### Cerebral Edema

Although cerebral edema is seen in up to 50% of patients with CVT, it is self-resolving in all but approximately 20% of those patients.[28] Patients whose cerebral edema does not resolve can develop intracranial hypertension and are at risk of permanent loss of vision. These patients should be treated with therapeutic LP despite the need to temporarily suspend anticoagulation.[30] Although there are no randomized trials supporting this treatment, there is consensus that treatment with acetazolamide is acceptable in these patients.[2,30] In a matched case-control analysis of patients in the ISCVT, 150 patients receiving steroids were compared to 150 patients not receiving steroids with similar clinical characteristics.[31] The study could not show any benefit from steroids, but because there was no standardized treatment dose, duration, or timing, and because the indications for steroids were various, no definite conclusions should be drawn.

With the advent of noninvasive interventions, surgical intervention in patients with CVT has become increasingly unnecessary. However, there is still a role for decompressive craniectomy in patients with cerebral edema and sufficient mass effect to threaten cerebral herniation. In one prospective study, 7 out of 10 patients with severe CVT who underwent decompressive craniectomy had a favorable outcome (mRS ≤3).[32] Two of the patients experienced herniation and died despite the surgical intervention. Four small studies have been published in recent years suggesting that there is considerable benefit to extensive decompressive craniectomy, with or without debridement.[32–35] In all of these studies, the patients received prophylactic doses of anticoagulant in the first 24 hours postoperatively, with full anticoagulation after the first day in almost all patients. A common concern for neurologists and neurosurgeons alike treating these patients is whether early anticoagulation in these patients is safe. In this group, totaling 25 patients, no late bleeding was reported. We conclude that early anticoagulation is safe and probably necessary (see case report in **Fig. 3**). Like thrombolysis, there is incomplete evidence for performing decompressive craniectomy, although it is a reasonable course of action to take when an experienced clinician determines that conservative management is not enough to prevent catastrophic deterioration.

In general, it is not possible to reliably predict clinical deterioration. To accomplish this, a predictive score that effectively defines a very high-risk group is needed. A risk score based on clinical features[36] and a risk score based on anatomic features[37] have been developed. The anatomic score lacks sufficient selectivity– some patients with high scores do very well–whereas the clinical risk score thus far developed lacks sensitivity. For the moment, worsening despite treatment or clinical severity even before treatment is initiated are in our opinion the only guides currently available in helping to decide when to initiate invasive therapy.

### Seizures

Seizures are a common presenting event in CVT. A total of 245 (40%) of the patients in the ISCVT presented initially with seizure.[3] Initial seizure was an independent predictor of further seizures in patients not treated with an antiepileptic drug (AED).[11] The study also demonstrated that patients with supratentorial venous thrombosis, especially of the superficial cortical veins or superior sagittal sinus, and those with puerperal CVT had a much higher likelihood of presenting with or having early seizures. On further analysis, 24 (51%) of 47 patients with a supratentorial lesion and seizure that were not treated with AED went on to have recurrent seizures and only 1 in 148 patients who were treated with AED had recurrent seizures, thus making a strong argument

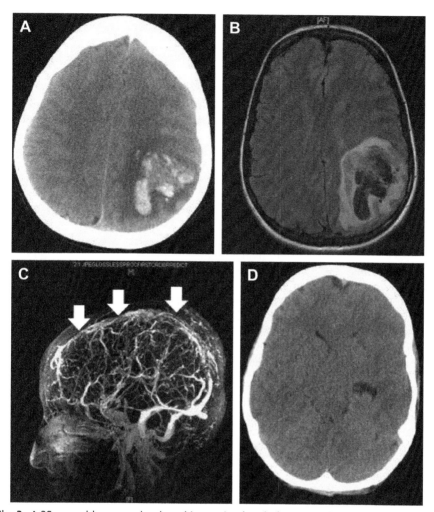

**Fig. 3.** A 28-year-old woman developed increasing headache over 4 days followed by right-sided weakness and mild aphasia. CT head (*A*) demonstrated a left parietal hemorrhage suspicious for venous infarction. MRI T2 FLAIR (*B*) showed intermixed blood products and bright T2 signal indicating hemorrhage and edema and consistent with hemorrhagic venous infarction, whereas MRV two-dimensional time-of-flight multi-image projection (*C*) showed a thinned, highly abnormal superior sagittal sinus with increased number of cortical veins (*arrows*). The patient was placed on intravenous unfractionated heparin and transferred to the authors' hospital. On arrival to the hospital, the patient was drowsy but arousable, with incomplete right hemiparesis and able to follow some commands. Within 5 hours of arrival, she became comatose and completely paretic. (*D*) Emergent CT head showed increased lesion volume (30%), enlarged left temporal horn, and effaced perimesencephalic cisterns. Emergent craniotomy was performed, patient was carefully anticoagulated postoperatively, and went on to do very well. She has returned to work as a research scientist, is without clinical deficit, but did develop poststroke epilepsy. Thrombotic risk factors included OCP use and homozygosity for MTHFR C677T polymorphism. Additionally, maternal history included deep vein thrombosis.

for AED treatment of patients with puerperal CVT and patients who present with seizure.[11] However, the study did not demonstrate sufficient efficacy of AED treatment in patients without both supratentorial CVT and seizures. Placing patients with supratentorial CVT and without seizure on an AED is not justified. Prophylactic treatment of selected patients with supratentorial lesions who are believed to be unstable may prove to be justified.

The incidence of late-onset seizures, usually defined as at least one month after initial presentation, was found to be low (5%–10.6%).[28] One study demonstrated that the strongest predictor of late seizures was an early hemorrhagic lesion.[38] Early onset seizures were also an important predictor for development of postacute seizures, those authors have suggested that patients presenting with hemorrhagic lesions and early onset seizures would benefit from a year of AED therapy.[28] It is estimated that 5% of patients go on to have epilepsy, defined as more than one late seizure.[2]

### Long-term Anticoagulation

The goal of long-term anticoagulation is to prevent the recurrence of CVT and systemic VTE (**Table 1**). The ISCVT trial noted an approximately 6.5% annual risk of any thrombotic event occurring.[3] Because there have not been adequate studies of long-term anticoagulation after CVT, the current guidelines are based on the established guidelines for anticoagulation following systemic VTE.[39,40] As such, the duration of anticoagulation after CVT is based on risk stratification determined by the presence of prothrombotic risk factors.

The hereditary, genetic, and acquired thrombophilias are separated into categories of varying severity. Patient with provoked CVT with transient risk factors such as dehydration, drugs (including OCPs), infection, trauma, and recent surgery, are treated for 3 months with anticoagulation after CVT.[2,41] Mild thrombophilia is defined as having either heterozygous prothrombin gene mutation, heterozygous factor V Leiden, or high levels of factor VIII, and the recommendations are 6 to 12 months of anticoagulation after CVT.[28] Severe thrombophilias include homozygous prothrombin gene mutation, homozygous factor V Leiden, protein C or protein S deficiency, antiphospholipid antibody syndrome, and antithrombin III deficiency. These entities carry such a high risk of recurrent VTE that indefinite treatment with anticoagulation is recommended.[2,39,40,41,42] Patients with a known malignancy and CVT should be started on LMWH for the first 3 to 6 months, followed by indefinite LMWH or vitamin K antagonist, at least until remission.[40,41] Patients who have a CVT during pregnancy or

| Table 1 | |
|---|---|
| **Long-term anticoagulation in CVT** | |
| **Risk Factor** | **Duration of Treatment** |
| Malignancy | Initially LMWH for 3–6 mo, followed by indefinite treatment with LMWH or Vitamin K antagonists, at least until remission |
| Transient thrombophilic state | 3 mo |
| Mild thrombophilia | 6–12 mo |
| Severe thrombophilia | Indefinite |
| Pregnancy or puerperium | LMWH for remainder of pregnancy and at least 6 wk postpartum, total 6 mo |

*Adapted from* Caprio F, Bernstein RA. Duration of anticoagulation after cerebral venous sinus thrombosis. Neurocrit Care 2012;16(2):335–42; with permission.

puerperium should continue LMWH for the duration of the pregnancy and at least 6 weeks postpartum for a total of at least 6 months of anticoagulation.[2,41]

## CLINICAL OUTCOMES IN ADULTS

Since the advent of both MRV for quick diagnosis and the widespread treatment with acute anticoagulation[43] it is widely accepted that CVT has come to have good outcomes when compared with other types of strokes. There is a concern, however, that measuring the outcomes in number of deaths and mRS scales is missing important long-term consequences of CVT, including neuropsychological and neuropsychiatric dysfunction.[2,44]

In the ISCVT, 21 (3.4%) of 624 patients died within the first 30 days of presentation; 6.8% after 6 months; and 8.3% at last follow-up (median of 16 months).[3] Predictors for mortality at 30 days include depressed consciousness, mental status disorder, thrombosis of the deep venous system, right hemispheric hemorrhage, and posterior fossa lesions.[1,2] Late deaths were often not caused by original CVT or recurrence, but were instead a consequence of underlying conditions, specifically malignancies.[2] Long-term follow-up in one study found that 6 (10%) out of 58 patients had poor outcome at a median of 50 months,[45] which suggests that a patient with CVT who survives the first few months will likely survive long term.

The ISCVT demonstrated good functional outcomes, with 79% of patients at long-term follow-up attaining an mRS score of 0 to 1, indicating no or minor residual symptoms.[3] This may contrast with findings in another study that found up to 75% of patients had residual symptoms, including motor deficits, visual field defects, seizures, and residual headaches.[43] Loss of vision was often secondary to optic atrophy, caused by persistent elevation of intracranial pressure.

## PEDIATRIC CVT

The Canadian Pediatric Ischemic Stroke Registry (CPISR) demonstrated that CVT occurs at a rate of 0.67 per 100,000 children per year,[17] although there is a concern that the diagnosis of CVT in children is missed and the rate is actually higher. This is slightly higher than the estimated 0.5 per 100,000 seen in adults, and the male/female ratio is closer to 1:1, compared with 1:3 in adults. A total of 43% of the children diagnosed with CVT were neonates, and 54% were younger than 1 year old. This increased risk for neonates is postulated to be caused by damage to the dural venous sinuses secondary to the molding of the skull bones during delivery, along with the general prothrombotic state and susceptibility to dehydration associated with the neonatal period[2] (**Box 3**). Although the presenting symptoms and signs in nonneonates were similar to those in adults, most neonates (71%) presented with seizures.[17] This is theorized to be caused by neonates' general propensity to have seizures, in addition to the potential selection bias inherent in neonates' inability to articulate other changes.

Like adults, the gold standard for diagnosis of CVT in pediatric populations is MRV and MRI with T2* (GRE) sequence, although some studies suggest that CTV is sometimes necessary for diagnosis when MRV is questionable.[2] The location of the thrombus was also similar to findings in adults, although there were significantly fewer hemorrhagic findings in nonneonates (23%) compared with neonates (35%) and adults (39%).[2,17]

In the CPISR, risk factors for CVT were found in all but four patients (2%), although in a subsequent study by Sebire and colleagues[46] that included an increased battery of genetic thrombophilias, all of the 42 children in the study demonstrated a clinical risk factor for CVT. A meta-analysis by Kenet and colleagues[47] of the various

**Box 3**
**Predisposing factors to CVT in the pediatric population**

*Prothrombotic state*
Factor V G1691 A mutation
Factor II G20210 A mutation
Protein C deficiency
Protein S deficiency
Anticardiolipin antibodies
Lipoprotein(a)
Antithrombin deficiency

*Drugs*
Asparaginase
Heparin (heparin-induced thrombocytopenia)
IgG (intravenous immunoglobulin)

*Infections*
Otitis
Mastoiditis
Sinusitis
Peritonsillar abscess
Endotoxemia
Trichinosis
Sepsis
Herpes zoster virus
Mucormycosis
Aspergillosis
Pneumococcal meningitis
Syphilis
HIV

*Vasculitides*
Systemic lupus erythematosus
Behçet disease
Polyarteritis nodosa
Sarcoidosis

*Other*
Cancer
Acute lymphoblastic leukemia
Nephrotic syndrome
Dehydration
Asphyxia

Maternal problems during pregnancy

Metabolic disorders

Vascular trauma

*Modified from* Refs.[47,51,52]

---

thrombophilias causing arterial ischemic stroke and CVT demonstrated that anti-thrombin deficiency had an odds ratio (OR) of 18.41, protein C deficiency had an OR of 6.30, protein S deficiency had an OR of 5.27, factor V G1691 A had an OR of 2.74, and factor II G20210 A had an OR of 1.95 for CVT. Analysis of the CPISR found that the risk factors were age dependent and often different from those found in adults. The most common risk factor in neonates was hypoxic encephalopathy; in preschool age children it was head and neck infections, such as otitis media, mastoiditis, and sinusitis. In older children the most common risk factors were chronic diseases, such as connective-tissue disorders.[17] The high rate of risk factor associations argues for complete work-up of possible genetic thrombophilia if no other causes are discovered.

In the child presenting with CVT, it is important to treat patients' symptoms, which includes administering adequate hydration, starting an appropriate AED if the child is seizing, and performing serial evaluations for elevated intracranial pressure, including periodic visual field and acuity testing. As in adults, acute treatment with anticoagulant in pediatric patients with CVT has not been studied in a randomized, controlled trial, although all the data, suggest it is safe and advantageous to treat nonneonatal pediatric patients presenting acutely with hemorrhagic and nonhemorrhagic CVT with either LMWH or UFH.[2,46,48] The data on endovascular thrombolysis are, similar to findings in adults, not statistically significant but endovascular intervention is believed to be a reasonable course of action in children with CVT without ICH who are rapidly deteriorating. A large European multicenter study on thromboembolism had 396 children with CVT and demonstrated that nonadministration of an anticoagulant before relapse had a hazard ratio of 11.2 for recurrent VTE, arguing for 3 to 6 months of prophylactic anticoagulation after CVT.[49]

For neonates, the treatment in the acute phase is not straightforward. No guidelines unreservedly recommend anticoagulation for neonates in the acute phase of CVT. One set of guidelines[50] recommends either anticoagulation or conservative management, with follow-up imaging to assess for propagation of the thrombus and initiation of anticoagulation at that time if it is found (**Box 4**). Another set of guidelines notes that "In neonates with acute CVT, treatment with LMWH or UFH may be considered.[2]" In the discussion of the results of the CPISR trial,[17] it is noted that the loose application of adult guidelines to neonates is "problematic," but later that "the study suggests that anticoagulant therapy is not associated with serious hemorrhage." The neurologist or pediatrician called to evaluate and treat a neonatal CVT is thus open to relying on clinical intuition on whether or not to treat with anticoagulation, and should not be faulted

---

**Box 4**
**Acute anticoagulation of pediatric CVT**

Neonates

  LMWH and UFH may be considered[2]

Nonneonates

  Treat with LMWH or UFH[2,46,48]

for either decision. A similar conclusion can be made about postacute anticoagulation, with the guidelines[2] suggesting that 6 weeks to 3 months of continued anticoagulation can be considered.

The CPISR trial demonstrated that, at long-term follow-up of an average of 1.6 years, 54% of children were normal, 38% had neurologic deficits, and 8% had died.[2,17] The deficits included motor impairment, developmental delay, speech impairment, and visual impairment.[17] Of the children who had died, half died directly from complications caused by the CVT and half from underlying disease.[17] Mortality was similar between neonates and nonneonates, although the rate of neurologic deficits at follow-up was only 34% in neonates.[2]

## REFERENCES

1. Bousser MG, Ferro JM. Cerebral venous thrombosis: an update. Lancet Neurol 2007;6(2):162–70.
2. Saposnik G, Barinagarrementeria F, Brown RD, et al. Diagnosis and management of cerebral venous thrombosis A statement for healthcare professionals from the American Heart Association/American Stroke Association. Stroke 2011;42(4):1158–92.
3. Ferro JM, Canhao P, Stam J, et al, ISCVT Investigators. Prognosis of cerebral vein and dural sinus thrombosis: results of the International Study on Cerebral Vein and Dural Sinus Thrombosis (ISCVT). Stroke 2004;35(3):664–70.
4. Stam J. Thrombosis of the cerebral veins and sinuses. N Engl J Med 2005;352:1791–8.
5. Wasay M, Kojan S, Dai AI, et al. Headache in cerebral venous thrombosis: incidence, pattern and location in 200 consecutive patients. J Headache Pain 2010;11(2):137–9.
6. de Bruijn SF, Stam J, Kappelle LJ. Thunderclap headache as first symptom of cerebral venous sinus thrombosis. CVST study group. Lancet 1996;348(9042):1623–5.
7. Slooter AJ, Ramos LM, Kappelle LJ. Migraine-like headache as the presenting symptom of cerebral venous sinus thrombosis. J Neurol 2002;249(6):775–6.
8. Todorov L, Laurito CE, Schwartz DE. Postural headache in the presence of cerebral venous sinus thrombosis. Anesth Analg 2005;101(5):1499–500.
9. Rodriguez S, Calleja S, Moris G. Cluster-like headache heralding cerebral venous thrombosis. Cephalalgia 2008;28(8):906–7.
10. Vestergaard K, Andersen G, Nielsen MI, et al. Headache in stroke. Stroke 1993;24(11):1621–4.
11. Ferro JM, Canhao P, Bousser MG, et al, ISCVT Investigators. Early seizures in cerebral vein and dural sinus thrombosis: risk factors and role of antiepileptics. Stroke 2008;39(4):1152–8.
12. Bladin CF, Alexandrov AV, Bellavance A, et al. Seizures after stroke: a prospective multicenter study. Arch Neurol 2000;57(11):1617.
13. Masuhr F, Busch M, Amberger N, et al. Risk and predictors of early epileptic seizures in acute cerebral venous and sinus thrombosis. Eur J Neurol 2006;13(8):852–6.
14. Idbaih A, Boukobza M, Crassard I, et al. MRI of clot in cerebral venous thrombosis: high diagnostic value of susceptibility-weighted images. Stroke 2006;37(4):991–5.

15. Marckmann P, Skov L, Rossen K, et al. Nephrogenic systemic fibrosis: suspected causative role of gadodiamide used for contrast-enhanced magnetic resonance imaging. J Am Soc Nephrol 2006;17(9):2359–62.
16. Leach JL, Fortuna RB, Jones BV, et al. Imaging of cerebral venous thrombosis: current techniques, spectrum of findings, and diagnostic pitfalls. Radiographics 2006;26(Suppl 1):S19–41 [discussion: S42–3].
17. deVeber G, Andrew M, Adams C, et al. Cerebral sinovenous thrombosis in children. N Engl J Med 2001;345(6):417–23.
18. Kimber J. Cerebral venous sinus thrombosis. QJM 2002;95(3):137–42.
19. Ferro JM, Canhao P, Stam J, et al. Delay in the diagnosis of cerebral vein and dural sinus thrombosis: influence on outcome. Stroke 2009;40(9):3133–8.
20. Owler BK, Parker G, Halmagyi GM, et al. Pseudotumor cerebri syndrome: venous sinus obstruction and its treatment with stent placement. J Neurosurg 2003;98(5):1045–55.
21. Lin A, Foroozan R, Danesh-Meyer HV, et al. Occurrence of cerebral venous sinus thrombosis in patients with presumed idiopathic intracranial hypertension. Ophthalmology 2006;113(12):2281–4.
22. Crassard I, Soria C, Tzourio C, et al. A negative D-dimer assay does not rule out cerebral venous thrombosis: a series of seventy-three patients. Stroke 2005; 36(8):1716–9.
23. Stroke Unit Trialists' Collaboration. Organised inpatient (stroke unit) care for stroke. Cochrane Database Syst Rev 2007;(4):CD000197.
24. Einhaupl KM, Villringer A, Meister W, et al. Heparin treatment in sinus venous thrombosis. Lancet 1991;338(8767):597–600.
25. de Bruijn SF, Stam J. Randomized, placebo-controlled trial of anticoagulant treatment with low-molecular-weight heparin for cerebral sinus thrombosis. Stroke 1999;30(3):484–8.
26. Coutinho JM, de Bruijn SF, deVeber G, et al. Anticoagulation for cerebral venous sinus thrombosis. Stroke 2012;43(4):e41–2.
27. van Dongen CJ, van den Belt AG, Prins MH, et al. Fixed dose subcutaneous low molecular weight heparins versus adjusted dose unfractionated heparin for venous thromboembolism. Cochrane Database Syst Rev 2004;(4): CD001100.
28. Einhaupl K, Stam J, Bousser MG, et al. EFNS guideline on the treatment of cerebral venous and sinus thrombosis in adult patients. Eur J Neurol 2010;17(10): 1229–35.
29. Dentali F, Squizzato A, Gianni M, et al. Safety of thrombolysis in cerebral venous thrombosis. A systematic review of the literature. Thromb Haemost 2010;104(5): 1055–62.
30. Ferro JM, Canhão P. Cerebral venous sinus thrombosis. In: Biller J, editor. Evidence-based management of stroke. 1st edition. Shrewsbury (United Kingdom): TFM Publishing Limited; 2011. p. 205–14.
31. Canhao P, Cortesao A, Cabral M, et al. Are steroids useful to treat cerebral venous thrombosis? Stroke 2008;39(1):105–10.
32. Zuurbier SM, Coutinho JM, Majoie CB, et al. Decompressive hemicraniectomy in severe cerebral venous thrombosis: a prospective case series. J Neurol 2012; 259(6):1099–105.
33. Theaudin M, Crassard I, Bresson D, et al. Should decompressive surgery be performed in malignant cerebral venous thrombosis? A series of 12 patients. Stroke 2010;41(4):727–31.

34. Coutinho JM, Majoie CB, Coert BA, et al. Decompressive hemicraniectomy in cerebral sinus thrombosis consecutive case series and review of the literature. Stroke 2009;40(6):2233–5.
35. Keller E, Pangalu A, Fandino J, et al. Decompressive craniectomy in severe cerebral venous and dural sinus thrombosis. Acta Neurochir Suppl 2005;94: 177–83.
36. Girot M, Ferro JM, Canhão P, et al. Predictors of outcome in patients with cerebral venous thrombosis and intracerebral hemorrhage. Stroke 2007;38(2): 337–42.
37. Zubkov AY, McBane RD, Brown RD, et al. Brain lesions in cerebral venous sinus thrombosis. Stroke 2009;40(4):1509–11.
38. Ferro JM, Correia M, Rosas MJ, et al, Cerebral Venous Thrombosis Portuguese Collaborative Study Group[Venoport]. Seizures in cerebral vein and dural sinus thrombosis. Cerebrovasc Dis 2003;15(1–2):78–83.
39. Lijfering WM, Brouwer JL, Veeger NJ, et al. Selective testing for thrombophilia in patients with first venous thrombosis: results from a retrospective family cohort study on absolute thrombotic risk for currently known thrombophilic defects in 2479 relatives. Blood 2009;113(21):5314–22.
40. Kearon C, Kahn SR, Agnelli G, et al. Antithrombotic therapy for venous thromboembolic disease: American College of Chest Physicians evidence-based clinical practice guidelines (8th edition). Chest 2008;133(Suppl 6):454S–545S.
41. Caprio F, Bernstein RA. Duration of anticoagulation after cerebral venous sinus thrombosis. Neurocrit Care 2012;16(2):335–42.
42. Crowther MA, Ginsberg JS, Julian J, et al. A comparison of two intensities of warfarin for the prevention of recurrent thrombosis in patients with the antiphospholipid antibody syndrome. N Engl J Med 2003;349(12):1133–8.
43. Breteau G, Mounier-Vehier F, Godefroy O, et al. Cerebral venous thrombosis 3-year clinical outcome in 55 consecutive patients. J Neurol 2003;250(1): 29–35.
44. Lindgren A. Long-term prognosis of cerebral vein and sinus thrombosis. Front Neurol Neurosci 2008;23:172–8.
45. English JD, Fields JD, Le S, et al. Clinical presentation and long-term outcome of cerebral venous thrombosis. Neurocrit Care 2009;11(3):330–7.
46. Sebire G, Tabarki B, Saunders DE, et al. Cerebral venous sinus thrombosis in children: risk factors, presentation, diagnosis and outcome. Brain 2005;128(Pt 3): 477–89.
47. Kenet G, Lutkhoff LK, Albisetti M, et al. Impact of thrombophilia on risk of arterial ischemic stroke or cerebral sinovenous thrombosis in neonates and children: a systematic review and meta-analysis of observational studies. Circulation 2010; 121(16):1838–47.
48. Kersbergen KJ, de Vries LS, van Straaten HL, et al. Anticoagulation therapy and imaging in neonates with a unilateral thalamic hemorrhage due to cerebral sinovenous thrombosis. Stroke 2009;40(8):2754–60.
49. Kenet G, Kirkham F, Niederstadt T, et al. Risk factors for recurrent venous thromboembolism in the European Collaborative Paediatric Database on Cerebral Venous Thrombosis: a multicentre cohort study. Lancet Neurol 2007;6(7): 595–603.
50. Monagle P, Chalmers E, Chan A, et al. Antithrombotic therapy in neonates and children: American College of Chest Physicians evidence-based clinical practice guidelines (8th edition). Chest 2008;133(Suppl 6):887S–968S.

51. Heller C, Heinecke A, Junker R, et al. Cerebral Venous Thrombosis in Children: A Multifacatorial Origin. Circulation 2003;108(11):1362–7.
52. Dafer R, Biller J. Cerebral Venous Thrombosis. In: Biller J, editor. Stroke in Children and Young Adults. 2nd Edition. Philadelphia: Saunders Elsevier; 2009. p. 233–48.

# Epilepsy
## New Drug Targets and Neurostimulation

Jorge J. Asconapé, MD

## KEYWORDS

- Epilepsy • Seizures • Antiepileptic drugs • Lacosamide • Rufinamide
- Ezogabine/ Retigabine • Retigabine • Perampanel • Neurostimulation

## KEY POINTS

- Epilepsy affects approximately 70 million people worldwide. Despite advances in the medical and surgical therapy of epilepsy, about 30% of patients do not achieve full seizure control.
- There is still a great a need for newer, more effective therapies.
- In the past 5 years new antiepileptic drugs (AEDs) have been approved for clinical use.
- Some of these drugs have unique, novel mechanisms of action; overall efficacy of these agents, however, seems similar to other AEDs.
- Neurostimulation, with the development of a variety of different devices and targets of stimulation, is a rapidly evolving field and will likely play an important role in management of severe epilepsy.

## INTRODUCTION

With an estimated incidence of 34 to 76 per 100,000 new cases per year, epilepsy affects about 70 million people worldwide.[1] About a third of patients with newly diagnosed epilepsy continue to have seizures despite antiepileptic drug (AED) therapy.[2] A recent study on outcome patterns of AED therapy in newly diagnosed epilepsy showed that 37% of patients had early, sustained seizure freedom; 22% had delayed but sustained seizure freedom; 16% fluctuated between periods of seizure freedom and relapse; and 25% never attained seizure freedom.[3] Overall, 68% of patients were seizure free, 62% on monotherapy.[3] Only a small proportion of patients with medication-resistant epilepsy are good candidates for surgical therapy. During the past two decades a large number of AEDs have been introduced. Many of these newer agents have proved safer, better tolerated, and easier to use than the "classic" drugs, but their impact in improving seizure control in medication-resistant epilepsy seems to have been modest at best.[4] Therefore, the need for newer therapies in epilepsy remains high.

Department of Neurology, Stritch School of Medicine, Loyola University Chicago, Maguire Center, Suite 2700, 2160 South First Avenue, Maywood, IL 60153, USA
E-mail address: jasconape@lumc.edu

Neurol Clin 31 (2013) 785–798
http://dx.doi.org/10.1016/j.ncl.2013.04.001
0733-8619/13/$ – see front matter © 2013 Elsevier Inc. All rights reserved.

AEDs with a novel mechanism of action have been recently approved for clinical use. Lacosamide (Vimpat) differs from traditional sodium channel blockers in that it works by prolonging the slow inactivated state of the channel. Retigabine/ezogabine is a first-in-class potassium channel opener. Perampanel (Fycompa), an α-amino-3-hydroxy-5-methyl-4-isoxazolepropionic acid (AMPA) antagonist, is the first drug in that class approved for clinical use. Rufinamide (Banzel), a more traditional sodium channel blocker, has also been added recently to the expanding list of AEDs.

Neurostimulation has been used experimentally for the treatment of epilepsy for more than four decades, starting with the pioneer studies on the effects of cerebellar stimulation in epileptic patients in the 1970s.[5] Vagus nerve stimulation, approved for use in Europe in 1994 and the United States and Canada in 1997, remains at present the only approved device for the treatment of epilepsy in the United States. For the past two decades deep brain stimulation (DBS) has been shown to be a safe and effective treatment of movement disorders, such as Parkinson disease, dystonia, and tremor. A large list of potential targets for neurostimulation in epilepsy, including deep brain structures, has been proposed and many are at different stages of clinical investigation (**Box 1**). Of this long list, two techniques have recently shown positive results in multicenter, randomized, double-blind studies in patients with medically intractable partial epilepsy: electrical stimulation of the anterior nucleus of the thalamus and responsive neurostimulation.[6,7]

A significant problem for the physician using neurostimulation in epilepsy, in essence an invasive procedure, has been the virtual lack of reliable predictors of good outcome.[8] A considerable proportion of patients treated with vagus nerve

---

**Box 1**
**Targets of neurostimulation for the treatment of epilepsy**

- Stimulation of cranial nerves
  - Vagus nerve stimulation
  - Trigeminal nerve stimulation
- Deep brain stimulation
  - Cerebellum
  - Thalamus
    - Anterior nucleus
    - Centromedian nucleus
  - Basal ganglia
    - Caudate nucleus
    - Subthalamic nucleus
    - Substantia nigra pars reticulata
- Stimulation of seizure focus
  - Repetitive transcranial magnetic stimulation
  - Invasive cortical stimulation
    - Hippocampus
    - Occipital
- Responsive stimulation

stimulation show minimal or no improvement in the frequency or severity of seizures. An external, noninvasive paradigm of stimulation, therefore, may be useful, if anything as a potential way of determining which patients may benefit from a more definitive implantation of a device. Among several targets for external (noninvasive) neurostimulation studied, bilateral external trigeminal stimulation has shown favorable results in early stages of clinical investigation.

## NEWER AEDS
### Lacosamide

Lacosamide was approved in 2008 by the US Food and Drug Administration (FDA) for the adjunctive treatment of partial-onset seizures in patients 17 years or older. The anticonvulsant properties of lacosamide were discovered in the 1980s through systematic testing in animal models of molecules chemically related to N-acetyl-D,L-alanine benzylamide. The efficacy profile of lacosamide in animal models predicted clinical effectiveness in partial and secondarily generalized tonic-clonic seizures. Lacosamide seems to exert its anticonvulsant effect by selectively enhancing the slow inactivation of voltage-gated sodium channels.[9] This effect is different from that of classic AEDs, such as phenytoin, carbamazepine, or lamotrigine, which modulate the fast inactivation of the sodium channel.

Lacosamide has a very favorable pharmacokinetic profile with complete absorption, linear kinetics, and low protein binding (**Table 1**). It has no significant pharmacokinetic interactions with other AEDs or with oral contraceptives. It does have, however, a significant pharmacodynamic interaction with other sodium channel blockers, such as phenytoin, carbamazepine, oxcarbazepine, and lamotrigine. The typical dose-dependent side effects shared by all sodium channel blocking drugs include dizziness,

| Table 1 Lacosamide | |
|---|---|
| Primary indication | Partial (focal) seizures |
| Mechanism of action | Selectively enhances slow inactivation of voltage-gated sodium channels |
| Oral bioavalability | Complete |
| Time to peak concentration ($T_{max}$) | 1 h (0.5–2.5 h) Food does not affect the rate or extent of absorption |
| Half-life | 13 h |
| Metabolism and excretion | About 60% of dose metabolized (CYP2C19), 40% excreted unchanged in the urine. No active metabolites. |
| Drug interactions | No significant pharmacokinetic interactions. Pharmacodynamic interaction with other sodium channel blockers[a] resulting in potentiation of dose-dependent side effects. |
| Protein binding | <15% |
| Dosing | 100–200 mg twice daily |
| Dosage forms and strengths | Tablets: 50 mg, 100 mg, 150 mg, 200 mg Oral solution: 10 mg/mL Injection: 200 mg/20 mL |
| Side effects | Dizziness, diplopia, blurred vision, headache, nausea, PR interval prolongation, atrial fibrillation, atrial flutter, multiorgan hypersensitivity |

[a] Sodium channel blockers: phenytoin, carbamazepine, oxcarbazepine, lamotrigine.

nausea, vomiting, blurred vision, diplopia, and ataxia. This toxicity is potentiated when lacosamide is used in combination with these drugs. Lacosamide shows much better tolerability if used in combination with non–sodium channel blockers, such as levetiracetam, topiramate, zonisamide, or valproate. Elimination is through a combination of metabolism (demethylation) and direct renal excretion (about 40% of the parent drug is recovered unchanged in the urine). Dose adjustments may be necessary in severe hepatic or renal disease. Lacosamide is efficiently extracted during hemodialysis; a supplementation of about 50% of the total daily dose is recommended after hemodialysis.

The clinical efficacy of lacosamide was demonstrated in three pivotal clinical trials in adult patients with partial seizures.[10–12] When all three trials are combined, the reduction in median seizure frequency per 28 days compared with baseline was 17.3%, 30.5%, and 37.3% for placebo, 200 mg/day, and 400 mg/day, respectively. The percent of patients achieving a greater than or equal to 50% reduction in the frequency of seizures was 22.3%, 36.5%, and 45% for placebo, 200 mg/day, and 400 mg/day, respectively. The dose of 600 mg/day had similar efficacy to the 400 mg/day, but with a higher incidence of side effects. The maximum dose approved by the US FDA was 400 mg/day.

Lacosamide is generally very well tolerated. Most common dose-dependent side effects observed in clinical trials include fatigue, dizziness, blurred or double vision, nausea, and vomiting. Serious cardiac toxicity is rare but may occur with the use of lacosamide. A dose-dependent PR interval prolongation has been observed. More rarely, asymptomatic first-degree atrioventricular block, atrial fibrillation, or atrial flutter was observed in the clinical trials. Lacosamide should be used with caution in patients with cardiac disease.

## Rufinamide

Rufinamide was introduced in the US market in 2008 for adjunctive treatment of seizures associated with the Lennox-Gastaut syndrome in patients 4 years or older. Lennox-Gastaut syndrome is a severe type of epilepsy with onset in childhood and characterized by intractable seizures and impaired mental development. Multiple seizures types including tonic, atonic, atypical absence, focal, or generalized tonic-clonic may occur. Seizures are typically very frequent, often observed on a daily basis.

Rufinamide, a triazole derivative, exerts its mechanism of action through modulation of the voltage-gated sodium channel, prolonging its inactivated state.[13] It has shown a broad spectrum of action in animal studies.[14] In clinical studies, it was effective in reducing the frequency of "drop attacks" (tonic or atonic seizures) and the total number of seizures in patients with Lennox-Gastaut syndrome.[15] Efficacy as adjunctive therapy in partial-onset seizures was modest.[16–18] Rufinamide did not receive approval from the FDA for use in partial seizures.

Rufinamide has a relatively favorable pharmacokinetic profile.[13] Its absorption after oral administration is complete at lower doses, but gradually decreases with doses higher than 1600 mg/day. It has low protein binding and a half-life of 6 to 10 hours. Rufinamide is eliminated almost completely by hydrolysis and carboxylation, independently of the cytochrome P-450 enzymatic system. It has no active metabolites and its pharmacokinetics is not significantly altered by renal insufficiency. Hemodialysis may reduce the exposure of rufinamide by about 30%. Rufinamide has a few but potentially significant drug-drug interactions as shown in **Table 2**. Caution is recommended with the concomitant use of valproate, a commonly used drug in Lennox-Gastaut syndrome, especially in children. The increase in phenytoin levels seems modest but it can be significant given the nonlinear pharmacokinetics of this drug. Rufinamide

| Table 2 Rufinamide | |
|---|---|
| Primary indication | Lennox-Gastaut syndrome |
| Mechanism of action | Prolongation of the inactivated state of the voltage-gated sodium channel |
| Oral bioavalability | 85% at 600 mg/d<br>Bioavailability decreases with increases in the dose |
| Time to peak concentration ($T_{max}$) | 4–6 h<br>Food increases absorption but, does not change the $T_{max}$ |
| Half-life | 6–10 h |
| Metabolism and excretion | Extensively metabolized by carboxylesterases. Metabolism independent of CYP P-450. No active metabolites.<br>About 2% excreted unchanged in the urine. |
| Drug interactions | Enzyme inducers[a] reduce rufinamide levels by 13.7%–46.3%. Valproate may increase rufinamide levels up to 70%, especially in children.<br>Rufinamide may increase phenytoin levels by 21%.<br>Rufinamide may produce a modest increase in the metabolism of oral contraceptives. |
| Protein binding | 34% |
| Dosing | 400–1600 mg twice daily |
| Dosage forms and strengths | Tablets: 200, 400 mg<br>Oral solution: 40 mg/mL |
| Side effects | Somnolence, dizziness, headache, nausea/vomiting, fatigue, shortening of the QT interval, multiorgan hypersensitivity |

[a] Enzyme inducers: carbamazepine, phenytoin, phenobarbital.

may induce the metabolism of oral contraceptives. A dose of 1600 mg for 2 weeks resulted in a mean decrease in the ethinyl estradiol and norethindrone area under the curve (AUC) of 22% and 14%, respectively.

In a well-designed clinical trial in patients with Lennox-Gastaut syndrome aged 4 to 30 years, rufinamide significantly reduced the median frequency of seizures compared with placebo (32.7% vs 11.7%; $P = .0015$).[15] The reduction in the median frequency of "drop attacks" was even more robust, with a 42.5% reduction in the rufinamide group versus a 1.4% increase in the placebo group ($P = .0001$). Most common side effects were somnolence and vomiting.

A mild shortening of the QT interval (up to 20 milliseconds) was observed with rufinamide use, and the drug should not be used in patients with familial short QT syndrome. Rare cases of hypersensitivity reaction have been reported.

Rufinamide can be started in children at a dose of 10 mg/kg in two divided doses and gradually increased up to a maximal dose of 45 mg/kg or 3200 mg/day. Adults may be started on 400 to 800 mg/day in two divided doses and increased to a maximum of 3200 mg/day.

### Ezogabine/Retigabine

Ezogabine (US adopted name, Potiga), known internationally by the nonproprietary name retigabine, is a new AED approved for adjunctive therapy for partial-onset seizures in patients aged 18 years and older. Its anticonvulsant properties were found by structural manipulation of the flupertine molecule, a nonopioid analgesic with weak anticonvulsant properties. It is a first-in-class potassium channel opener, with a mechanism of action different than other AEDs. Ezogabine stabilizes in the open position the voltage-gated potassium channels (Kv7.2-Kv7.5; corresponding genes KCNQ2-KCNQ5), decreasing neuronal hyperexcitability by membrane hyperpolarization.[19]

Ezogabine has a favorable pharmacokinetic profile (**Table 3**). It is rapidly absorbed after oral administration with peak levels in about 1.5 hours. It has negligible protein binding and a relatively short half-life of 7 to 11 hours. Ezogabine is metabolized to a monoacetylated derivative (NAMR), which is biologically active.[20] The elimination of ezogabine is mainly through renal excretion, with 36% of an oral dose recovered in the urine as unchanged parent drug and 18% as NAMR. In patients with moderate to severe renal impairment (creatinine clearance <50 mL/min) dose adjustments are probably necessary. There is also a significant increase in the exposure of ezogabine in the presence of moderate or severe liver failure. Ezogabine has no significant effect on the pharmacokinetics of other AEDs and does not affect the metabolism of oral contraceptive ethinyl estradiol/norgestrel. Phenytoin and carbamazepine moderately decrease the exposure of ezogabine. More importantly, ezogabine may increase digoxin levels through an NAMR-mediated, concentration-dependent inhibition of the P-glycoprotein–mediated digoxin transport. Crystals with a bilirubin-like appearance are detected in the serum and urine of patients receiving ezogabine. This may result in discoloration or turbidity of the urine; it may also produce a false elevation of bilirubin levels in serum or urine caused by interference with laboratory essays.

Ezogabine demonstrated efficacy as adjunctive therapy in partial-onset seizures in three well-designed clinical trials.[21–23] Daily doses of 900 and 1200 mg, in three equally divided doses, were statistically superior to placebo in achieving a median percent reduction in monthly seizure frequency. A daily dose of 600 mg showed a statistically significant difference in one study[22] but not in another.[21] The most commonly adverse events leading to drug discontinuation in the clinical trials included dizziness,

| Table 3 Ezogabine (retigabine) | |
| --- | --- |
| Primary indication | Partial (focal) seizures |
| Mechanism of action | Enhances transmembrane potassium currents mediated by the Kv7.2 to 7.5 (KCNQ) family of ion channels |
| Oral bioavalability | 60% Food slows the rate of absorption but not the extent. |
| Time to peak concentration ($T_{max}$) | 0.5–2 h |
| Half-life | 7–11 h |
| Metabolism and excretion | Extensively metabolized; acetylation (NAT2) and glucuronidation (mainly UTG1A4). Main metabolite (NAMR) is biologically active but less potent. CYP P-450 not involved in metabolism of ezogabine. |
| Drug interactions | Ezogabine may increase digoxin serum concentrations. Phenytoin and carbamazepine may reduce exposure of ezogabine. Alcohol ingestion enhances exposure of ezogabine |
| Protein binding | <15% |
| Dosing | 200–400 mg 3 times daily |
| Dosage forms and strengths | Tablets: 50, 200, 300, 400 mg |
| Side effects | Dizziness, somnolence, confusion, psychosis, hallucinations, urinary retention, prolongation of QT interval. |

somnolence, headache, fatigue, confusion, dysarthria, and urinary tract infection. Most of these adverse events were dose-dependent. Hallucinations and psychosis have been reported in about 2% of patients. Urinary retention was observed in 29 of 1365 patients (approximately 2%) during the clinical trials, with five of them requiring catheterization. This effect is likely caused by an ezogabine effect on bladder potassium channels (mainly $K_v7.4$, and to a lesser extent $K_v7.1$ and $K_v7.5$).[24]

Ezogabine is usually started at a dose of 100 mg three times daily, and the dose gradually increased in weekly intervals until a total daily dose of 600 to 900 mg is reached in 4 to 6 weeks. The maximal approved total daily dose by the FDA is 1200 mg. A more conservative dosing is recommended in the elderly or in patients with a heavy medication load.

## Perampanel

Perampanel was approved by the FDA in 2012 for adjunctive use of partial-onset seizures in patients aged 12 years and older. Perampanel is an orally active, highly selective, noncompetitive AMPA receptor antagonist. Glutamate is the main excitatory neurotransmitter in the brain and plays an important role in the generation and spread of seizures. Glutamate receptors are found in excitatory synapses and can be divided into ionotropic and metabotropic. There are three types of ionotropic receptors: (1) AMPA, (2) N-methyl-D-aspartate, and (3) kainate. AMPA receptors play an essential role in the generation of physiologic excitatory postsynaptic potentials and in the pathologic paroxysmal depolarization shift observed in epileptic neurons.[25] AMPA receptors seem to be also involved in the development and expression of amygdala kindling in animal models of epilepsy.[26] Perampanel inhibits the AMPA-induced increases in free calcium ion concentrations in cortical neurons, reducing neuronal excitability.[27]

Perampanel has a favorable pharmacokinetic profile (**Table 4**). It is well absorbed after oral administration.[28] It is highly bound to serum proteins (95%–96%), mainly albumin and $\alpha_1$-acid glycoprotein. Perampanel is extensively metabolized by oxidation and subsequent glucuronidation. Oxidative metabolism is primarily mediated by

| Table 4 Perampanel | |
| --- | --- |
| Primary indication | Partial (focal) seizures |
| Mechanism of action | Selective, noncompetitive (allosteric) AMPA-type glutamate receptor antagonist |
| Oral bioavalability | Complete |
| Time to peak concentration ($T_{max}$) | 1 h (0.5–2.5). Food slows the rate of absorption, but not the extent. |
| Half-life | 66–90 h |
| Metabolism and excretion | Extensively metabolized by oxidation and glucuronidation (CYP 3A4 and 3A5). No active metabolites. |
| Drug interactions | Carbamazepine and phenytoin reduce the exposure of perampanel. A dose of 12 mg/day of perampanel reduces the exposure of levonorgestrel by approximately 40% |
| Protein binding | 95% |
| Dosing | 4–12 mg once daily |
| Dosage forms and strengths | Tablets: 2, 4, 6, 8, 10, 12 mg |
| Side effects | Somnolence, dizziness, fatigue, vertigo, ataxia, weight gain, irritability, hostility, aggression |

CYP3A4 with a minor contribution from CYP3A5. The mean half-life is 105 hours allowing for a once-daily dose. Perampanel accumulates in the presence of liver failure and dose adjustments may be necessary. A 1.8-fold and 3.3-fold increase in the AUC of free perampanel in mild and moderate liver failure, respectively, was found compared with healthy control subjects. Mild renal failure does not affect the disposition of perampanel significantly and dose adjustments are not necessary. Perampanel disposition has not been formally studied in moderate or severe renal insufficiency. Perampanel has a favorable drug interaction profile. Enzyme inducers, such as phenytoin and carbamazepine, reduce the exposure of perampanel, reducing the AUC approximately in half. CYP3A4 inhibitors, such as rifampin or St. John's wort, may prolong the elimination of perampanel. A dose of perampanel of 12 mg/day for 21 days resulted in a decrease in the $C_{max}$ and AUC of levonorgestrel of 42% and 40%, respectively. No significant effect on oral contraceptives metabolism was seen at doses of 4 and 8 mg/day.

Three phase III studies provide class I evidence that perampanel, at doses of 4 to 12 mg, is effective and well tolerated as adjunctive therapy in patients with refractory focal seizures.[29-31] Combined results of the trials showed a median percent reduction in the frequency of monthly seizures of about 14%, 23%, 29%, and 26.5% for the placebo, perampanel 4-mg, 8-mg, and 12-mg groups, respectively. The percent of patients achieving a greater than or equal to 50% reduction in seizure frequency was 20%, 28.5%, 35%, and 35% for the placebo, perampanel 4-mg, 8-mg, and 12-mg groups, respectively. Doses of 2 mg/day were not effective.[31] A clear dose-response curve was observed between doses of 4 and 8 mg, with the 12-mg dose apparently providing no clear added efficacy. However, a trend toward more patients achieving a greater than or equal to 75% or a 100% seizure reduction on 12 mg/day of perampanel was observed in one study, suggesting that some patients may obtain an additional benefit.[30] The overall efficacy and tolerability of perampanel was maintained after 1 year.[32] Most common adverse effects reported in the clinical trials included dizziness, somnolence, fatigue, irritability, ataxia, falls, and headache. With the exception of headache, side effects were dose-dependent. The package insert of perampanel includes a boxed warning for "serious psychiatric and behavioral reactions including aggression, hostility, irritability, anger, and homicidal ideation and threats..." Most common psychiatric adverse events observed in the clinical trials are shown in **Table 5**.

**Table 5**
**Psychiatric and behavioral side effects of perampanel**

|  | Placebo n = 442% | Perampanel | | |
|---|---|---|---|---|
|  |  | 4 mg n = 172% | 8 mg n = 431% | 12 mg n = 255% |
| Irritability | 3 | 4 | 7 | 12 |
| Anxiety | 1 | 2 | 3 | 4 |
| Aggression | 1 | 1 | 2 | 3 |
| Anger | <1 | 0 | 1 | 3 |
| Confusional state | <1 | 1 | 1 | 2 |
| Euphoric mood | 0 | 0 | <1 | 2 |
| Mood altered | <1 | 1 | <1 | 2 |

Adverse reactions in pooled double-blind trials in patients with partial-onset seizures. Reactions ≥2% of patients in 12 mg-perampanel group.

Perampanel can be administered once daily given its prolonged half-life. A starting dose of 2 mg/day at bedtime is recommended. Patients comedicated with enzyme-inducing drugs may be started at 4 mg/day. Daily dose may be increased by 2 mg at weekly intervals until a dose of 4 to 8 mg is achieved. A maximal dose of 12 mg has been approved by the FDA.

## NEUROSTIMULATION
### Electrical Stimulation of the Anterior Nucleus of the Thalamus

The anterior nucleus of the thalamus is connected to several structures that are commonly involved in seizures. It receives projections from the hippocampus, mostly arising from the subiculum, by way of the fornix → mammillary bodies → mammillo-thalamic tract (Vicq d'Azyr bundle), and has efferent connections to the cingulate cortex and entorhinal cortex. Stimulation of the anterior nucleus inhibits chemically induced seizures in animal models.[33-35] Pioneer studies by Cooper and Upton[36] in humans in the 1980s demonstrated a reduction in seizure frequency and electroencephalogram spikes in five of six patients undergoing chronic bilateral stimulation. Several other unblinded, pilot studies have demonstrated positive effects of anterior nucleus stimulation in patients with intractable epilepsy, with an average reduction in the frequency of seizures of approximately 50%.[37-42]

A positive multicenter, double-blind, randomized trial of bilateral electrical stimulation of the anterior nuclei of the thalamus (SANTE study; Medtronic, Minneapolis, MN) has been completed in patients with focal epilepsy.[6] The device used is similar to the one used for DBS in patients with Parkinson disease. The stimulating leads are placed stereotactically in both anterior nuclei. The two pulse generators are contained in one device unit that is implanted subcutaneously in one side of the chest. The pattern of stimulation used in epilepsy, however, differs from the one used in movements disorders in that it is intermittent rather than continuous. A total of 110 patients with medically refractory partial seizures, including secondarily generalized seizures, were randomized.[6] Half received stimulation and the other half did not during a 3-month blinded phase. After 3 months, all patients received unblinded stimulation. In the last month of the blinded phase the stimulated group had a 29% greater reduction in seizures than the placebo group ($P = .002$). By 2 years, there was a 56% median percent reduction of seizures, 54% of patients had a greater than or equal to 50% reduction in seizure frequency, and 14 subjects were seizure free for at least 6 months. By 5 years, 69% of patients had a greater than or equal to 50% reduction in seizure frequency, median reduction in seizure frequency was also 69%, and 16% of patients were seizure free for at least 6 months.[43] Side effects reported more frequently in the stimulation group included depression and memory loss. Five deaths were observed during the study, none attributed directly to the procedure.[6] Five patients (4.5%) had intracranial hemorrhage detected by neuroimaging, but none were symptomatic. Implant site infection was found in 14 subjects (12.7%), but none involved brain parenchyma. Acute, transient worsening of seizures related to the stimulation was observed in two patients.

As a result of the SANTE trial, anterior thalamic stimulation for the treatment of focal and secondarily generalized seizures has been approved for clinical use in Canada and the European Union. It remains investigational in the United States.

### Responsive Neurostimulation

The ability of electrical stimulation to suppress epileptiform discharges was elegantly demonstrated by Penfield and Jasper[44] in their studies on direct cortical stimulation in humans in the 1950s. With the widespread use of intracranial recordings and bedside cortical stimulation for the evaluation of candidates for epilepsy surgery, the possibility of aborting a seizure by applying direct electrical stimulation on the seizure focus could be tested. A closed-loop system with software designed to detect spontaneous seizures and automatically respond with electrical stimulation was successfully developed.[45,46] As a result, an implantable, programmable system (Responsive Neurostimulator System; Neuro Pace, Mountain View, CA) was designed for chronic use for the treatment of focal seizures.[47] The system's operation is analogous to the feedback control in automatic implantable cardiac defibrillators. The device is implanted in the skull and is connected to one or two intracranial depth or strip electrodes, each with one to four contacts. Seizure detection is achieved by three configurable detection algorithms that are tailored to the patient's individual ictal electrographic pattern. The stimulation is also adjustable in terms of frequency and amplitude.

A large multicenter trial using the Responsive Neurostimulation System was completed recently.[7] A total of 191 patients with medically intractable partial epilepsy were implanted. One month after implantation, patients were randomized 1:1 to either stimulation (treatment) or no-stimulation (sham) groups. Safety and efficacy were assessed during a 12-week blinded period followed by and 84-week open-label period during which all patients received stimulation. There was a 37.9% mean reduction in seizure frequency in the treatment group versus a 17.3% reduction in the sham group ($P = .012$). In the third month of stimulation the difference was more pronounced with a 41.5% and 9.4% reduction in the treatment and sham groups, respectively ($P = .008$). There was no difference between the groups in reported adverse events. The therapeutic effect was sustained. At 1 year the mean reduction in seizure frequency and the percent of patients achieving a greater than or equal to 50% reduction in seizure frequency was 44% each; at 2 years it was 53% and 55%, respectively. There was significant improvement in the quality of life scales and no evidence of deterioration in mood or neuropsychological function. Overall rate of intracranial hemorrhage was 4.7% (9 of 191 subjects). Of those nine cases, two-thirds were related to the procedure itself (three epidural hematomas, two intraparenchymal hemorrhages, and one subdural hematoma). The other three cases were seizure-related traumatic subdural hematomas. Implant or incision infection was observed in 5.2% of subjects (40% of which required explantation of the system). There were no infections of the brain or skull.

Overall, these results are fairly similar to those of the anterior nucleus of the thalamus trial, both in terms of efficacy and safety. Responsive neurostimulation, as opposed to DBS, requires a precise localization of the seizure focus or foci. Candidates include patients that have undergone an invasive evaluation with intracranial electrodes for epilepsy surgery and are deemed poor candidates for a resection. Potential scenarios include a discreet seizure focus in an eloquent cortical area or two bilateral independent foci (eg, in patients with bilateral mesial temporal sclerosis).[48] For obvious reasons the use of this device is limited to tertiary epilepsy centers.

### External Trigeminal Stimulation

External trigeminal nerve stimulation has reduced seizure frequency in patients with drug-resistant epilepsy in an open-label trial, with an efficacy similar to that of vagus nerve stimulation.[49] A technique that allows for external (noninvasive) trigeminal stimulation (TNS; Neuro Sigma, Westwood, CA) is currently under investigation. A subcutaneous implantable device has also been evaluated by the same manufacturer. The external device provides bilateral stimulation of the supraorbitary nerves by using a removable helmet. Recently, positive results were observed in a phase II, randomized, double-blind, active-control trial in patients with drug-resistant epilepsy.[50] Subjects were randomized to active treatment (eTNS, 120 Hz) or control (eTNS, 2 Hz). Subjects in the active treatment group experienced a significant improvement in the responder rate ($\geq$50% reduction in the frequency of seizures) during the 18-week acute treatment period (responder rate 40.5% at 18 weeks vs 17.8% at 6 weeks; $P = .01$). At all times during the study the treatment group showed a statistically significant improvement compared with the control group. External trigeminal stimulation may prove a useful device for the treatment of refractory epilepsy, and potentially a predictor of outcome for other forms of neurostimulation.

## SUMMARY

Epilepsy affects about 70 million people worldwide. Despite recent advances in therapy, about a third of these patients continue to have seizures. Newer, innovative approaches to the treatment of epilepsy are still greatly needed.

New AEDs have been introduced in the past 5 years, some with novel mechanisms of action. Lacosamide, ezogabine (retigabine), and perampanel are indicated for the treatment of partial seizures as adjunctive therapy. Rufinamide has shown efficacy in reducing drop attacks (tonic and atonic seizures) in patients with Lennox-Gastaut syndrome. Overall efficacy of these agents seems similar to other AEDs currently being used, although comparative trials are not available.

Neurostimulation, with the development of a variety of different devices and targets of stimulation, is a rapidly evolving field and will likely play an important role in management of severe epilepsy. For several years vagus nerve stimulation played an important role in the palliative management of intractable seizures. DBS of the anterior nucleus of the thalamus and responsive neurostimulation have shown good efficacy and tolerability in well-designed clinical trials. The efficacy of these therapies is slightly superior to that of vagus nerve stimulation, but the potential for serious complications is much higher. The indication for these techniques, in terms of patient selection and timing, still remains unclear and more research is needed to make solid evidence-based decisions. External (noninvasive) trigeminal stimulation seems promising not only as a therapy per se but also as a potential predictor of outcome. With other modalities of neurostimulation, such as hippocampal stimulation, occipital stimulation, and transcranial magnetic stimulation in advanced stages of investigation, it is clear that neurostimulation is a rapidly expanding and, it is hoped, promising field for patients with epilepsy.

## REFERENCES

1. Ngugi AK, Kariuki SM, Bottomley C, et al. Incidence of epilepsy: a systematic review and meta-analysis. Neurology 2011;77:1005–12.
2. Kwan P, Brodie MJ. Early identification of refractory epilepsy. N Engl J Med 2000;342:314–9.
3. Brodie MJ, Barry SJ, Bamagous GA, et al. Patterns of treatment response in newly diagnosed epilepsy. Neurology 2012;78:1548–54.
4. Löscher W, Schmidt D. Modern antiepileptic drug development has failed to deliver: ways out of the current dilemma. Epilepsia 2011;52:657–78.
5. Cooper IS, Amin I, Riklan M, et al. The effect of chronic cerebellar stimulation upon epilepsy in man. Trans Am Neurol Assoc 1973;98:192–6.
6. Fisher R, Salanova V, Witt T, et al. Electrical stimulation of the anterior nucleus of thalamus for treatment refractory epilepsy. Epilepsia 2010;51:899–908.

7. Morrell MJ, RNS System in Epilepsy Study Group. Responsive cortical stimulation for the treatment of medically intractable partial epilepsy. Neurology 2011; 77:1295–304.
8. Elliot RE, Morsi A, Kalhorn SP, et al. Vagus nerve stimulation in 436 consecutive patients with treatment-resistant epilepsy: long-term outcomes and predictors of response. Epilepsy Behav 2011;20:57–63.
9. Errington AC, Stöhr T, Heers C, et al. The investigational anticonvulsant lacosamide selectively enhances slow inactivation of voltage-gated sodium channels. Mol Pharmacol 2008;73:157–69.
10. Ben-Menachem E, Biton V, Jatuzis D, et al. Efficacy and safety of oral lacosamide as adjunctive therapy in adults with partial-onset seizures. Epilepsia 2007;48:1308–17.
11. Halász P, Kälviäinen R, Mazurkiewicz-Beldzińska M, et al. Adjunctive lacosamide for partial-onset seizures: efficacy and safety results from a randomized controlled trial. Epilepsia 2009;50:443–53.
12. Chung S, Sperling M, Biton V, et al. Lacosamide: efficacy and safety as oral adjunctive treatment in adults with partial-onset seizures [abstract 3.197]. Presented at the American Epilepsy Society Annual Meeting. Philadelphia, December 3, 2007.
13. Perucca E, Cloyd J, Critchley D, et al. Rufinamide: clinical pharmacokinetics and concentration-response relationships in patients with epilepsy. Epilepsia 2008;49:1123–41.
14. White HS, Franklin MR, Kupferberg HJ, et al. The anticonvulsant profile of rufinamide (CGP 33101) in rodent seizure models. Epilepsia 2008;49:1213–20.
15. Glauser T, Kluger G, Sachdeo R, et al. Rufinamide for generalized seizures associated with the Lennox-Gastaut syndrome. Neurology 2008;70:1950–8.
16. Brodie MJ, Rosenfeldt WE, Vázquez B, et al. Rufinamide for the adjunctive treatment of partial seizures in adults and adolescents. Epilepsia 2009;50: 1899–909.
17. Palhagen S, Canger R, Henriksen O, et al. Rufinamide: a double-blind, placebo-controlled proof of principle trial in patients with epilepsy. Epilepsy Res 2001;43: 115–24.
18. Cheng-Hakimian A, Anderson GD, Miller JW. Rufinamide: pharmacology, clinical trials, and role in clinical practice. Int J Clin Pract 2006;60(11):1497–501.
19. Gunthorpe MJ, Large CH, Sankar R. The mechanism of action of retigabine (ezogabine), a first-in-class K+ channel opener for the treatment of epilepsy. Epilepsia 2012;53(3):412–24.
20. Hempel R, Schupke H, McNeilly PJ, et al. Metabolism of retigabine (D-23129), a novel anticonvulsant. Drug Metab Dispos 1999;27:613–22.
21. Porter RJ, Partiot A, Sachdeo R, et al. Randomized, multicenter, dose-ranging trial of retigabine for partial-onset seizures. Neurology 2007;68:1197–204.
22. Brodie MJ, Lerche H, Gil-Nagel A, et al. Efficacy and safety of adjunctive ezogabine (retigabine) in refractory partial epilepsy. Neurology 2010;75:1817–24.
23. French JA, Abou-Khalil BW, Leroy RF, et al. Randomized, double-blind, placebo-controlled trial of ezogabine (retigabine) in partial epilepsy. Neurology 2011;76:1555–63.
24. Brickel N, Gandhi P, VanLandingham K, et al. The urinary safety profile and secondary renal effects of retigabine (ezogabine): a first-in-class antiepileptic drug that targets KCNQ (Kv7) potassium channels. Epilepsia 2012;53(4): 606–12.
25. Uchida K. Excitatory amino acid receptors appear to mediate paroxysmal depolarizing shifts in rat neocortical neurons in vitro. Brain Res 1992;577:151–4.

26. Rogawski MA, Kurzman PS, Yamaguchi SI, et al. Role of AMPA and GluR5 kainate receptors in the development and expression of amygdale kindling in the mouse. Neuropharmacology 2001;40:28–35.

27. Hanada T, Hashizume Y, Tokuhara N, et al. Perampanel: a novel, orally active, noncompetitive AMPA-receptor antagonist that reduces seizure activity in rodent models of epilepsy. Epilepsia 2011;52(7):1331–40.

28. Templeton D. Pharmacokinetics of perampanel, a highly selective AMPA-type glutamate receptor antagonist following once- and multiple-daily dosing [abstract]. Epilepsia 2010;51(Suppl 4):70.

29. French JA, Krauss GL, Biton V, et al. Adjunctive perampanel for refractory partial-onset seizures: randomized phase III study 304. Neurology 2012;79: 589–96.

30. French JA, Krauss GL, Steinhoff BJ, et al. Evaluation of adjunctive perampanel in patients with refractory partial-onset seizures: results of randomized global phase III study 305. Epilepsia 2013;54(1):117–25.

31. Krauss GL, Serratosa JM, Villanueva V, et al. Randomized phase III study 306: adjunctive perampanel for refractory partial-onset seizures. Neurology 2012;78: 1408–15.

32. Krauss GL, Perucca E, Ben-Menachem E, et al. Perampanel, a selective, noncompetitive α-amino-3-hydroxy-5-methyl-4-isoxazolepropionic acid receptor antagonist, as adjunctive therapy for refractory partial-onset seizures: interim results from phase III, extension study 307. Epilepsia 2013;54(1):126–34.

33. Mirski MA, Rossell LA, Terry JB, et al. Anticonvulsant effect of anterior thalamic high frequency electrical stimulation in the rat. Epilepsy Res 1997;28: 89–100.

34. Takebayashi S, Hashizume K, Tanaka T, et al. The effect of electrical stimulation and lesioning of the anterior thalamic nucleus on kainic acid-induced focal cortical seizure status in rats. Epilepsia 2007;48:348–58.

35. Takebayashi S, Hashizume K, Tanaka T, et al. Anticonvulsant effect of electrical stimulation and lesioning of the anterior thalamic nucleus on kainic acid-induced focal limbic seizures in rats. Epilepsy Res 2007;74:163–70.

36. Cooper IS, Upton AR. The effect of chronic stimulation of cerebellum and thalamus upon neurophysiology and neurochemistry of cerebral cortex. In: Lazorthes Y, Upton AR, editors. Neurostimulation: an overview. New York: Futura; 1985. p. 207–11.

37. Sussman NM, Goldman HW, Jackel A, et al. Anterior thalamic stimulation in medically intractable epilepsy. Part II. Preliminary clinical results. Epilepsia 1988;29:677.

38. Hodaie M, Wennberg RA, Dostrovsky JO, et al. Chronic anterior thalamus stimulation for intractable epilepsy. Epilepsia 2002;43:603–8.

39. Kerrigan JF, Litt B, Fisher RS, et al. Electrical stimulation of the anterior nucleus of the thalamus for the treatment of intractable epilepsy. Epilepsia 2004;45: 346–54.

40. Lee KJ, Jang KS, Shon YM. Chronic deep brain stimulation of subthalamic and anterior thalamic nuclei for controlling refractory partial epilepsy. Acta Neurochir Suppl 2006;99:87–91.

41. Lim SN, Lee ST, Tsai YT, et al. Electrical stimulation of the anterior nucleus of the thalamus for intractable epilepsy: a long-term follow-up study. Epilepsia 2007; 48:342–7.

42. Osorio I, Overman J, Giftakis J, et al. High frequency thalamic stimulation for inoperable mesial temporal epilepsy. Epilepsia 2007;48:1561–71.

43. Salanova V, Fisher R, SANTE Study Group. Long term efficacy of the SANTE trial (stimulation of the anterior nucleus of the thalamus for epilepsy) [abstract 1.272]. Presented at the American Epilepsy Society Annual Meeting. San Diego (CA), December 1, 2012.

44. Penfield W, Jasper H. Electrocorticography. In: Penfield W, Jasper H, editors. Epilepsy and the functional anatomy of the human brain. Boston: Little, Brown; 1954. p. 692–738.

45. Kossoff EH, Ritzl EK, Politsky JM, et al. Effect of an external responsive neurostimulation on seizures and electrographic discharges during subdural electrode monitoring. Epilepsia 2004;45:1560–7.

46. Osorio I, Frei MG, Sunderam S, et al. Automated seizure abatement in humans using electrical stimulation. Ann Neurol 2005;57:258–68.

47. Sun FT, Morrell MJ, Wharen RE Jr. Responsive cortical stimulation for the treatment of epilepsy. Neurotherapeutics 2008;5:68–74.

48. Miller JW. Responsive cortical stimulation: the 21% solution? Epilepsy Curr 2012;12(3):97–8.

49. DeGiorgio CM, Murray D, Markovic D, et al. Trigeminal nerve stimulation for epilepsy: long-term feasibility and efficacy. Neurology 2009;72:936–8.

50. DeGiorgio C, Soss J, Cook I, et al. Phase II double blind randomized controlled trial of trigeminal nerve stimulation in 50 subjects with drug resistant epilepsy [abstract 1.040]. Presented at the American Epilepsy Society Annual Meeting. San Diego (CA), December 1, 2012.

# Surgical Treatment of Parkinson Disease: Past, Present, and Future

Andrew P. Duker, MD*, Alberto J. Espay, MD, MSc

## KEYWORDS

- Parkinson disease • Deep brain stimulation • Patient selection
- Beta band oscillations

## KEY POINTS

- The surgical treatment of Parkinson disease (PD) has progressed from destructive and lesional procedures to focused and targeted brain stimulation.
- The effects of deep brain stimulation (DBS) typically mirror the benefits of levodopa, however with the benefit of reducing motor fluctuations and off time, as well as decreasing dyskinesia.
- The 2 main targets for DBS in PD, the subthalamic nucleus (STN) and internal segment of the globus pallidus (GPi), appear to give similar outcomes, although individual patient factors and surgeon expertise may be important.
- Developing concepts in DBS, including closed loop paradigms and segmented electrodes, promise to further refine this therapy.

## INTRODUCTION

The surgical treatment of Parkinson disease (PD) has evolved sporadically over the past century. Early attempts at relieving parkinsonian symptoms included bilateral posterior cervical rhizotomy by Leriche in 1912[1] and later by others in an attempt to improve rigidity and tremor. Later surgeries focused on interruption of the pyramidal tracts (motor cortex,[2] cervical spinal cord,[3] and cerebral peduncle).[4] Surgery on the

Disclosures: Dr Duker has nothing to disclose. Dr Espay is supported by the K23 career development award (NIMH, 1K23MH092735); has received grant support from CleveMed/Great Lakes Neurotechnologies and Michael J Fox Foundation; personal compensation as a consultant/scientific advisory board member for Solvay (Abbot/Abbvie), Chelsea Therapeutics, TEVA, Impax, Merz, Solstice Neurosciences, Eli Lilly, and USWorldMeds; and honoraria from Novartis, UCB, TEVA, the American Academy of Neurology, and the Movement Disorders Society. He serves as Associate Editor of Movement Disorders and Frontiers in Movement Disorders and is on the editorial board of The European Neurologic Journal.
Department of Neurology and Rehabilitation Medicine, James J. and Joan A. Gardner Center for Parkinson's Disease and Movement Disorders, University of Cincinnati Neuroscience Institute, University of Cincinnati, 260 Stetson Street, Suite 2300, Cincinnati, OH 45267-0525, USA
* Corresponding author.
E-mail address: Andrew.Duker@uc.edu

basal ganglia for PD, particularly the pallidofugal fibers, was initially explored by Meyers in 1951,[5] and given support by the favorable outcome on a parkinsonian patient whose anterior choroidal artery was serendipitously ligated by Cooper when performing a pedunculotomy.[6] With the advent of stereotactic surgery, reports by Spiegel and colleagues[7] and others on the benefits of pallidotomy began to surface, and eventually thalamotomy was found to reduce parkinsonian tremor. In the 1960s, levodopa was found to dramatically improve the symptoms of PD[8] and there was a temporary hiatus in the surgical treatment of PD. Despite the profound efficacy of levodopa, complications, such as dyskinesias and motor fluctuations, prompted a renewed interest in the surgical treatment of PD in the early 1990s, primarily through the previously used lesional surgeries. Although stimulation of the deep structures of the brain had been performed previously,[9] the modern era of chronic deep brain stimulation (DBS) was led by the reports of Benabid and colleagues,[10] first of the ventral intermediate nucleus of the thalamus (Vim), then later the subthalamic nucleus (STN)[11] and the internal segment of the globus pallidus (GPi).[12] Thalamic DBS was approved by the US Food and Drug Administration in 1997 for the treatment of tremor associated with essential tremor and PD, and STN and pallidal DBS in 2002 for the treatment of PD. In a short time, DBS became an established treatment for advanced PD. Evidence has accumulated supporting the long-term efficacy of DBS, and at the same time new technology has continued to refine the procedure.

**Case study**

A 66-year-old man presents to the Movement Disorders Center for evaluation and treatment of worsening symptoms from his PD. He had the onset of right-hand resting tremor at the age of 58 years, followed by micrographia, decreased dexterity when typing, then later slowness and shuffling of gait. He ultimately had good improvement with levodopa for several years. Over time, however, the duration of benefit from his medication doses shortened, and he required increasing doses of medication to obtain the same benefit. Adjunctive medications including a catechol-O-methyl transferase inhibitor, dopamine agonist, and a monoamine oxidase-B inhibitor yielded modest improvement, but motor fluctuations became progressively more difficult to control, alternating between "on" periods with good function and "off" periods marked by freezing of gait and near-immobility. Sleep was disrupted by painful off-period symptoms returning in the middle of the night. Moderate to severe dyskinesia complicated his functioning in the "on" periods, partially attenuated by the addition of amantadine. Depression was present but adequately treated with an antidepressant.

## PATIENT SELECTION

The Core Assessment Program for Intracerebral Transplantations (CAPIT) was developed and published in 1992,[13] in an attempt to standardize patient selection, inclusionary criteria, and reporting of outcomes in studies of intracerebral transplantation (originally, fetal dopamine neurons). This protocol was later updated and adapted to both ablative and neurostimulation procedures in the Core Assessment Program for Surgical Interventional Therapies (CAPSIT) protocol.[14] From this protocol, and with experience over time, a set of standardized evaluations have evolved, identifying candidates who will derive lasting benefits from the procedure, while being cognitively, emotionally, and socially prepared for DBS.[15] It is important for centers to evaluate patients in a standardized fashion to accurately identify those patients in whom the benefits of the surgery will outweigh the potential risks. A decision-making algorithm may be helpful (**Fig. 1**).

DBS performed in a patient with an atypical parkinsonism may not benefit and, in fact, may accelerate the symptomatic decline of these conditions.[16] Therefore, a

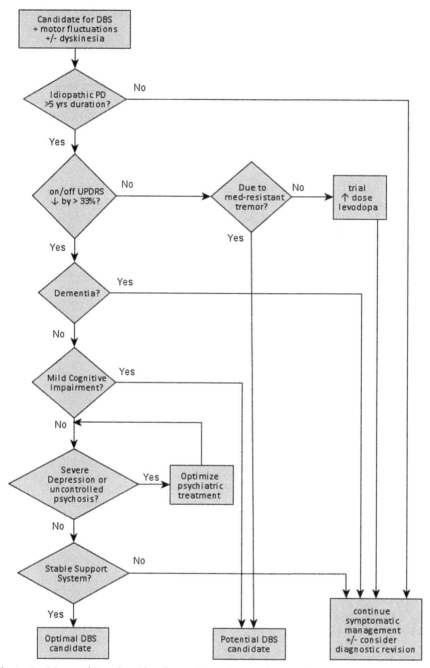

**Fig. 1.** Decision-making algorithm for patient selection for DBS surgery in PD.

diagnosis of idiopathic PD is a prerequisite for consideration of functional neurosurgery. Disability that requires consideration for DBS after a disease duration of 5 years or less suggests the presence of a PD mimic, most often an atypical parkinsonism, such as the parkinsonian variant of multiple system atrophy. A preoperative evaluation of levodopa responsiveness is mandatory, with a 33% decrease in the Unified Parkinson's Disease Rating Scale (UPDRS) part III motor score often suggested as the threshold beyond which surgical benefits materialize. DBS mostly benefits symptoms that are improved with levodopa, with the possible exception of medication-resistant tremor (in which benefit from DBS may exceed that of medication). The presurgical evaluation helps to establish a patient's realistic expectations from surgery.

Preoperative cognitive assessments should be performed to exclude patients with dementia. In addition, behavioral assessments are necessary to identify significant depression, given the small but serious risk of attempted suicide reported in some cases.[17] Finally, a sufficient social support network is essential to help care for the patient during the postoperative and stimulation titration process, which can take several months.

An "appropriate DBS candidate" may come from 3 major categories. The previously mentioned case, a cognitively intact patient with idiopathic PD, good response to levodopa, but with motor fluctuations, including shortened duration of benefit from the medication and bothersome dyskinesia despite optimal medical management, should be considered for DBS. Alternatively, a patient with well-controlled PD except for medication-resistant tremor may also benefit from the procedure. Finally, patients with poor symptom control because of inability to tolerate adequate doses of levodopa may also benefit from surgical intervention. Except in the latter, less common scenario, response to levodopa remains the best predictor for surgical response, as magnitude of benefit to DBS matches but does not outperform that of levodopa response.

## SURGICAL TARGET SELECTION

Thalamic stimulation is effective at reducing tremor in PD, and although the benefit is sustained, Vim DBS does not address bradykinesia or other PD symptoms, which invariably progress over time.[18,19] Preferred targets include the STN and GPi, and the choice between them depends on individual patient factors and the experience of the surgeon. STN stimulation has consistently across studies been shown to allow for greater reduction in dopaminergic medication postoperatively. GPi stimulation is often more effective at reducing dyskinesia directly, unaccounted for by a reduction in dopaminergic medications. Although there is some suggestion that GPi DBS is "safer" from a neurocognitive standpoint,[20] leading some to suggest this target for cognitively impaired patients who are otherwise good candidates,[21] controlled clinical trials have not demonstrated significant cognitive differences in outcomes between the 2 targets.

## OPERATIVE PROCEDURE

The location of the surgical target is typically chosen preoperatively on magnetic resonance imaging (MRI) by the neurosurgeon, based on visual landmarks. Coregistration with a standardized brain atlas can also be used. Brain mapping software determines the 3-dimensional coordinates of the target, which can then be entered into a frame secured to the patient's skull. If a frameless system is used, the angle and depth of the target is calculated with respect to skull fiducial markers. After burr hole placement, a microelectrode is slowly passed along the trajectory, and the depth of the target is identified based on microelectrode recording. The stimulating macroelectrode is then placed (**Fig. 2**) and tested intraoperatively to verify the threshold for side effects (depending on the target, these can include paresthesias, muscle contraction, conjugate eye deviation, visual phosphenes). The macroelectrode is secured into

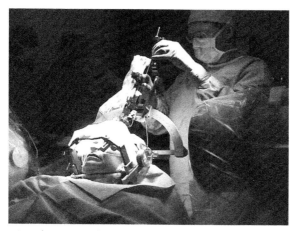

**Fig. 2.** Intraoperative placement of the DBS electrode.

position and the contralateral target is approached in a similar manner if a bilateral procedure is being performed. The electrodes are then connected to an implantable pulse generator (IPG), often in a separate procedure.

## POSTOPERATIVE PROGRAMING

Initial programing of the DBS stimulators often takes place several weeks after implantation, to permit the "lesion effect" of improved function following lead implantation to dissipate, allowing for easier identification of symptoms and improvements from stimulation. The quadripolar electrode has contacts spaced 1.5 mm or 0.5 mm apart depending on the lead used, and stimulation can be delivered in a monopolar (one active electrode contact as cathode with the IPG as anode) or bipolar (different electrode contacts used for both cathode and anode) fashion. The most effective electrode contact configuration gives the greatest benefit with the least amount of side effects due to current spread to surrounding structures. Stimulation amplitude is started at a low setting and increased gradually over time, which can allow for a reduction in medication. Programing optimization can take up to 4 to 6 months and may require multiple adjustment sessions.

## OUTCOMES

STN and GPi DBS have been shown in several randomized controlled clinical trials to be superior to medical management alone.[22–24] Patients receiving DBS gained on average 4.4 to 4.6 hours of "on" time without troublesome dyskinesia, had 1.0 to 2.6 fewer hours per day of "on" time with troublesome dyskinesia, and 2.4 to 4.2 fewer hours per day of "off" time. Quality of life, off-medication UPDRS motor scores, and sleep have also been reported to improve. Recent randomized trials comparing STN to GPi DBS showed no differences in motor function between groups, in both unilateral[25] and bilateral[26] stimulation. Given the similar outcome, it has been recommended that individual patient factors (eg, STN if greater medication reduction is desired, GPi if greater antidyskinetic effect is pursued) and surgeon preference dictate target selection. Another randomized trial did find a significant difference in motor scores as a secondary outcome favoring STN compared with GPi DBS, but no difference in the primary outcomes of functional health (disability score) or cognitive, mood, or behavioral effects.[27]

## DBS COMPLICATIONS

The incidence of serious adverse events related to DBS varies depending on the study. In 3 large multicenter trials,[24,26,27] intracranial or intracerebral hemorrhage occurred in 2% of patients, ischemic stroke in 0% to 1%, implantation site infection in 3% to 8%, and seizures in 0% to 3%. A postoperative confusional state was also seen in up to 21% in one of the trials,[26] although this required additional hospitalization in only 2%. Lead fracture and device malfunction are also possible complications, which can cause loss of clinical benefit.[28]

The prevalence of suicidal ideation may increase after DBS, with a multicenter retrospective survey finding a rate of 0.90% suicide attempts and 0.45% suicide completions.[29] Declines in cognition in longitudinal follow-up have been documented[30,31]; however, it remains unclear whether DBS hastens this decline. Smaller series initially suggested that DBS may have a negative impact on frontal executive functioning, in some patients leading to a "mental state comparable to progressive supranuclear palsy."[32] However, larger studies comparing patients receiving DBS to best medical management found overall cognitive scores (eg, Mattis dementia rating scale) to be similar, although found declines in verbal fluency (both semantic and phonemic), working memory, and processing speed.[23,33] Verbal fluency has been the most consistently decreased outcome following STN DBS across many studies and meta-analyses.[34]

## EMERGING CONCEPTS
### Axial Features of PD

Although DBS is very helpful in reducing motor fluctuations and dyskinesia, it may be less effective in treating certain axial symptoms, such as freezing of gait and falls, and, indeed, these symptoms are often less responsive to dopaminergic therapy as well. DBS of the pendunculopontine nucleus (PPN), known from animal research to be an important center for locomotion, has been studied as one treatment approach for these resistant symptoms. Thus far, data from only small open-label trials are available,[35–38] and although all of the trials reported improvement in duration of freezing and falls, blinded assessments in one trial[37] did not show improvements. Limiting factors in these studies were the small sample size (4–6 patients in each study) and the challenge of targeting a location that can be difficult to visualize on MRI sequences and does not as of yet have a clearly defined microelectrode recording signature. Further research is needed to determine if the PPN will fulfill the promise of a target to improve postural instability and other axial symptoms.

### Early Versus Late DBS

Although DBS is currently recommended for patients with PD with at least 5 years of disease duration and motor disability that does not improve with optimization of medication therapy, there has been growing interest in examining whether earlier implantation of DBS may be associated with larger and longer-lasting improvements in quality of life, before social and occupational activities are threatened.[39] A recent clinical trial of 251 patients with PD and "early" motor complications (after a mean disease duration of 7.5 years) randomized to STN DBS plus medical therapy or medical therapy alone, demonstrated greater quality of life, as measured by the Parkinson's Disease Questionnaire (PDQ-39), in the DBS plus medical therapy group after 2 years, compared with the medical therapy alone group.[40] However the definition of "early" has been subject to debate and the long-term efficacy (and potential disease modification) of earlier implantation remains unknown.

### Intermediate-Frequency Stimulation

High-frequency stimulation has long been held as the necessary mechanism for DBS-based improvement since it was first investigated.[10] Later research confirmed that stimulation frequencies more than 130 Hz were the most effective in the STN.[41] Frequencies less than 20 Hz appear to worsen bradykinesia,[41,42] but there is some evidence that frequencies in the 60-Hz to 80-Hz range could improve freezing and gait,[43] although the duration of this benefit may be transient.[44]

### Rate Versus Pattern of Neuronal Firing

Updated models of basal ganglia physiology suggest that motor benefit from DBS results from changes in the pattern of neuronal firing, particularly related to the synchronicity of intrinsic neuronal oscillations in the basal ganglia, rather than simple changes to the firing rate.[45] This synchronicity can manifest as an increase in the power of specific frequencies of local field potentials (LFPs) when recording from particular nuclei within the basal ganglia. In the STN and GPi, LFP oscillations in the beta band frequency (11–30 Hz) are associated with worsened motor function in the off-medication state,[46] and the power of these oscillations is attenuated by voluntary movement, and dopamine,[47,48] suggesting that the beta band may be "pathologic" in PD. It has been demonstrated that DBS also attenuates the beta band synchrony,[49] leading to research into "closed-loop" or adaptive DBS.[50] Suppression of oscillatory activity through a closed-loop paradigm was more effective than standard open-loop stimulation in controlling parkinsonian motor symptoms in the MPTP-treated African green monkey.[51] Other advances in DBS technology, such as segmented electrodes, may provide the ability to "steer" the direction of stimulation and shape the electrical field to better encompass desired structures but exclude spread to fibers contributing to side effects of stimulation.[52,53]

## SUMMARY

DBS surgery is a very effective treatment for the appropriately selected patient with PD and can afford decreased motor fluctuations, reduced "off" time, and improvement in dyskinesia. Outcomes for STN and GPi targets appear to be largely similar, and the choice of target is best made based on individual patient factors and surgeon preference. The inner workings of the basal ganglia, or the "dark basement" of the mind as Wilson referred to them,[54] are slowly yielding their secrets, led in large part by research based on surgically implanted patients. Adaptive, "closed-loop" DBS and new technologies, including segmented electrodes, may help to further refine and improve this procedure.

## REFERENCES

1. Leriche R. Ueber Chirurgischen Eingriff bei Parkinson's scher Krankheit. Neurologische Zeitblaetter 1912;13:1093–6.
2. Klemme RM. Surgical treatment of dystonia, paralysis agitans and athetosis. Arch Neurol Pysch 1940;44:926.
3. Putnam TJ. Relief from unilateral paralysis agitans by section of the pyramidal tract. Arch Neurol 1938;40:1049–50.
4. Walker AE. Cerebral pedunculotomy for the relief of involuntary movements. II. Parkinsonian tremor. J Nerv Ment Dis 1952;116(6):766–75.
5. Meyers R. Surgical experiments in the therapy of certain "extrapyramidal" diseases: a current evaluation. Acta Psychiatr Neurol Suppl 1951;67:1–42.

6. Cooper IS. Ligation of the anterior choroidal artery for involuntary movements; parkinsonism. Psychiatr Q 1953;27(2):317–9.
7. Spiegel EA, Wycis HT, Marks M, et al. Stereotaxic apparatus for operations on the human brain. Science 1947;106(2754):349–50.
8. Cotzias GC, Van Woert MH, Schiffer LM. Aromatic amino acids and modification of parkinsonism. N Engl J Med 1967;276(7):374–9.
9. Hariz MI, Blomstedt P, Zrinzo L. Deep brain stimulation between 1947 and 1987: the untold story. Neurosurg Focus 2010;29(2):E1.
10. Benabid AL, Pollak P, Louveau A, et al. Combined (thalamotomy and stimulation) stereotactic surgery of the VIM thalamic nucleus for bilateral Parkinson disease. Appl Neurophysiol 1987;50(1–6):344–6.
11. Limousin P, Pollak P, Benazzouz A, et al. Effect of parkinsonian signs and symptoms of bilateral subthalamic nucleus stimulation. Lancet 1995;345(8942):91–5.
12. Siegfried J, Lippitz B. Bilateral chronic electrostimulation of ventroposterolateral pallidum: a new therapeutic approach for alleviating all parkinsonian symptoms. Neurosurgery 1994;35(6):1126–9.
13. Langston JW, Widner H, Goetz CG, et al. Core assessment program for intracerebral transplantations (CAPIT). Mov Disord 1992;7(1):2–13.
14. Defer GL, Widner H, Marié RM, et al. Core assessment program for surgical interventional therapies in Parkinson's disease (CAPSIT-PD). Mov Disord 1999;14(4):572–84.
15. Lang A, Widner H. Deep brain stimulation for Parkinson's disease: patient selection and evaluation. Mov Disord 2002;17(Suppl 3):s94–101.
16. Shih LC, Tarsy D. Deep brain stimulation for the treatment of atypical parkinsonism. Mov Disord 2007;22(15):2149–55.
17. Doshi PK, Chhaya N, Bhatt MH. Depression leading to attempted suicide after bilateral subthalamic nucleus stimulation for Parkinson's disease. Mov Disord 2002;17(5):1084–5.
18. Benabid AL, Pollak P, Gao D, et al. Chronic electrical stimulation of the ventralis intermedius nucleus of the thalamus as a treatment of movement disorders. J Neurosurg 1996;84(2):203–14.
19. Rehncrona S, Johnels B, Widner H, et al. Long-term efficacy of thalamic deep brain stimulation for tremor: double-blind assessments. Mov Disord 2003;18(2):163–70.
20. Rodriguez-Oroz MC, Obeso JA, Lang AE, et al. Bilateral deep brain stimulation in Parkinson's disease: a multicentre study with 4 years follow-up. Brain 2005;128(Pt 10):2240–9.
21. Rouaud T, Dondaine T, Drapier S, et al. Pallidal stimulation in advanced Parkinson's patients with contraindications for subthalamic stimulation. Mov Disord 2010;25(12):1839–46.
22. Deuschl G, Schade-Brittinger C, Krack P, et al. A randomized trial of deep-brain stimulation for Parkinson's disease. N Engl J Med 2006;355(9):896–908.
23. Weaver FM, Follett K, Stern M, et al. Bilateral deep brain stimulation vs best medical therapy for patients with advanced Parkinson disease: a randomized controlled trial. JAMA 2009;301(1):63–73.
24. Williams A, Gill S, Varma T, et al. Deep brain stimulation plus best medical therapy versus best medical therapy alone for advanced Parkinson's disease (PD SURG trial): a randomised, open-label trial. Lancet Neurol 2010;9(6):581–91.
25. Okun MS, Fernandez HH, Wu SS, et al. Cognition and mood in Parkinson's disease in subthalamic nucleus versus globus pallidus interna deep brain stimulation: the COMPARE trial. Ann Neurol 2009;65(5):586–95.

26. Follett KA, Weaver FM, Stern M, et al. Pallidal versus subthalamic deep-brain stimulation for Parkinson's disease. N Engl J Med 2010;362(22):2077–91.
27. Odekerken VJ, Van Laar T, Staal MJ, et al. Subthalamic nucleus versus globus pallidus bilateral deep brain stimulation for advanced Parkinson's disease (NSTAPS study): a randomised controlled trial. Lancet Neurol 2013;12(1):37–44.
28. Guridi J, Rodriguez-Oroz MC, Alegre M, et al. Hardware complications in deep brain stimulation: electrode impedance and loss of clinical benefit. Parkinsonism Relat Disord 2012;18(6):765–9.
29. Voon V, Krack P, Lang AE, et al. A multicentre study on suicide outcomes following subthalamic stimulation for Parkinson's disease. Brain 2008; 131(Pt 10):2720–8.
30. Schüpbach WM, Chastan N, Welter ML, et al. Stimulation of the subthalamic nucleus in Parkinson's disease: a 5 year follow up. J Neurol Neurosurg Psychiatry 2005;76(12):1640–4.
31. Weaver FM, Follett KA, Stern M, et al. Randomized trial of deep brain stimulation for Parkinson disease: thirty-six-month outcomes. Neurology 2012;79(1):55–65.
32. Saint-Cyr JA, Trépanier LL, Kumar R, et al. Neuropsychological consequences of chronic bilateral stimulation of the subthalamic nucleus in Parkinson's disease. Brain 2000;123(Pt 10):2091–108.
33. Witt K, Daniels C, Reiff J, et al. Neuropsychological and psychiatric changes after deep brain stimulation for Parkinson's disease: a randomised, multicentre study. Lancet Neurol 2008;7(7):605–14.
34. Parsons TD, Rogers SA, Braaten AJ, et al. Cognitive sequelae of subthalamic nucleus deep brain stimulation in Parkinson's disease: a meta-analysis. Lancet Neurol 2006;5(7):578–88.
35. Stefani A, Lozano AM, Peppe A, et al. Bilateral deep brain stimulation of the pedunculopontine and subthalamic nuclei in severe Parkinson's disease. Brain 2007;130(Pt 6):1596–607.
36. Moro E, Hamani C, Poon YY, et al. Unilateral pedunculopontine stimulation improves falls in Parkinson's disease. Brain 2010;133(Pt 1):215–24.
37. Ferraye MU, Debû B, Fraix V, et al. Effects of pedunculopontine nucleus area stimulation on gait disorders in Parkinson's disease. Brain 2010;133(Pt 1):205–14.
38. Khan S, Gill SS, Mooney L, et al. Combined pedunculopontine-subthalamic stimulation in Parkinson disease. Neurology 2012;78(14):1090–5.
39. Espay AJ, Vaughan JE, Marras C, et al. Early versus delayed bilateral subthalamic deep brain stimulation for Parkinson's disease: a decision analysis. Mov Disord 2010;25(10):1456–63.
40. Schuepbach WM, Rau J, Knudsen K, et al. Neurostimulation for Parkinson's disease with early motor complications. N Engl J Med 2013;368(7):610–22.
41. Moro E, Esselink RJA, Xie J, et al. The impact on Parkinson's disease of electrical parameter settings in STN stimulation. Neurology 2002;59(5):706–13.
42. Eusebio A, Chen CC, Lu CS, et al. Effects of low-frequency stimulation of the subthalamic nucleus on movement in Parkinson's disease. Exp Neurol 2008; 209(1):125–30.
43. Moreau C, Defebvre L, Destée A, et al. STN-DBS frequency effects on freezing of gait in advanced Parkinson disease. Neurology 2008;71(2):80–4.
44. Ricchi V, Zibetti M, Angrisano S, et al. Transient effects of 80 Hz stimulation on gait in STN DBS treated PD patients: a 15 months follow-up study. Brain Stimul 2012;5(3):388–92.
45. Brown P, Marsden CD. What do the basal ganglia do? Lancet 1998;351(9118): 1801–4.

46. Brown P. Oscillatory nature of human basal ganglia activity: relationship to the pathophysiology of Parkinson's disease. Mov Disord 2003;18(4):357–63.

47. Levy R, Ashby P, Hutchison WD, et al. Dependence of subthalamic nucleus oscillations on movement and dopamine in Parkinson's disease. Brain 2002; 125(Pt 6):1196–209.

48. Cassidy M, Mazzone P, Oliviero A, et al. Movement-related changes in synchronization in the human basal ganglia. Brain 2002;125(Pt 6):1235–46.

49. Bronte-Stewart H, Barberini C, Koop MM, et al. The STN beta-band profile in Parkinson's disease is stationary and shows prolonged attenuation after deep brain stimulation. Exp Neurol 2009;215(1):20–8.

50. Marceglia S, Rossi L, Foffani G, et al. Basal ganglia local field potentials: applications in the development of new deep brain stimulation devices for movement disorders. Expert Rev Med Devices 2007;4(5):605–14.

51. Rosin B, Slovik M, Mitelman R, et al. Closed-loop deep brain stimulation is superior in ameliorating parkinsonism. Neuron 2011;72(2):370–84.

52. Martens HC, Toader E, Decré MM, et al. Spatial steering of deep brain stimulation volumes using a novel lead design. Clin Neurophysiol 2011;122(3):558–66.

53. Chaturvedi A, Foutz TJ, McIntyre CC. Current steering to activate targeted neural pathways during deep brain stimulation of the subthalamic region. Brain Stimul 2012;5(3):369–77.

54. Wilson S. Modern problems in neurology. London: Arnold & Company; 1928.

# Deep Brain Stimulation in Nonparkinsonian Movement Disorders and Emerging Technologies, Targets, and Therapeutic Promises in Deep Brain Stimulation

Douglas Anderson, MD[a],*, Ninith Kartha, MD[b]

## KEYWORDS

- Deep brain stimulation • Movement disorders • Essential tremor • Dystonia
- Tourette syndrome

## KEY POINTS

- Nonparkinsonian movement disorders can be associated with disabling and debilitating symptoms and signs, and using deep brain stimulation (DBS) for treatment in intractable and severe cases can have positive effects on patients' lives.
- However, the use of DBS in nonparkinsonian movement disorders is difficult because of the small numbers of patients with these disorders, the shortage of clinical trials to guide therapy, complex regulatory and ethical issues related to the use of DBS in young patients (when it might be indicated), rare conditions despite the severity of presentation, and potential side effects and complications.
- Partly because of the reversibility of DBS therapy, research and innovation in this field has been extensive, both in technological improvement and also in application to other neural network disorders.

## INTRODUCTION

The increased use of deep brain stimulation (DBS) in movement disorders has a well-documented history, emerging from the practice of ablative stereotactic surgery for movement disorders with microelectrode recording for lesion site confirmation.[1,2] The change to continuous high-frequency stimulation was initiated by observations

Disclosures: The authors have nothing to disclose.
[a] Department of Neurological Surgery, Loyola University Medical Center, 2150 South 1st Avenue, Room 2700, Maywood, IL 60153, USA; [b] Department of Neurology, Loyola University Medical Center - Stritch Medical School, 2150 South 1st Avenue, Maywood, IL 60153, USA
* Corresponding author.
E-mail address: dander1@lumc.edu

Neurol Clin 31 (2013) 809–826
http://dx.doi.org/10.1016/j.ncl.2013.03.008
0733-8619/13/$ – see front matter © 2013 Elsevier Inc. All rights reserved.

reported by Hassler and colleagues[3] and Ohye and colleagues.[4] Benabid and colleagues[5-7] in a series of clinical papers[4,8] laid the foundation for the growth of an expanding neurologic and neurosurgical research and clinical enterprise that continues today.

The success of DBS for Parkinson disease (PD) and, to a lesser extent, other movement disorders, has been a surprising disruptive technology, requiring close collaboration between neurologists and neurosurgeons to monitor the evolution of DBS treatments in concert with new medical strategies. In addition, the investment made by the medical technology industry and governmental scrutiny and regulation have created a complex web of ethics, economics, medical research, and clinical practice.

The best clinical scientific evidence in the literature concerning patient selection, targets, and outcomes comes from experience with DBS for PD.[9,10] Clinicians and researchers have drawn from that experience, expanding DBS applications to other movement disorders and several other conditions that confront the neurologist and neurosurgeon. However, most of that information comes as case reports or small open-label nonrandomized trials of DBS applied to less common neurologic conditions or DBS targets. It comprises a less clear scientific body of evidence to justify routine practice. Nonetheless, there exists a growing literature describing the rapid evolution of new DBS targets, technologies, strategies, and techniques. These efforts comprise a testament to the ingenuity and knowledge of neurologic and neurosurgical predecessors whose work has been translated from proposed ablative procedures to DBS but also the evolution of knowledge concerning pathologic neural networks, and, ultimately, the shortcomings of available interventions. Many of the disorders for which DBS is directed have groups of patients experiencing intractable conditions that have failed available therapies.

The promise of DBS research and practice is based on the concept that modulation of pathophysiologic neural networks can alter brain activity in a therapeutic way, thereby treating intractable neurologic conditions defined by such neural network derangements.[11] Use of DBS is spurred on by its reversibility, its success in the treatment of PD, and the inadequacy of treatments for certain intractable neurologic conditions. It is balanced by its invasiveness and the potential for surgical complications such as hemorrhage, infection, and biophysical failure of electrodes or circuits. More complex are complications or unintended side effects caused by the inaccuracy of DBS placement and/or the stimulation of structures outside of the intended target. However, unintended side effects may lead to new understanding of target structure and related circuitry function. An example of this phenomenon has been reported and was based on observations during the course of subthalamic nucleus (STN) stimulation for PD. Unexpected improvements in patients with concomitant obsessive-compulsive disorder (OCD) led to an additional trial of STN stimulation for intractable OCD.[12]

---

**Case study**

A 55-year-old man with a history of coronary artery disease, hypertension, hyperlipidemia, coronary artery bypass graft, and surgical repair of an aortic dissection with prosthetic aortic valve replacement had acute onset of vertical diplopia, left eyelid ptosis, and mild right-sided weakness. He had been noncompliant with a prophylactic oral anticoagulation regimen at the time of symptom onset. Seven months later he presented with neurologic findings consistent with Benedikt syndrome. In addition to cranial nerve III signs, he had developed a coarse, high-amplitude, low-frequency action and postural tremor of the right upper extremity with a milder resting component. The right lower extremity showed similar but less severe findings. There was also a right pronator drift and impaired dexterity of rapid fine movements of the right hand. Magnetic resonance imaging (MRI) showed findings consistent with an infarction of the medial left thalamus, left cranial nerve III fascicles, red nucleus (RN), right cerebral peduncle, and bilateral cerebellar hemispheres. The cause was likely thromboembolic and the patient was unresponsive to pharmacotherapy. He described his tremor as the most disabling aspect of his poststroke symptoms. As determined by the Washington Heights-Inwood Genetic Study of ET (WHIGET) Tremor Rating Scale, he scored 4/4 tremor severity preoperatively. The decision was made to attempt DBS implantation in the posterior subthalamic area for the intractable and debilitating right-sided tremor with favorable results.[13]

## PATIENT SELECTION ISSUES

This case study is used to illustrate several complex issues concerning DBS as it applies to the treatment of non-PD movement disorders but also to several other disorders. In the case study described, Investigational Review Board consultation was performed before this operation. The DBS equipment was used off label. The use of DBS for PD and essential tremor (ET), has US Food and Drug Administration (FDA) approval. For intractable OCD, dystonia and Gilles de la Tourette syndrome (GTS), the FDA has issued a humanitarian device exemption (HDE). For other disorders such as treatment-resistant major depression, clinical trials are active. Funding for small populations of patients with unusual movement disorders is scarce. The transition from DBS innovation and research to clinical practice has been rapid but there remain several problems. Patterns of use in the United States show that patients receiving DBS for PD and ET in 2007 compared with 2000 are older and sicker but experience fewer complications (3.8% in 2000 vs 2.8% in 2007). Also, in 2000, 75% of procedures were performed in multidisciplinary centers with well-established programs, whereas in 2007 that number decreased to 50%.[14]

Continued innovation requires appropriate ethical frameworks, guidelines for the variety of clinical and research opportunities, and an awareness of past mistakes. The field of neuroethics has emerged,[15] defining the potential problems with DBS and other forays into the clinical treatment of neurologic and neuropsychiatric conditions.[16] This is a complicated task, but the persistent numbers of patients with neural network disorders and attendant conditions is reason for careful but constructive and progressive ethical deliberation. Patient selection and candidacy require agreement concerning standard but condition-specific definitions of intractability in neurologic conditions. Also, because well-designed clinical trials define patients who might benefit from DBS in a disease such as PD, it is incumbent on clinicians to provide patients with appropriate information and neurosurgical collaboration. At present, DBS may be appropriate for earlier use in PD, in lieu of long trials of polydrug therapies.[1] As research continues in newer areas such as treatment-resistant depression, it is necessary to understand the degree to which patients understand the process of clinical research. A recent study examined severely depressed patients' capability to give informed consent. The thesis was based on a concern that patients with severe depression might lack the judgment required of clinical trial participants. The study concluded that patients with treatment-resistant depression showed "very good performance across all domains of decisional capacity."[17] However, therapeutic misconception was notable in their responses and remained a concern. It might be true that most patients (especially with a treatment-resistant neurologic disorder), when offered participation in a clinical trial, have some inherent degree of misconception as to the potential for therapeutic benefit. Perhaps, as has been reported in other analyses of this sort for other patient populations, it is unrealistic to expect from patients an altruistic motive for entering any clinical trial.

At present, the ways in which DBS is being introduced and studied, at least in the United States, pose several problematic issues. There are clearly difficult fiscal and regulatory barriers[18] to the practice and ongoing research of DBS. These barriers include many areas in the development of DBS including the availability of research funding, biophysical improvement of DBS hardware, application of DBS for unusual and rare conditions, and regulatory delays. There are a few ways that clinicians can introduce new applications for DBS into the clinical armamentarium. The FDA has used the status of HDE to make available DBS therapy for patients with intractable OCD. The HDE is a designation that anticipates fewer than 4000 patients per year as candidates for treatment. Criticisms of this designation center on the potential for a "market driven regulatory strategy that could be applied to other conditions to the detriment of scientific discovery, patient safety, and research integrity."[19] However, as it stands, there exists an impasse between insurance carriers who refuse to pay for such treatment, citing its experimental character despite the FDA's language as to what the HDE definition entails, such that few DBS procedures for intractable OCD are being performed. Clinicians occasionally use standard DBS equipment in off-label designations. Although this is common across several classes of therapeutic interventions, the practice as it applies to DBS, especially for neuropsychiatric conditions, is fraught with difficulties and pitfalls.[18] Innovative clinical practice and collaboration with medical industry have been major factors in the development of DBS but it seems that governmental regulatory reform is essential for the practice of DBS to proceed in the most useful, efficacious, humane, and scientifically acceptable way. Fins and colleagues[16] provide an excellent summary of these issues. In the meantime, Hariz[20] points out that 9 separate DBS targets have been tried in GTS, 8 for OCD, and 5 for depression.

## PATIENT OVERVIEW AND MANAGEMENT GOALS

For each patient with a non-PD movement disorder, there are several considerations that are taken into account. Three of the most common non-PD movement disorders are reviewed.

### ET

Essential tremor is the most common pathologic tremor disorder, with a prevalence rate of 0.4% to 5%.[21] ET is typically manifested as a postural and kinetic tremor of the distal upper extremities, but a rest component can be present and the legs and midline regions (head, face, tongue, and voice) also can be affected.[22] With progression, tremor amplitude increases and frequency decreases, causing functional disability and often psychosocial distress.[23] The most effective oral therapies are propranolol and primidone, but an estimated 25% to 55% of patients are medication refractory and may be candidates for surgical management[24,25] DBS is approved by the FDA for use in the treatment of medically refractory ET. The preferred target is the ventral intermediate nucleus of the thalamus (VIM). DBS has several advantages compared with thalamotomy (surgical lesioning), including reversibility because of smaller lesion size, the ability to adjust stimulation settings to optimize efficacy and minimize side effects, and the ability to perform bilateral procedures safely.[5,26] Disadvantages include the expense of procedure, requirement for reliable long-term follow-up, hardware-related complications (infection, lead wire malfunction or breakage) and battery replacement every 2 to 5 years if the device is left on continuously. Patients with ET typically can turn off their implantable pulse generator at night, extending the life of the battery up to 7 to 10 years.[27]

Appropriate patient selection and realistic expectations are important factors determining surgical outcome. ET is a clinical diagnosis and should be confirmed by a thorough history and neurologic examination that excludes causative drugs and identifies other movement disorders (dystonic or cerebellar outflow tremor, atypical parkinsonism, myoclonus). Tremor should be disabling with surgery presenting an acceptable risk/benefit ratio. Tremor rating scales can be used to help quantify tremor severity and disability for preoperative assessment and to determine postoperative effectiveness. Unilateral stimulation should be considered if disability is only associated with tremor of 1 hand, usually the dominant hand. Maximum tolerated doses of propranolol and primidone should be attempted to establish medically refractory status. Factors such as age, medical comorbidities, and cognitive impairment should be taken into account and may influence the decision to pursue unilateral or bilateral stimulation. Patients should be educated on the nature of the surgical procedure, the perioperative and postoperative risks, and the need for regular long-term follow-up.

Thalamic stimulation is generally safe and effective in improving tremor outcomes but is given a level C recommendation because of a lack of double-blind placebo-controlled trials supporting its efficacy.[24] Improvement in tremor rating scale scores is seen after implantation compared with baseline, presumably as a lesion effect, and after stimulation is turned on compared with when the device is turned off.[25] Upper limb tremor scores can improve by 70% to 90% and although unilateral stimulation primarily affects contralateral tremor, a milder ipsilateral effect may also occur.[27–29] Head and voice tremors show less predictable response to therapy than limb tremors and typically require bilateral stimulation for maximal effect.[30,31] Limited data are available on effects of stimulation on health-related quality of life and long-term effects of stimulation. One study of 27 patients showed that DBS contributed to improvement in activities of daily living including writing, grooming tasks, eating, drinking, and cooking from 6 to 26 months following surgery, and patients also reported significant improvement in emotional reactions and participation in social life and hobbies.[32] Another study found a reduction in limb tremor severity in 10 of 13 patients at 6-year to 7-year follow-up. Hand functions, measured by spiral and line drawing and pouring tasks, remained significantly better in the stimulation-on state compared with baseline and the stimulation-off state at both 2 and 6 to 7 years after surgery with no evidence of significant disease progression.[33] However, other studies have shown a loss of tremor control over time, which may be caused by several factors including tolerance to stimulation, progression of disease, improper lead placement, and misdiagnosis.[34–37] Adjustment of stimulation settings may help if tolerance is the main cause of decline.

Adverse events associated with DBS are mild and can be caused by perioperative or hardware-related complications and stimulation side effects.[26,36] Stimulation side effects include dysarthria, paresthesias, dystonia, and imbalance, which are symptoms that may be reduced or resolved by adjustment of stimulation settings. Perioperative complications include intracerebral hemorrhage, ischemic stroke, infection, and depression. Decline in cognitive function and mood following DBS is less common in patients with ET than in PD but a decrease in verbal fluency may occur and suicide following VIM DBS has been reported.[27,38] Dysarthria and gait instability are more common after bilateral than unilateral stimulation.[28]

### Dystonia

Dystonia is a disorder characterized by involuntary and sustained, often torsional, muscle contractions resulting in twisting and repetitive movements and abnormal postures.[39] Because dystonia can vary in clinical presentation and cause, treatment is tailored toward individual patients and can involve alleviating symptoms or treating secondary causes.[40] Treatment options include physical therapy, anticholinergic agents and muscle relaxants, and botulinum toxin in focal or segmental dystonia. DBS is approved by the FDA for use in medically refractory dystonia under an HDE and is now the preferred surgical therapy because of its lower risk of side effects compared with pallidotomy and the ability to adjust stimulation settings.[40]

Several studies have established the efficacy of bilateral stimulation of the globus pallidus interna (GPi) in the treatment of primary generalized and segmental dystonia.[41–43] In a multicenter, prospective study of 22 patients with primary generalized dystonia, GPi DBS improved mean dystonia movement scores by 51% and one-third of patients improved by more than 75% compared with preoperative scores on a commonly used dystonia rating scale.[41] Benefit was seen at 3 months and sustained at 1 year in most patients, although 4 had limited improvement or worsening, and no definite predictors of response were identified, possibly because of small sample size. Other studies have identified possible predictors of better outcome, including younger age, presence of DYT1 gene-positive status, shorter disease duration, and presence of phasic or mobile dystonia as opposed to tonic contractions and fixed postures[44–46] Although phasic movements may respond immediately or within days of surgery, tonic contractions and sustained postures may display a delayed response in which symptoms improve gradually over a course of weeks or months.[47] Symptomatic and functional improvements are typically maintained in the long term. One study following 9 patients with both primary and secondary forms of dystonia showed benefit maintained up to 10 years after surgery.[48] In a long-term follow-up of the multicenter trial discussed earlier, motor, quality-of-life, and cognitive and depression scores observed at 1 year remained stable at 3 years and there was no evidence of tolerance to the effects of long-term DBS.[49]

DBS is also effective in the treatment of cervical dystonia (CD) in botulinum toxin–refractory patients with features such as head tremor, prominent phasic component, sagittal or lateral shifts, and anterocollis.[47] After surgery, patients show greater than 50% improvements in motor, disability, and pain scores.[50,51] A prospective, single-blind study of 10 patients with severe medication-resistant CD showed significant and sustained improvement in head and neck postures over a 1-year period with 59% improvement in the total Toronto Western Spasmodic Torticollis Rating Scale (TWSTRS) score, 24% improvement in a quality-of-life measure, and 58% improvement in a depression score. Although there was variability in the magnitude of response, 90% of the patients improved after therapy.[50] Patients with Meige syndrome (a combination of upper and lower facial and oromandibular dystonia) may also benefit from GPi DBS. Small studies and case reports have shown greater than 50% improvement in rating scales in patients with idiopathic cranial CD[52–54]; however, efficacy is not established.

Investigation of DBS in secondary dystonia is also limited to small studies and case reports, and these have generally shown a less pronounced response to stimulation than primary dystonia,[47] although improvement has been documented in several disorders. A study of 9 patients with tardive dystonia (TD) showed benefit within a week of stimulation, which was maintained for longer than1 year, with 83% improvement in motor scores, although the clinical assessment was nonblinded.[55] Another study also documented improvement of TD symptoms in 5 patients within 12 to 72 hours of stimulation,[56] which contrasts with the delayed effect typically seen in primary dystonia. There are case reports of efficacy of GPi DBS in other forms of secondary dystonia, including myoclonus dystonia,[57] posttraumatic hemidystonia,[58] and pantothenate kinase–associated neurodegeneration.[59]

The potential side effects associated with DBS for dystonia include the perioperative, hardware-related, and stimulation-related side effects seen in ET. In one study of 16 patients, 2 committed suicide, although a definite connection to DBS could not be determined.[60] Another potential complication is a rebound phenomenon in which dystonia may be severely exacerbated if the stimulation is rapidly or inadvertently stopped.[61] However, the incidence of cognitive side effects is lower than that seen in PD, and, in general, studies have shown a low frequency of complications and serious adverse effects.[62,63]

## GTS

GTS is a childhood-onset disorder characterized by a combination of chronic motor and vocal tics, often associated with obsessive-compulsive symptoms and disturbances of attention.[64] Although DBS is not currently FDA-approved for this indication, several case reports and case series have investigated the effects of stimulation in medically refractory patients with severe and disabling tics. Several guidelines have been outlined that generally recommend limiting surgical intervention to adult subjects with severe and disabling tics who have failed conventional medical therapy and reasonable behavioral interventions and whose psychological comorbidities are adequately managed[65–67]; however, general consensus on the criteria for patient selection and the best target for stimulation has yet to be established. Stimulation targets that have been investigated include the anterior internal capsule,[68] nucleus accumbens and internal capsule,[69] centromedian thalamus-parafascicular complex,[70,71] and GPi,[72] with reported tic reduction of 41% to 88% as well as reported decrease in affective and obsessional symptoms and self-injurious behavior. The differences in the degree of improvement and impact on behavioral symptoms are difficult to determine because of small sample sizes and variability in patient selection criteria, rating methods, and surgical technique.[72] Clarifying these aspects of DBS for GTS is an area for future research.

## SURGICAL TARGETS AND OPERATIVE NUANCES
### VIM

Neurologic conditions: ET, unilateral disabling kinetic tremor in multiple sclerosis.[73,74]

Target coordinates as per literature review
- X: 12.3 mm, 13 to 15 mm, 11.5 mm lateral from the anterior commissure (AC) to posterior commissure (PC) line (11 mm lateral to the wall of the third ventricle)
- Y: 6.3 to 6.5 mm anterior to the PC, best target being the anterior margin of VIM in the anteroposterior plane[75]
- Z: 0 (at the level of AC-PC line)

DBS settings commonly cited in recent literature
Low-intensity current: 0.2 to 2.0 mA. Frequency: greater than 100 Hz.

### Recent Advances in Treatment Optimization

VIM DBS for severe ET developed from microelectrode recording (MER) and continues to rely on that technology for accurate target localization and electrophysiologic documentation. However, MER increases the invasiveness of the procedure.[76] Magnetic resonance diffusion tensor imaging (DTI) theoretically can predict the most likely site for successful DBS in tremor surgery from thalamocortical projection density. The tremor neural network has been elucidated by selecting initial DTI seed locations, set at the theoretically most effective stimulation site within VIM where the DTI images show thalamic connections to the primary motor cortex. These projections seem to play a key role in successful stimulation.[77]

### Posterior Subthalamic Area, Including Thalamic Fasciculus, Zona Incerta, Prelemniscal Radiation, and Lenticular Fasciculus

Neurologic conditions: ET,[78] combined resting and intention tremor[13]

Target coordinates as per literature review
   These areas are presented together because of the proximity of their respective anatomic coordinates.
   X: 8 to 10 mm lateral, 12 + 1.8 mm,[79] 10.9 ± .8 mm lateral to AC-PC
   Y: 3 to 5 mm posterior to the midcommissural point, −5.5 + 1.9 mm, 3 mm anterior to the PC, 7.6 ± 1.2 mm posterior to the midcommissural point[79]
   Z: −3 to 4; −1.2 + 2.9 mm, −3.9 ± 1.7 mm inferior to the AC-PC plane defined on axial T2-weighted imaging, slightly posteromedial to the STN, at the level of maximal diameter of the RN[79]

DBS settings most commonly cited in recent literature
   Amplitude, 2.6 V; pulse width, 120 microseconds; frequency, 185 Hz

### Recent Advances in Treatment Optimization

There is growing evidence that DBS for ET is more successful with the posterior sub-thalamic area as the target compared with VIM.[80] This target was used for a combined tremor following midbrain infarction associated with Benedikt syndrome.[13]

### Caudal Zona Incerta

Neurologic condition: alternative target for PD with tremor,[79–81] multiple sclerosis–associated tremor, ET.

Target coordinates as per literature review
   X: 13 to 15 mm lateral to midline
   Y: 4.5 to 6.5 mm posterior to midcommissural point
   Z: 0 to 5 mm inferior to AC-PC plane

   Blomstedt and colleagues[79] describes the target as being at the same axial level as the STN posteromedial to the tail of the STN (X, 10–12) at the level of RN maximum diameter (approx Z, −4).

### Recent Advances in Treatment Optimization

Kerl and colleagues[78] described localization with 3 T MRI and T2 fluorescence in situ hybridization (FLASH) two-dimensional (2D) sequences with 40-Hz bandwidth, for accurate localization of the caudal zona incerta (cZI). Blomstedt describes cZI as a more efficient treatment of ET.[79–81]

### GPi

Neurologic conditions: PD, dystonia,[41] CD,[82] DYT1 primary torsion dystonia (PTD),[83] GTS,[84] chorea-acanthosis,[85,86] Huntington disease,[86] Lesch-Nyhan syndrome,[87] and intractable status dystonicus.[88]

Target coordinates cited in literature
   X: 20 to 23 mm lateral to the AC-PC line
   −Y: 2 to 3 mm anterior to the midcommissural point
   −Z: 2 to 5 mm below the AC-PC line

DBS settings cited in recent literature: variable. for GTS, 1 V, 130 Hz, Pulse width (PW) 30 60 microseconds.[47]
For dystonia: 130 Hz, PW 450 microseconds, monopolar mode, 1 to 2.5 V.

### Recent Advances in Treatment Optimization

GPi is best visualized in 3-T MRI axial view and to a lesser degree, coronal on T2 FLASH 2D images; TR 625 milliseconds, Te 25 2D fast low-angle shot MRI with standard bandwidth of 40 kHz. Subregions within the GPi include posteroventral (motor) and anteromedial (limbic) portions of the nucleus.[89] DBS in children has been a complicated topic, but Markun and colleagues[83] describe the benefit for early intervention and the sustained benefit of DBS GPi in children with PTD. A report claims that multiple electrode placements can improve outcomes in generalized dystonia if initial results with 1 electrode are suboptimal or if recurrent symptoms are noted.[90]

### Centromedian Parafascicular Nuclear Complex (Crossing Point Between the Centromedian, Substantia Periventricularis, and Nucleus Ventralis–Oralis Internus)

Neurologic conditions: GTS.[72,91,92]

Target coordinates as per literature review
   X: 5 to 10 mm lateral
   Y: 4 to 8 mm posterior to the midcommissural line
   Z: 0

DBS settings cited in recent literature: bipolar mode, 4 to 6 V, 125 Hz, PW 210 microseconds.

### Recent Advances in Treatment Optimization

This work still consists of small case series.

### Nucleus Accumbens

Neurologic condition: GTS[69] (previous work has centered around the nucleus accumbens as a target for DBS treatment of intractable OCD).

Target coordinates as per literature review
   X: 2.5 mm lateral to the third ventricular wall
   X: 2.5 mm anterior to the posterior commissure
   Z: 2 mm inferior to the commissural line

### Cerebellar Stimulation

Neurologic condition: dystonia (previous work in cerebellar stimulation by Cooper and colleagues[93] for movement disorder has attracted renewed interest because of the finding that basal ganglia communicate with the cerebellum.[94,95]

## DIRECTIONS IN RESEARCH AND INNOVATION

A more precise understanding of how DBS alters activity within neural circuits to achieve therapeutic effect is an area that has gained some traction in recent years.[96] Delong and Wichman[97] describe DBS's role as a focal and functionally specific modification of disease-related brain circuits, as opposed to modification of the disease process. However, recent reports have described changes in temporal lobe metabolism and increased connectivity, suggesting a possible example of disease process modification.[98] DBS as applied to movement disorder acts to regularize activity within the motor circuit thereby reducing the passage of pathologic information from the pallidum.[96] DBS can affect local cells around the electrode, afferent inputs into the DBS region, and fibers of passage, complicating the effort to determine the mechanism of action for each disease process or condition. The new technologies of optogenetics coupled with solid-state optics to drive or inhibit distinct neural circuit elements in an animal model of PD have begun to answer these important questions.[99,100] Optical deconstruction focuses on specific elements of the neural circuit via "single component microbial light activated regulators of trans-membrane conduction and ... in vivo light delivery, to ultimately understand different elements in the disease neuro-circuit."[100] In an animal model of PD, it has been shown that therapeutic effects can be ascribed to selective stimulation of afferent axons projecting into the STN. DBS in the region of STN activated descending gamma-aminobutyric acid fibers from the striatum and GP traveling in fiber bundles surrounding the STN, suggesting wider neurochemical modulation resulting in network-wide changes in neural activity.[99] In almost all DBI target regions there exist several subregions that interact with other dissociable brain networks.

Improving the accuracy of DBS electrode placement has been aided by advances in neuroimaging, advances in intraoperative electrophysiology, development of responsive DBS systems, novel stimulation strategies, and development of better hardware and software.

Advances in neuroimaging continue to positively affect DBS. High-tesla and multimodal MRI can improve identification and refine target accuracy.[89,101,102] DTI may aid in the identification of fiber tracts that might be affected by stimulation.[103,104] DTI images of the STN and surrounding tissue medium have been used to model estimates of electrical conductivity. Using previously published effective stimulation parameters, activation profiles can be constructed for various settings of the DBS system. One study found that activation could spread outside the borders of the dorsal STN and resulted in activation of the zona incerta, fields of Forel, and portions of the internal capsule. Models suggest that 1-mm adjustments of the electrode placement result in substantial effects on the neural response to DBS, via direct and indirect effects.[105] Although MER have been the mainstay in defining the longest and lateral (most preferred) aspects of the STN,[105] another study poses the possibility of dispensing with microelectrode recording in STN placement. They concluded that STN DBS under general anesthesia with routine stereotactic verification did not have a negative effect on efficacy or safety.[101]

Intraoperative electrophysiology MER has long been the methodology of choice for accurate localization of DBS targets for movement disorder.[106] Performing and interpreting MER remains a qualitative and demanding technique. New methodologies that automatically combine MER information with a three-dimensional atlas may refine target identification.[107] Additional work has been focused on quantifying the intraoperative STN MER mapping for identification of subregions within the STN.[108] In STN DBS placement, Seifried and colleagues[105] described using 5 concentrically situated microelectrodes as the target was approached, identifying a bursting and more oscillatory pattern in the dorsal (the preferred) versus ventral STN.

Responsive DBS systems that both monitor for pathologic neural activity and respond with appropriately timed stimulation when abnormal rhythms are detected are a source of considerable interest. Reports define 2 fundamental requirements: (1)

recording and identifying of causal pathophysiologic network patterns (beta frequency band oscillations recorded at the stimulation target seem to be a possibility), and[109] (2) closed-loop feedback stimulation of the target circuits whose activation can interfere with the emerging pathologic pattern. These systems are being studied and developed predominantly in the context of epilepsy and movement disorders, but identification of recordable brain signals associated with clinical disorders might allow for feedback control of several other neurologic and neuropsychiatric conditions.[110]

Documenting metabolic changes related to both neurologic condition and also treatment effects can be accomplished with functional MRI (fMRI)[111] and/or positron emission tomography (PET).[98] Processing this information requires substantial time and expertise. Postoperative MRI data continue to have artifact and electrode concerns.

The development of stimulation strategies includes current-controlled devices with independent electrode energy sources. This technology has the capability of current steering, which can theoretically target distinct neural populations for preferential activation. Shaping the DBS signal via current-controlled devices with a goal of improved clinical benefit and avoidance of unwanted side effects has recently been described.[112] However, measureable clinical benefit remains to be documented in a clinical trial. The first clinical trial with a current-constant mode of delivery showed improvement in motor function compared with control groups, but awaits additional clinical trials comparing outcomes with the constant-voltage DBS of the predominant systems, which presently do not have selective electrode energy sources.[113]

Functional hardware and software have been developed. Automated trajectory planning systems, integrated with MRI anatomic data, have been developed to improve target precision and avoid critical brain structures including small vessels, theoretically decreasing the likelihood of surgery-related complications.[114] Silicon-based microelectrode arrays have been developed for long-term neural recording and stimulation, thus avoiding magnetic artifact and potential complications associated with postoperative confirmatory and fMRI imaging.[115] Transventricular routes to DBS targets have been associated with increased complications, prompting the development of implantable guide tubes to avoid the problems of passage, noted especially during peri-aqueductal grey and pedunculopontine nucleus electrode placement.[102] Larson[116] reviewed several other techniques and technological innovations presently being developed and evaluated to further improve the patient's surgical experience while undergoing DBS implantation (and stereotactic gene transfer techniques).

### Treatment Resistance/Complications

Functional neurosurgery programs that are active in DBS therapies have reported in-hospital complication rates of 0.8% to 1.2%.[2-4] Surgical complications associated with DBS throughout the literature are predominantly temporary, but are common. Hemorrhage, both asymptomatic (5%–10%) and more serious (0%–3%), and infection (~10% rates of device or wound infection) remain the most problematic complications, but the incidence is low and other issues do arise. Most serious adverse events reported in trials are resolved within 6 months. Treatment-related adverse events are associated with target and surrounding anatomic structures and tracts. It is possible to treat some wound dehiscences and/or infections with partial hardware removal and antibiotics in the presence of infection and debridement alone with antibiotics in dehiscence without overt infection.[117]

Technical malfunctions of DBS electrodes are reported to occur in 3.2% of cases (36/1142 electrodes). Problems include short circuits, disconnections, and loose contacts, and can lead to poor results with DBS therapy. Impedance measurements can be diagnostic for many of these complications.[118]

T2-weighted signal abnormality can be seen in up to 6.3% of patients having DBS, as reported in a series of 239 implants in 139 patients in the absence of hemorrhage or infection. This unusual finding is best described as idiosyncratic vasogenic edema. Most patients remained asymptomatic, whereas 3 out of 14 experienced transient symptoms. One patient required and responded to steroid treatment.[119]

## SUMMARY/DISCUSSION

DBS faces several challenges as it evolves as an adjunctive procedural therapy in the treatment of movement disorders and several other neurologic and neuropsychiatric conditions. At the same time, it holds promise for diverse neurologic intervention and investigation.[120] Because of its status as a device, the regulatory procedures and funds necessary for research and development can be arduous and sometimes overwhelming. It took a reported 10 years and millions of dollars to complete a study (blinded, randomized controlled trial) to determine the relative efficacy of DBS GPi versus STN in the treatment of PD. Legislative and regulatory reform are necessary for DBS to flourish.[19] Appropriate patient selection, timing of surgery, target sites, electrode design, electrode settings, and so forth are questions yet to be answered. The definitions of intractable, treatment resistance, and the like remain open to individual interpretation. However, surprising results and benefits for patients with several disorders are being reported in the literature with increasing frequency. As knowledge accrues, DBS will confront increasingly complex ethical problems, but also, very likely, therapeutic success.

## REFERENCES

1. Deuschl G, Schade-Brittinger C, Krack P, et al. A randomized trial of deep-brain stimulation for Parkinson's disease. N Engl J Med 2006;355:896–908.
2. Benabid AL, Chabardes S, Torres N, et al. Functional neurosurgery for movement disorders: a historical perspective. Prog Brain Res 2009;175:379–91.
3. Hassler R, Riechart T, Munginger F, et al. Physiological observations in stereotactic operations in extrapyramidal motor disturbances. Brain 1960;83:337–50.
4. Ohye C, Kubota K, Hooper HE, et al. Ventrolateral and subventrolateral thalamic stimulation. Arch Neurol 1964;11:427–34.
5. Benabid AL, Pollak P, Gervason C, et al. Long-term suppression of tremor by chronic stimulation of the ventral intermediate thalamic nucleus. Lancet 1991; 337:403–6.
6. Benabid AL, Pollak P, Louveau A, et al. Combined (thalamotomy and stimulation) stereotactic surgery of the Vim thalamic nucleus for bilateral Parkinson disease. Appl Neurophysiol 1987;50:344–6.
7. Benabid A, Pollak P, Gao D. Chronic electrical stimulation of the ventralis intermedius nucleus of the thalamus as a treatment of movement disorders. J Neurosurg 1996;84:203–14.
8. Limousin P, Krack P, Pollak P, et al. Electrical stimulation of the subthalamic nucleus in advanced Parkinson's disease. N Engl J Med 1998;339:1105–11.
9. Follett K, Weaver F, Stern M, et al. Pallidal versus subthalamic deep-brain stimulation for Parkinson's disease. N Engl J Med 2010;362:2077–91.
10. Weaver F, Follett K, Stern M, et al. Bilateral deep brain stimulation vs best medical therapy for patients with advanced Parkinson disease a randomized controlled trial. JAMA 2009;301:63–73.

11. Johnson MD, Miocinovic S, McIntyre CC, et al. Mechanisms and targets of deep brain stimulation in movement disorders. Neurotherapeutics 2008;5(2):294–308.
12. Mallet L, Polosan M, Jaafari N, et al. Subthalamic nucleus stimulation in severe obsessive compulsive disorder. N Engl J Med 2008;359:2121–34.
13. Bandt K, Anderson D, Biller J. Deep brain stimulation as an effective treatment option for post-midbrain infarction-related tremor as it presents with Benedikt syndrome. J Neurosurg 2008;109:635–9.
14. Pilitsis J, Burrows A, Peters ML, et al. Changing practice patterns of deep brain stimulation in Parkinson's disease and essential tremor. Stereotact Funct Neurosurg 2012;90:25–9.
15. Wind J, Anderson D. From prefrontal leucotomy to deep brain stimulation: the historical transformation of psychosurgery and the emergence of neuroethics. Neurosurg Focus 2008;25(1):E10, 1–5.
16. Fins J, Dorfman G, Pancrazio J. Challenges to deep brain stimulation: a pragmatic response to ethical, fiscal, and regulatory concerns. Ann N Y Acad Sci 2012;1265:80–90.
17. Fisher C, Dunn L, Christopher P, et al. The ethics of research on deep brain stimulation for depression: decisional capacity and therapeutic misconception. Ann N Y Acad Sci 2012;1265:69–79.
18. Tomycz N, Cheng B, Cantella D, et al. Pursuing new targets and indications for deep brain stimulation: considerations for device-related clinical research in the United States [letter to the editor]. Neuromodulation 2011;14:389–92.
19. Fins J, Mayberg H, Nuttin B, et al. Misuse of the FDA's humanitarian device exemption in deep brain stimulation for obsessive-compulsive disorder. Health Aff 2011;30(2):302–11.
20. Hariz M. Twenty-five years of deep brain stimulation: celebrations and apprehensions. Mov Disord 2012;27:930–3.
21. Louis ED, Ottman R, Hauer WA. How common is the most common adult movement disorder? Estimates of the prevalence of essential tremor throughout the world. Mov Disord 1998;13:5–10.
22. Deuschl G, Bain P, Brin M. Consensus statement of the Movement Disorders Society on tremor. Mov Disord 1998;13(Suppl 3):2–23.
23. Busenbark KL, Nash J, Nash S, et al. Is essential tremor benign? Neurology 1991;41:1982–3.
24. Zesiwicz TA, Elble R, Louis ED, et al. Practice parameter: therapies for essential tremor: report of the Quality Standards Subcommittee of the American Academy of Neurology. Neurology 2005;64:2008–20.
25. Louis ED. Clinical practice. Essential tremor. N Engl J Med 2001;345:887–91.
26. Della Flora E, Perera C, Cameron AL, et al. Deep brain stimulation for essential tremor: a systematic review. Mov Disord 2010;25:1550–9.
27. Schuurman PR, Bosch DA, Bossuyt PM, et al. A comparison of continuous thalamic stimulation and thalamotomy for suppression of severe tremor. N Engl J Med 2000;342:461–8.
28. Limousin P, Speelman JD, Gielen F, et al. Multicentre European study of thalamic stimulation in parkinsonian and essential tremor. J Neurol Neurosurg Psychiatry 1999;66(3):289–96.
29. Ondo W, Almaguer M, Jankovic J, et al. Thalamic deep brain stimulation: comparison between unilateral and bilateral placement. Arch Neurol 2001;58(2):218–22.
30. Putzke JD, Uitti RJ, Obwegeser AA, et al. Bilateral thalamic deep brain stimulation: midline tremor control. J Neurol Neurosurg Psychiatry 2005;76(5):684–90.

31. Pahwa R, Lyons KL, Wilkinson SB, et al. Bilateral thalamic stimulation for the treatment of essential tremor. Neurology 1999;53:1447–50.
32. Hariz GM, Lindberg M, Bergenheim AT. Impact of thalamic deep brain stimulation on disability and health-related quality of life in patients with essential tremor. J Neurol Neurosurg Psychiatry 2002;72:47–52.
33. Rehncrona S, Johnels B, Widner H, et al. Long-term efficacy of thalamic deep brain stimulation for tremor: double-blind assessments. Mov Disord 2003; 18(2):163–70.
34. Deuschl G, Raethjen J, Hellriegel H, et al. Treatment of patients with essential tremor. Lancet Neurol 2011;10:148–61.
35. Blomstedt P, Hariz GM, Hariz MI, et al. Thalamic deep brain stimulation in the treatment of essential tremor. Br J Neurosurg 2007;21:504–9.
36. Pilitsis JG, Metman LV, Toleikis JR, et al. Factors involved in long-term efficacy of deep brain stimulation of the thalamus for essential tremor. J Neurosurg 2008; 109:640–6.
37. Troster A, Fields J, Pahwa R, et al. Neuropsychological and quality of life outcome after thalamic stimulation for essential tremor. Neurology 1999;53(8): 1774–80.
38. Okun M, Rodriguez R, Mikos A, et al. Deep brain stimulation and the role of the neuropsychologist. Clin Neuropsychol 2007;21(1):162–89.
39. Fahn S, Bressman SB, Marsden CD. Classification of dystonia. Adv Neurol 1998;78:1–10.
40. Jankovic J. Treatment of dystonia. Lancet Neurol 2006;5:864–72.
41. Vadailhet M, Vercueil L, Houeto JL, et al. Bilateral deep brain stimulation of the globus pallidus in primary generalized dystonia. N Engl J Med 2005;352: 459–67.
42. Kupsch A, Benecke R, Muller J, et al. Pallidal deep-brain stimulation in primary generalized or segmental dystonia. N Engl J Med 2006;355:1978–90.
43. Isaias IU, Alterman RL, Tagliati M. Deep brain stimulation for primary generalized dystonia: long-term outcomes. Arch Neurol 2009;66(4):465–70.
44. Coubes P, Cif L, El Fertit H, et al. Electrical stimulation of the globus pallidus internus in patients with primary generalized dystonia: long-term results. J Neurosurg 2004;101(2):189–94.
45. Coubes P, Roubertie A, Vayssiere N, et al. Treatment of DYT1-generalized dystonia by stimulation of the internal globus pallidus. Lancet 2000;355:2220–1.
46. Isaias IU, Alterman RL, Tagliati M. Outcome predictors of pallidal stimulation in patients with primary dystonia: the role of disease duration. Brain 2008; 131(Pt 7):1895–902.
47. Albanese A, Barnes MP, Bhatia KP, et al. A systematic review on the diagnosis and treatment of primary (idiopathic) dystonia and dystonia plus syndromes: report of an EFNS/MDS-ES Task Force. Eur J Neurol 2006;13:433–44.
48. Loher TJ, Capelle HH, Kaelin-Lang A, et al. Deep brain stimulation for dystonia: outcome at long-term follow up. J Neurol 2008;255:881–4.
49. Vidhailet M, Vercueil L, Houeto JL. Bilateral pallidal deep brain stimulation in primary generalized dystonia: a prospective three-year follow-up study. Lancet Neurol 2007;6:223–9.
50. Kiss ZH, Doig-Beyaert K, Eliasziw M, et al. The Canadian multicenter study of deep brain stimulation for cervical dystonia. Brain 2007;130:2879–86.
51. Hung SW, Hamani C, Lozano AM, et al. Long-term outcome of bilateral pallidal deep brain stimulation for primary cervical dystonia. Neurology 2007;68(6): 457–9.

52. Houser M, Waltz T. Meige syndrome and pallidal deep brain stimulation. Mov Disord 2005;20:1203–5.

53. Ostrem JL, Marks WJ, Volz MM, et al. Pallidal deep brain stimulation in patients with cranial-cervical dystonia (Meige syndrome). Mov Disord 2007;22(13): 1885–91.

54. Blomstedt P, Tisch S, Hariz MI. Pallidal deep brain stimulation in the treatment of Meige syndrome. Acta Neurol Scand 2008;118(3):198–202.

55. Gruber D, Trottenberg T, Kivi A, et al. Long-term effects of pallidal deep brain stimulation in tardive dystonia. Neurology 2009;73:53–8.

56. Trottenberg T, Volkmann J, Deuschl G, et al. Treatment of severe tardive dystonia with pallidal deep brain stimulation. Neurology 2005;64:344–6.

57. Trottenberg T, Meissner W, Kabus C, et al. Neurostimulation of the ventral intermediate thalamic nucleus in inherited myoclonus-dystonia syndrome. Mov Disord 2001;16:769–71.

58. Loher TJ, Hasdemir MG, Burgunder JM, et al. Long-term follow-up study of chronic globus pallidus internus stimulation for posttraumatic hemidystonia. J Neurosurg 2000;92(3):457–60.

59. Shields D, Sharma N, Gale J, et al. Pallidal stimulation for dystonia in pantothenate kinase-associated neurodegeneration. Pediatr Neurol 2007;37(6):442–5.

60. Foncke EM, Schuurman PR, Speelman JD. Suicide after deep brain stimulation of the internal globus pallidus for dystonia. Neurology 2006;66:142–3.

61. Krauss JK, Yianni J, Loher TJ, et al. Deep brain stimulation for dystonia. J Clin Neurophysiol 2004;21:18–30.

62. Pillon B, Ardouin C, Dujardin K, et al. Preservation of cognitive function in dystonia treated by pallidal stimulation. Neurology 2006;66(10):1556–8.

63. Halbig TD, Gruber D, Kopp UA, et al. Pallidal stimulation in dystonia: effects on cognition, mood, and quality of life. J Neurol Neurosurg Psychiatry 2005;76:1713–6.

64. Kurlan R. Tourette's syndrome. N Engl J Med 2010;363:2332–8.

65. Mink J, Walkup J, Frey K, et al. Patient selection and assessment recommendations for deep brain stimulation in Tourette syndrome. Mov Disord 2006;21(11): 1831–8.

66. Ackermans L, Temel Y, Visser-Vandewalle V. Deep brain stimulation in Tourette's syndrome. Neurotherapeutics 2008;5(2):339–44.

67. Cavanna AE, Eddy CM, Mitchell R, et al. An approach to deep brain stimulation for severe treatment-refractory Tourette syndrome: the UK perspective. Br J Neurosurg 2011;25(1):38–44.

68. Flaherty AW, Williams ZM, Amirnovin R, et al. Deep brain stimulation of the anterior internal capsule for the treatment of Tourette syndrome: technical case report. Neurosurgery 2005;57(Suppl 3):E403.

69. Kuhn J, Lenartz D, Mai JK, et al. Deep brain stimulation of the nucleus accumbens and the internal capsule in therapeutically refractory Tourette syndrome. J Neurol 2007;254:963–5.

70. Servello D, Porta M, Sassi M, et al. Deep brain stimulation in 18 patients with severe Gilles de la Tourette syndrome refractory to treatment: the surgery and stimulation. J Neurol Neurosurg Psychiatry 2008;79(2):136–42.

71. Dehning S, Mehrkens J, Muller N, et al. Therapy-refractory Tourette syndrome: beneficial outcome with globus pallidus internus deep brain stimulation. Mov Disord 2008;23(9):1300–2.

72. Piedad JC, Rickards HE, Cavanna AE. What patients with Gilles de la Tourette syndrome should be treated with deep brain stimulation and what is the best target? Neurosurgery 2012;71:173–92.

73. Hosseini H, Mandat T, Mandat T, et al. Unilateral thalamic deep brain stimulation for disabling kinetic tremor in multiple sclerosis. Neurosurgery 2012;70(1):66–9.

74. Hassan A, Ahlskog JE, Rodriguez M, et al. Surgical therapy for multiple sclerosis tremor: a 12 year follow-up study. Eur J Neurol 2012;19:764–8.

75. Papavassiliou E, Rau G, Heath S, et al. Thalamic deep brain stimulation for essential tremor: relation of lead location to outcome. Neurosurgery 2008; 62(Suppl 2):884–94.

76. Zrinzo L, Foltynie T. Reducing hemorrhagic complications in functional neurosurgery: a large case series and systematic literature review. J Neurosurg 2012; 116:84–94.

77. Klein JC, Barbe MT, Seifried C, et al. The Tremor Network targeted by successful VIM deep brain stimulation in humans. Neurology 2012;78:787–95.

78. Kerl H, Gerigk L, Huck S, et al. Visualisation of the zona incerta for deep brain stimulation at 3.0 tesla. Clin Neuroradiol 2012;22:55–68.

79. Blomstedt P, Sandvik U, Linder J, et al. Deep brain stimulation of the subthalamic nucleus versus the zona incerta in the treatment of essential tremor. Acta Neurochir 2011;153:2329–35.

80. Sandvik U, Koskinen L, Lundquist A, et al. Thalamic and subthalamic deep brain stimulation for essential tremor: where is the optimal target? Neurosurgery 2012; 70:840–6.

81. Fytagordis A, Sandik U, Astron M, et al. Long term follow-up of deep brain stimulation of the caudal zona incerta for essential tremor. J Neurol Neurosurg Psychiatry 2012;83:258–62.

82. Skogseid M, Ramm-Pettersen J, Volkmann J, et al. Good long-term efficacy of pallidal stimulation in cervical dystonia: a prospective, observer-blinded study. Eur J Neurol 2012;19:610–5.

83. Markun L, Starr P, Air E, et al. Shorter disease duration correlates with improved long-term deep brain stimulation outcomes in young-onset DYT1 dystonia. Neurosurgery 2012;71:325–30.

84. Cannon E, Silburn P, Coyne T, et al. Deep brain stimulation of anteromedial globus pallidus interna for severe Tourette's syndrome. Am J Psychother 2012;169:860–6.

85. Li P, Huang R, Song W, et al. Deep brain stimulation of the globus pallidus internal improves symptoms of chorea-acanthocytosis. Neurol Sci 2012;33:269–74.

86. Edwards T, Zrinzo L, Limousin P, et al. Deep brain stimulation in the treatment of chorea. Mov Disord 2011;27:357–63.

87. Deon L, Kalichman M, Booth C, et al. Pallidal deep-brain stimulation associated with complete remission of self-injurious behaviors in a patient with Lesch-Nyhan syndrome: a case report. J Child Neurol 2012;27:117–20.

88. Wolcott B, Nahed BV, Kahle K, et al. Deep brain stimulation for medically refractory life threatening status dystonicus in children. J Neurosurg Pediatr 2012;9: 99–102.

89. Nolte I, Gerigk L, Al-Zghloul M, et al. Visualization of the internal globus pallidus: sequence and orientation for deep brain stimulation using a standard installation protocol at 3.0 tesla. Acta Neurochir 2012;154:481–94.

90. Cif L, Gonzalez-Martinez V, Vasques X, et al. Staged implantation of multiple electrodes in the internal globus pallidus in the treatment of primary generalized dystonia. J Neurosurg 2012;116:1144–52.

91. Visser-Vandewalle V, Temel Y, Boon P, et al. Chronic bilateral thalamic stimulation: a new therapeutic approach in intractable Tourette syndrome. J Neurosurg 2003; 99:1094–100.

92. Krauss JK, Pohle T, Weigel RA, et al. Deep brain stimulation of centre median-parafascicular complex in patients with movement disorders. J Neurol Neurosurg Psychiatry 2002;72:546–8.
93. Cooper IS, Upton AR, Amin I. Chronic cerebellar stimulation (CCS) and deep brain stimulation (DBS) in involuntary movement disorders. Appl Neurophysiol 1982;45(3):209–17.
94. Hoshi E, Tremblay L, Féger J, et al. The cerebellum communicates with the basal ganglia. Nat Neurosci 2005;8:1491–3.
95. Bostan AC, Dum RP, Strick PL, et al. The basal ganglia communicate with the cerebellum. Proc Natl Acad Sci U S A 2010;107:8452–6.
96. McIntyre C, Savasta M, Walter B, et al. How does deep brain stimulation work? Present understanding and future questions. J Clin Neurophysiol 2004;1:40–50.
97. Delong M, Wichmann T. Deep brain stimulation for movement and other neurologic disorders. Ann N Y Acad Sci 2012;1265:1–8.
98. Smith GS, Laxton W, Tang-Wai D, et al. Increased cerebral metabolism after one year of deep brain stimulation in Alzheimer disease. Arch Neurol 2012;69(9):1141–3.
99. Gradinaru V, Mogri M, Thompson K, et al. Optical deconstruction of parkinsonian neural circuitry. Science 2009;324:354–9.
100. Krook-Magnuson E, Armstrong C, Oijala M, et al. On-demand optogenetic control of spontaneous seizures in temporal lobe epilepsy. Nat Commun 2013;4:1376.
101. Nakajima T, Zrinzo L, Foltynie T, et al. MRI-guided subthalamic nucleus deep brain stimulation without microelectrode recording: can we dispense with surgery under local anaesthesia? Stereotact Funct Neurosurg 2011;89:318–25.
102. Khan S, Javed S, Park N, et al. A magnetic resonance imaging-directed method for transventricular targeting of midline structures for deep brain stimulation using implantable guide tubes. Neurosurgery 2010;66:234–7.
103. Krieg S, Buchmann N, Gempt J, et al. Diffusion tensor imaging fiber tracking using navigated brain stimulation – a feasibility study. Acta Neurochir 2012;154:555–63.
104. Yamada K, Akazawa K, Yuen S, et al. MR imaging of the ventral thalamic nuclei. AJNR Am J Neuroradiol 2010;31:732–5.
105. Seifried C, Weise L, Hartmann R, et al. Intraoperative microelectrode recording for the delineation of subthalamic nucleus topography in Parkinson's disease. Brain Stimul 2012;5:378–84.
106. Sterio D, Zonenshayn M, Mogilner A, et al. Neurophysiological refinement of subthalamic nucleus targeting. Neurosurgery 2002;50:58–69.
107. Lujan JL, Noecker AM, Butson CR, et al. Automated 3-dimensional brain atlas fitting to microelectrode recordings from deep brain stimulation surgeries. Stereotact Funct Neurosurg 2009;87:229–40.
108. Novak P, Przybyszewski A, Barborica A, et al. Localization of the subthalamic nucleus in Parkinson disease using multi unit activity. J Neurol Sci 2011;310(1–2):44–9.
109. Little S, Brown P. What brain signals are suitable for feedback control of DBS in PD. Ann N Y Acad Sci 2012;1265:9–24.
110. Berenyi A, Belluscio M, Mao D, et al. Closed loop control of epilepsy by transcranial electrical stimulation. Science 2012;337:735–7.
111. Anderson JS, Dhatt HS, Ferguson MA, et al. Functional connectivity targeting for deep brain stimulation in essential tremor. AJNR Am J Neuroradiol 2011;32:1963–8.

112. Chaturvedi A, Foutz T, McIntyre C. Current steering to activate targeted neural pathways during deep brain stimulation of the subthalamic region. Brain Stimul 2012;5:369–77.
113. Okun M, Gallo B, Mandybur G, et al. Subthalamic deep brain stimulation with a constant-current device in Parkinson's disease: an open-label randomized controlled trial. Lancet Neurol 2012;11:140–9.
114. Essert C, Haegelen C, Lalys F, et al. Automatic computation of electrode trajectories for deep brain stimulation: a hybrid symbolic and numerical approach. Int J Comput Assist Radiol Surg 2012;7:517–32.
115. Han M, Manoonkitiwongsa P, Wang C, et al. In vivo validation of custom-designed silicon-based microelectrode arrays for long-term neural recording and stimulation. IEEE Trans Biomed Eng 2012;59:346–54.
116. Larson P. Minimally invasive surgery for movement disorders. Neurosurg Clin N Am 2010;21:691–8.
117. Fenoy AJ, Simpson RK. Management of device related wound complications in deep brain stimulation surgery. J Neurosurg 2012;116:1324–32.
118. Allert N, Markou M, Miskiewicz AA, et al. Electrode dysfunctions in patients with deep brain stimulation: a clinical retrospective study. Acta Neurochir 2011;153:2342–9.
119. Englot DJ, Glastonbury CM, Larson P. Abnormal T2-weighted MRI signal surrounding leads in a subset of deep brain stimulation patients. Stereotact Funct Neurosurg 2011;89:311–7.
120. Hyam J, Kringelbach M, Silburn P, et al. The autonomic effects of deep brain stimulation– a therapeutic opportunity. Nat Rev Neurol 2012;8:391–400.

# Update on Therapeutic Options for Multiple Sclerosis

Matthew McCoyd, MD

## KEYWORDS

- McDonald criteria • Fingolimod (Gilenya) • Teriflunomide (Aubagio)
- BG-12 (Tecfidera) • Natalizumab (Tysabri) • Alemtuzumab (Lemtrada) • Vitamin D

## KEY POINTS

- Physicians and their patients with multiple sclerosis (MS), a disease that predominantly affects young people and commonly leads to disability, now have an increasing armamentarium of therapeutic options at their disposal to combat the condition.
- The diagnostic criteria for MS have been recently updated and now include simplified radiologic findings to satisfy the classical dissemination in space (DIS) and dissemination in time (DIT); however, the diagnosis still rests on the clinical presentation.
- The recently approved and emerging therapies seem to offer greater efficacy than the "platform" therapies that were first introduced starting in the 1990s (although with limited head-to-head data) and also may have more complex side effect profiles for physicians to navigate.
- Although a single "cause" of MS has not been identified, there is increasing evidence that vitamin D deficiency likely plays a role in MS and that supplementation of vitamin D is both safe and potentially beneficial in the treatment of MS.

## INTRODUCTION

MS has been part of the human condition likely since the beginning of time. Literature from the early the 1300s describing the medical maladies of St Lidwina of Holland paint a picture that is highly characteristic of relapsing-remitting MS by today's review. Her physicians, at a loss for effective options, treated her ailments by wrapping her head in candlewick. In the mid-1800s, the clinical features of MS were well described by Charcot and the pathologic features beautifully detailed by Dr Robert Carswell. Despite increasing medical knowledge and understanding of the disease, treatments lagged far behind. Charcot's outlook on treatment in the 1800s was, unfortunately, true for greater than a century: "After what precedes, need I detain you longer over the question of remedies? The time has not yet come when such a subject can be seriously considered. I can only tell you of some experiments, the results of which have, unfortunately, not been very encouraging."

Neurology Residency Training Program, Loyola University Medical Center, Building 105, Room 2700, 2160 South First Avenue, Maywood, IL 60153, USA
E-mail address: mmccoyd@lumc.edu

Neurol Clin 31 (2013) 827–845
http://dx.doi.org/10.1016/j.ncl.2013.03.010     neurologic.theclinics.com

Into this void many advocated various treatments and remedies, some well meaning and others with more dubious intentions. "Failure to make headway with effective treatment…did not prevent rampant speculation or extensive therapeutic experimentation. As a result, multiple sclerosis soon acquired a regrettable reputation for maverick medicine based on shameless exploitation of its capricious natural history, which flattered the uncritical and those devoted to extrapolation from anecdotal experience."[1] Sadly, with an understandable desire for a "cure" from patients and families, this practice of "medicine" has not been eradicated to this day.

It was not until the early 1990s that, after decades of study, the first effective disease-modifying agent for the treatment of relapsing forms of MS, interferon beta-1b (IFNB), was approved based on the data from its clinical study.[2,3] The study was able to show a statistically significant reduction in relapses, time to first and second exacerbation, and the disease burden detected by magnetic resonance imaging (MRI).[2,3] Although not a cure, it was a major breakthrough that led to great, and well-deserved, excitement within the MS community. "IFNB is not the long-awaited cure for MS. Almost all patients on medication had attacks eventually, and one in four deteriorated. But half a loaf is better than no bread, and should treatment with IFNB translate into extra years of gainful employment and quality life, if only for some, that would be sweet indeed."[4]

Today, we stand on the precipice of changing landscape in MS therapies. Several new medications have been approved by the US Food and Drug Administration (FDA) in the United States, and several more are awaiting a final decision or are completing phase 3 clinical trials. The question facing physicians, patients, and families is not just a question of remedies but how to navigate the increasingly complex effective treatment options for MS.

### Updates in Diagnostic Criteria for Multiple Sclerosis

Although the primary focus of this review is on recent updates in therapeutic options, at least a short review of the recent changes in the diagnostic criteria is prudent. The bedrock of the diagnosis still lies in the clinical context of the patient's presentation and physical examination findings, suggesting relapsing pathologic condition of the central nervous system (CNS). Little has changed from the clinical perspective of diagnosis since the "Schumacher Criteria" was first introduced in 1965: objective evidence on neurologic examination or by history of dysfunction of 2 or more separate parts of the nervous system reflecting predominantly white matter pathologic condition separated by a reasonable period without a more reasonable explanation.[5] However, although the clinical context is still the single most critical component in diagnostic consideration, cranial and spinal cord MRI has become an indispensable paraclinical study. Since the initial paper reviewing the MRI findings in patients with MS demonstrated "abnormalities on a scale not previously seen except at necropsy" was published in the Lancet 1981 and led the investigators to correctly conclude "the potential of NMR in the diagnosis of MS needs little emphasis," MRI has become increasingly critical to the diagnosis.[6] Although only briefly mentioned in the 1983 "Poser Criteria,"[7] MRI took on a critical role in the 2001 "McDonald criteria" for the diagnosis of MS, allowing for an earlier diagnosis in those who experienced a clinically isolated syndrome (CIS) before the second clinical event.[8]

The McDonald Criteria were revised in 2005[9] and more recently in 2010.[10] The major change in the 2010 criteria is regarding MRI criteria for dissemination in space (DIS) and dissemination in time (DIT). The previous criteria (Modified Barkhof/Tintore criteria)[11,12] for DIS and DIT were believed to be too difficult to apply consistently by nonimaging specialists.[10] Under the current McDonald criteria, DIS utilizes the

"Swanton criteria."[13] DIS can now be shown by the presence of 1 T2 lesion in 2 of 4 critical areas: juxtacortical, periventricular, infratentorial, and spinal cord (with lesions within a symptomatic region excluded in patients with brainstem or spinal cord syndromes). DIT can be confirmed by the presence of a new T2 lesion at any time, irrespective of the timing of the baseline MRI, or an asymptomatic gadolinium-enhancing (GdE) lesion not due to non-MS pathology at any time. This revision is based on the concept that if both enhancing and nonenhancing lesions are seen on the same scan, they did not develop during the same demyelinating event and therefore indicate 2 or more separate demyelinating events.[14] The panel emphasized that the criteria should only by applied to those who have experienced a typical CIS or progressive paraparesis/cerebellar/cognitive syndrome in the setting of suspected primary progressive MS. Interestingly, the panel did not include cerebrospinal fluid (CSF) analysis as part of the diagnostic algorithm. The panel "reaffirmed that positive CSF findings (elevated IgG index or two or more oligoclonal bands) can be important to support the inflammatory demyelinating nature of the underlying condition, to evaluate alternative diagnosis and to predict CDMS." However, CSF was not included because the panel believed that "further liberalizing the MRI requirement in CSF-positive patients is not appropriate, as CSF status was not evaluated for its contribution to Magnetic Imaging in Multiple Sclerosis (MAGNIMS) criteria for DIS and DIT."[10]

The current criteria have clearly simplified and streamlined the diagnosis of MS, likely increasing the number of patients who will be diagnosed with the disease or at least allowing them to be diagnosed at a much earlier time. It is not clear what impact this will have on the "perception" of MS (because those with milder disease, and possibly better outcomes, will be included). It is particularly important to consider the diagnostic criteria in place at the time of the various disease-modifying therapy pivotal trials. The patients who took part in the 1993 IFNB clinical trial were somewhat different than those involved in more recent studies, having slightly more severe and longer-running MS. Indeed, the overall event rate has decreased in MS clinical trials— in both the treatment and placebo arms.[14,15] Patients with more benign disease have been recruited into MS clinical trials over the last decade compared to the "original" pivotal trials, in part due to improvements in MRI technology and use, the availability of proven therapies, and changes in the demographics of MS.[16]

### Pathogenesis of Multiple Sclerosis

Although the pathogenesis of MS is incompletely understood, a brief review of the generally accepted simplistic theories of MS may be helpful in understanding the role of some of the new treatment options for MS. It is generally, although not universally, held that MS is an immune-mediated inflammatory disease.[17,18] A widely held concept is that MS occurs when certain environmental exposures (such as viruses), or lack thereof (of adequate sunlight/vitamin D), trigger the activation of CNS autoreactive T cells in genetically susceptible individuals (although no causative genes have been identified and the disease does not seem to be purely genetic), which leads to a CNS inflammatory disease.[19] The target of the immune-mediated response is believed to be cellular components of the CNS that are normally shielded by the immunologic privilege in part provided by the blood–brain barrier (BBB).[20] Antigen-presenting cells (APCs) may "present" CNS self-antigen fragments to CNS-reactive T cells in cervical lymph nodes that drain the brain or may present foreign antigens with characteristics similar to CNS self-antigens ("molecular mimicry").[19] Activated T cells may then exit the lymph nodes and upregulate molecules that facilitate migration across the BBB.[19] Once within the CNS, autoreactive immune cells participate in a proinflammatory-mediated process that leads to demyelination and eventual axonal injury.[21]

Within this context, it would seem to make sense that the treatment of MS would be directed at altering the function of the dysregulated immune system. This approach can be achieved by aggressive immune suppression (which has generally not proven to be effective[4,19]), sequestering autoreactive T cells within lymph nodes, preventing their trafficking across the BBB, and/or altering their response within the CNS.

### Recently Approved Therapies for Multiple Sclerosis: Fingolimod, Teriflunimide and Tecfidera

Fingolimod (Gilenya), a once daily oral tablet, was approved by the FDA for the treatment of relapsing forms of MS on September 22, 2010. Fingolimod is believed to work by sequestering autoreactive T cells and B cells within lymph nodes, preventing their migration into the CNS before they even enter the peripheral blood stream.[22] Fingolimod is a sphingosine-1-phosphate (S1P) receptor (S1PR) modulator.[23] There are 5 identified S1PRs subtypes. T and B cells express $S1P_1$ primarily and $S1P1_{3-5}$ less so. Lymphocytes migrate along an S1P gradient to egress from lymph nodes. The binding of fingolimod to $S1P_1$ results in the internalization and degradation of the receptor, effectively sequestering the cells within the lymph nodes.

Fingolimod was approved based on 2 randomized double-blind phase 3 clinical trials: FREEDOMS (FTY720 Research Evaluating Effects of Daily Oral Therapy in Multiple Sclerosis)[24] and TRANSFORMS (Trial Assessing Injectable Interferon vs FTY720 Oral in Relapsing-Remitting Multiple Sclerosis).[25] FREEDOMS was a 24-month placebo-controlled trial that enrolled patients with relapsing-remitting MS aged 18 to 55 years with Expanded Disability Status Scale (EDSS) scores of 0 to 5.5, who had either one or more relapses in the previous 1 year or 2 or more relapses in the previous 2 years, to receive either fingolimod at a dose of 0.5 mg or 1.25 mg daily or placebo at a 1:1:1 ratio.[24] The primary end point was the annualized relapse rate (ARR). Secondary end points included the time to confirmed disability progression (an increase of 1 point in EDSS score [or half point if the baseline EDSS was 5.5]) confirmed after 3 months and absence of relapse, time to disability progression confirmed after 6 months, and MRI measures of inflammation, burden of disease, and tissue destruction. Of the 1272 enrolled patients, 1033 completed the study. Patients participated at 138 centers in 22 countries.

The ARR was 0.18 for the 0.5 mg dose, 0.16 for the 1.25 mg dose, and 0.40 for the placebo arm, representing relative reductions of 54% and 60%, respectively. The cumulative probability of disability progression confirmed over 3 months was 17.7% for the 0.5 mg dose, 16.6% for the 1.25 mg dose, and 24.1% for the placebo group. The cumulative probability of disability progression confirmed over 6 months was 12.5% for the 0.5 mg dose, 11.5% for the 1.25 mg dose, and 19% for placebo.

The treatment arms (0.5 mg and 1.25 mg arms) also had significantly fewer GdE lesions at 6, 12, and 24 months, as well as fewer new or enlarged T2 lesions.

The TRANSFORMS study was a 12-month double-blind double-whammy study. Patients with MS with a recent history of at least 1 relapse were randomized to receive fingolimod, 1.25 mg or 0.5 mg, or interferon beta-1a at a weekly intramuscular dose of 30 μg. The primary end point was the ARR. Secondary end points included the number of new or enlarged T2 lesions and progression of sustained disability at 3 months.[25] Inclusion criteria were similar to those of the FREEDOMS study. A total of 1292 patients were recruited at 172 centers from 18 countries; 1153 completed the study.

The ARRs were 0.20 for the 1.25 mg dose, 0.16 for the 0.5 mg dose, and 0.33 for the interferon group, relative risk reductions (RRR) of 38% and 52% compared with the interferon group. Patients receiving fingolimod had significantly fewer new or enlarged T2 and GdE lesions. There were no significant differences in confirmed disability progression.

A third randomized double-blind placebo-controlled trial, FREEDOMS II, was recently completed.[26] The 24-month study with 1083 patients was a multicenter trial, with a largely US cohort (95%).[27] About 75% of patients had undergone prior treatment. A total of 778 patients completed the study. The primary end point was the reduction in the ARR. Fingolimod, 0.5 mg, reduced the ARR by 48% (ARR ratio: 0.52) compared with placebo. There was no significant difference in disability progression. In all 5 clinical studies (phase 3 studies: FREEDOMS, FREEDOMS II, and TRANSFORMS; phase 2 studies: D2201, D1201), the 0.5 mg dose of fingolimod reduced the ARR by 48% to 54% versus placebo.[28]

Adverse events were similar in the 2 trials (FREEDOMS and TRANSFORMS). There were 2 deaths in the FREEDOMS trial, 2 during the TRANSFORMS trial, and 2 after the trial concluded. In the FREEDOMS trial, 2 of the deaths were in the placebo arm (1 due to a pulmonary embolism and the other from a traffic accident). The cause of death in the fingolimod group was suicide; the patient was receiving the 1.25 mg dose. The 2 deaths in the TRANSFORMS trial also occurred in the 1.25 mg arm. One death was related to disseminated primary varicella zoster virus (VZV) infection. The patient had no history of chicken pox, had negative value of baseline VZV antibody titer, and was exposed to a child with chicken pox while receiving a course of corticosteroids for an MS relapse. Baseline VZV antibody titers are recommended in patients considering fingolimod. For those who have no history of chicken pox and test negative for VZV antibody titer, pretreatment immunization is recommended. The second death was related to herpes simplex encephalitis. The patient received intravenous methylprednisolone after initially presenting for a presumed MS relapse. Two patients, also receiving the 1.25 mg dose, died after the conclusion of the TRANSFORMS trial. One patient died because of complications from aspiration pneumonia (baseline EDSS 5.0) 6 months after the trial ended; the patient had discontinued fingolimod after 11 months and was not on the medication at the time of death. The other patient died as a result of metastatic breast cancer 10 months after the trial concluded.[25] There were no deaths in either trial among patients receiving the 0.5 mg dose.

Fingolimod administration is associated with T-cell lymphopenia. However, despite concerns for significant infectious processes, to date there has been no such signal. Certain infections were seen more commonly in those receiving active treatment in the phase 3 clinical trials. Lower respiratory tract infections were seen more commonly with fingolimod (9.6% receiving 0.5 mg vs 6.0% receiving placebo). In April 2012, a patient receiving fingolimod was diagnosed with progressive multifocal leukoencephalopathy (PML). However, the patient had been on natalizumab for 3 years and tested positive for John Cunningham virus (JCV) antibody, prompting the switch.[29] The patient was diagnosed with PML within a few months of discontinuing natalizumab. It was not apparent at the time this manuscript was submitted whether fingolimod had or had not contributed to the infection. Overall, the infectious signal seems to be low. Integrated safety results from fingolimod phase 2 and phase 3 clinical studies have not shown an increased risk of infections.[30] "Although serious infections and neoplastic complications might be anticipated with a drug that dramatically reduces the number of lymphocytes, this was not seen in the fingolimod development program. The overall incidence of infection, including severe and serious infections, was comparable between control groups and those receiving fingolimod 0.5 mg."[23]

Cardiac side effects have been recognized with the use of fingolimod both during the clinical trials and after the drug came to market. Transient dose-related decreases in heart rate (HR) occur after the first dose.[24] Based on the finding in clinical trials, 6-hour first dose observation (FDO) was recommended. Decreases were generally mild and usually within the first 6 hours, with the second decrease occurring as late as 20 hours later. Sitting systolic blood pressure (BP) dropped by 4.12 mm Hg and sitting diastolic BP dropped by 2.97 mm Hg during FDO. The average sitting HR measured by apical pulse decreased by 6.97 beats per minute (BPM) during FDO and 6.81 BPM in registry trials. Maximal decreases occurred around 5 hours after first dose.[31] A 57-year old man in the United States died within 24 hours of receiving the first dose. The cause of death could not be identified and there was not thought to be clear evidence that the drug played a role in the death. The patient did have "extensive brainstem lesions" and was taking two BP medications (metoprolol and amlodipine). There were several deaths reported in patients in Europe receiving fingolimod. Of these, 3 were due to sudden heart attacks, 1 was from bradycardia, and 6 cases were unexplained. There is no evidence that fingolimod was related to the deaths. The FDA evaluated the cases and could not definitively conclude that fingolimod was related to any of the deaths.[32] The FDA did recommend that fingolimod be contraindicated for any patient with recent (6 months) occurrence of myocardial infarction, unstable angina, stroke, transient ischemic attack (TIA), decompensated heart failure requiring hospitalization, class III or IV heart failure, history of Mobitz type II second or third degree atrioventricular block or sick sinus syndrome (unless the patient has a pacemaker), baseline QT interval of 500 ms or more, or treatment with class Ia or class III antiarrhythmic drugs.[33]

Macular edema, a condition defined by fluid accumulation within the central retina or macula, was also noted in clinical trials, albeit rarely (0.5% in TRANSFORMS, 0.6% in FREEDOMS).[34] The overall incidence with the 0.5 mg dose in all phase 2 and phase 3 trials, including FREEDOMS II, was 0.4%. Most of the cases occurred within the first three months of starting therapy. Most resolved within 6 months after treatment was discontinued.[24] Unlike optic neuritis (ON), macular edema is usually painless and is not associated with a rapid alternating pupillary defect, and patients usually experience metamorphopsia. It is recommended that patients undergo a baseline ophthalmologic examination and a second examination after 3 to 4 months. Patients with a history of diabetes mellitus or uveitis are at an increased risk of macular edema.

Teriflunomide (Aubagio) is a once-daily oral medication that has been FDA approved for the treatment of relapsing forms of MS. Teriflunomide is the active metabolite of leflunomide. Leflunomide was approved in 1998 for the treatment of rheumatoid arthritis (trade name: Arava). This drug reversibly inhibits dihydroorotate dehydrogenase, a mitochondrial enzyme involved in pyrimidine synthesis for DNA replication.[35] The drug limits stimulated T-cell and B-cell activation, proliferation, and function in response to autoantigens. Slowly dividing or resting cells, which rely on the salvage pathway for pyrimidine synthesis, are relatively unaffected by teriflunomide.[36]

Teriflunomide's pivotal trial, the Teriflunomide Multiple Sclerosis Trial (TEMSO), was a randomized double-blind placebo-controlled parallel group study. A total of 1088 patients from 127 centers in 21 countries were randomized, and 1086 patients received treatment (placebo, teriflunomide, 7 mg, or teriflunomide, 14 mg). A total of 796 patients in this group completed the study, with a similar proportion of patients in each arm completing the study (71.3% for placebo, 74.9% for the 7 mg dose, and 73.3% for the 14 mg dose). Patients eligible for enrollment were those aged 18 to 55 years, who met McDonald criteria (2005) for the diagnosis of MS, had relapsing forms of MS (with or without progression), had an EDSS of 5.5 or less, and had at least 2 relapses within the past 2 years or 1 relapse within the previous 1 year (but none in the 60 days before randomization). The primary end point was determining the efficacy of teriflunomide in reducing the ARR (the number of confirmed relapses per patient-year). Key secondary end points included determining the efficacy of teriflunomide in delaying the progression of disability (defined as an increase from baseline

EDSS of at least 1.0 point, and of 0.5 points for those with an EDSS $\geq$5.5) and total lesion volume on MRI.

Teriflunomide reduced the ARR at 7 mg and 14 mg doses when compared with placebo (0.54 for placebo, 0.37 for both 7 mg and 14 mg doses of teriflunomide), with a 31% relative reduction in relapse rate. The time to first relapse was longer and the number of relapse-free patients was higher. There was a 23.7% RRR for confirmed disability progression for 7 mg teriflunomide and 29.8% reduction for 14 mg teriflunomide when compared with placebo (27.3% for placebo, 21.7% for 7 mg dose, 20.2% for the 14 mg dose). Patients in both teriflunomide treatment arms had few GdE lesions and fewer unique active lesions (new T2 or GdE lesions).

The effectiveness, safety, and tolerability of teriflunomide was compared with that of 3 times weekly subcutaneous interferon beta-1a (Rebif) in the phase 3 TENERE (A Study Comparing the Effectiveness and Safety of Teriflunomide and Interferon Beta-1a in Patients with Relapsing Multiple Sclerosis) trial. The trial included 324 patients. The primary end point was the risk of treatment failure, defined as the occurrence of a confirmed relapse or permanent discontinuation for any cause, whichever came first. No statistical superiority was observed between the 2 treatments. The estimated ARR of teriflunomide, 14 mg, (0.259) was similar to the relapse rate in the interferon arm (0.216). The rate of permanent treatment discontinuation was higher in the interferon arm (21.8%) than the teriflunomide 7 mg arm (8.2%) and 14 mg arm (10.9%). An additional phase 3 multicenter double-blind placebo-controlled clinical trial, the TOWER (Teriflunomide Oral in People with Relapsing Multiple Sclerosis) study, also compared teriflunomide to placebo. The study included 1169 patients in 26 countries. The study showed a 36.3% reduction in the ARR (0.319) for those treated with teriflunomide, 14 mg, compared with placebo (0.501), the primary end point. About 52% of treated patients were relapse free as opposed to 38% in the placebo arm. There was a 31.5% reduction in the risk of 12-week sustained disability.[37] Teriflunomide is also being studied in a CIS trial, TOPIC (Phase III Study with Teriflunomide Versus Placebo in Patients with First Clinical Symptoms of Multiple Sclerosis). The study is expected to be completed in June 2013.[38]

Common adverse effects with an increased incidence in the teriflunomide groups compared with placebo group included diarrhea, nausea, hair thinning or decreased hair density, and elevated alanine aminotransferase levels. Hair thinning was generally mild or moderate in intensity, with the maximum hair loss occurring in the first 6 months, and was distributed evenly over the scalp (vs patchy). Most cases of hair loss resolved while the patient was on therapy.[39] Mean reductions in neutrophil and lymphocyte count baseline values were small in magnitude but slightly more notable in the 14 mg arm than in the 7 mg or placebo arm. No serious opportunistic infections were observed. Screening for latent tuberculosis is recommended because the medication can reactivate the disease. A total of 3 cases of serious pyelonephritis were reported in the 14 mg group. No deaths were reported.

Teriflunomide has been labeled a pregnancy category X medication for both women and men, although there are no cases of known birth defects associated with the drug. The pregnancy rating is based on leflunomide's (Arava) pregnancy category. The pregnancy category was assigned based on the mechanism of action of the drug (interference with DNA and RNA synthesis) as well as on animal studies in pregnant rats and rabbits, which demonstrated an increased risk for congenital malformations, and not based on human cases.[40] Two separate studies did not demonstrate an increase in the rate of major malformations or a specific pattern of major malformations in children of women exposed to leflunomide before or after conception.[41,42] There were 11 pregnancies during the TEMSO trial. There were 4 spontaneous abortions (1 in the placebo arm and 3 in the high-dose teriflunomide group) and 6 induced abortions. One patient in the high-dose group was treated for 31 days of pregnancy and delivered a healthy baby. Over the entire teriflunomide clinical program, 65 pregnancies were reported in 63 patients across 8 clinical studies. Of the 65 pregnancies, 43 occurred in patients exposed to teriflunomide. There were 20 induced abortions, 8 spontaneous abortions, 12 healthy newborns, 2 "ongoing pregnancies," and 1 "outcome pending." No structural defects or functional deficits have been reported to date.[43,44] The rate of spontaneous abortions was similar to that of the general population.

The medication can be rapidly cleared with cholestyramine or activated charcoal. Teriflunomide has a long terminal half-life (~19 days) because it is highly protein bound and is slowly eliminated from the plasma (taking up to 6 months).[36] Treatment with cholestyramine has been shown to decrease teriflunomide concentrations by 97% or more after 11 days of administration and reduce the elimination half-life of teriflunomide to 2 to 3 days.[36] The drug does not need to be given on 11 consecutive days unless there is a need for rapid elimination. Teriflunomide levels can be checked to confirm drug clearance.

BG-12 (Tecfidera, dimethyl fumarate or Tecfidera) is a twice-daily oral medication that has been investigated for use in relapsing forms of MS. BG-12 is thought to activate the nuclear 1 factor-like 2 antioxidant response pathway, the primary cellular defense against the cytotoxic effects of oxidative stress.[45] Fumaric acid esters may decrease leukocyte passage through the BBB and exert neuroprotective properties by the activation of antioxidative pathways.[46] BG-12 may also suppress proinflammatory cytokine production or directly inhibit proinflammatory pathways.[45] Fumarates have been used for 2 decades to treat psoriasis.[47]

BG-12 was studied in 2 phase 3 trials: DEFINE and CONFIRM. DEFINE (Determination of the Efficacy and Safety of Oral Fumarate in Relapsing-Remitting Multiple Sclerosis) was a randomized double-blind placebo-controlled 2-year trial that compared 2 doses of BG-12 to placebo. Eligible patients were those aged 18 to 55 years, diagnosed with relapsing MS by the McDonald criteria, with baseline EDSS of 0 to 5.0, with a documented clinical relapse within 12 months before randomization, or with at least 1 GdE lesion on MRI 6 weeks before randomization. A total of 1237 patients from 198 sites in 28 countries were randomized and 1234 received treatment; 952 completed the study (78% in placebo and 77% in BG-12 arms). Patients were randomized 1:1:1 to receive BG-12 at a dose of 240 mg twice daily, 240 mg 3 times daily, or placebo. The primary end point was the proportion of patients who had a relapse by 2 years. Secondary end points included the numbers of GdE lesions and of new or enlarging T2 hyperintense lesions, the ARR, and the time to progression of disability.

BG-12 significantly reduced the proportion of patients who had at least 1 relapse by 2 years. About 27% of the patients on twice daily and 26% of patients in the 3 times daily group, when compared with 46% in the placebo group, had a relapse at 2 years. Patients receiving treatment had a 49% to 50% reduction in the risk of relapse compared with placebo. Time to first relapse was prolonged from 38 weeks in the placebo arm to 87 and 91 weeks in the BG-12 groups. The ARR was 0.17 in the twice daily BG-12 group and 0.19 in the 3 times daily group compared with 0.36 in the placebo group, relative reductions of 53% and 48%.

BG-12 reduced the risk of confirmed disability progression that was sustained for 12 weeks by 38% in the twice daily group and 34% in the 3 times daily group. Compared with placebo, BG-12 reduced the number of new or enlarging lesions by 85% with the twice daily regimen and 74% with the 3 times daily regimen. GdE lesions were reduced by 90% (twice daily) and 73% (3 times daily). About 93% of patients in the twice daily arm were free from GdE lesions at 2 years.

The CONFIRM (Comparator and an Oral Fumarate in Relapsing-Remitting Multiple Sclerosis) trial was a randomized, multicenter (200 sites in 28 countries), double-blind, 2-year trial that evaluated the efficacy of and safety of BG-12. A rater-blinded active agent, glatiramer acetate (Copaxone) was included as a reference comparator (patients were aware of their treatment). A total of 1430 patients were enrolled, and 1417 patients were included in the intention-to-treat population. Patients were randomized 1:1:1:1 to receive oral placebo, BG-12, 240 mg twice daily or 3 times daily, or daily subcutaneous glatiramer acetate. The primary efficacy end point was the annualized relapse rate at 2 years. Secondary end points included the number of new or enlarging hyperintense T2 lesions, new hypointense lesions on T1, proportion of patients with a relapse, and time to disability progression. Tertiary end points included a comparison of the relative benefits and risks of BG-12 or glatiramer acetate versus placebo.[48]

BG-12 twice daily and 3 times daily led to a reduction in the ARR relative to placebo of 44% and 50% (0.22 and 0.20 vs 0.40), respectively. Glatiramer acetate reduced the ARR by 29% versus placebo (0.29 vs 0.40). The risk of a relapse was reduced by 34% with twice daily BG-12, 45% with 3 times daily BG-12, and 29% with glatiramer acetate. Disability progression was not statistically reduced with any of the treatments.

The number of new or enlarging T2 lesions was reduced with twice daily BG-12 by 71%, 3 times daily BG-12 by 73%, and glatiramer acetate by 54%. New hypointense T1 lesions were reduced by 57% by twice daily BG-12, by 65% by 3 times daily BG-12, and by 41% by glatiramer acetate. The percentage of patients free from new or enlarging T2 lesions was 27% for twice daily BG-12, 31% for 3 times daily BG-12, and 24% for glatiramer acetate (compared with12% for placebo). The odds of having more GdE lesions was reduced by twice daily BG-12 by 74%, by 3 times daily BG-12 by 65%, and by glatiramer acetate by 61%.

Adverse events that occurred more frequently in patients receiving BG-12 in both studies included flushing, gastrointestinal (GI) events (diarrhea, nausea, upper abdominal pain, and vomiting), upper respiratory tract infections, erythema, proteinuria, and pruritis. The incidence of flushing and GI events was the highest in the first month of treatment and declined thereafter. Flushing occurred in 35% of the twice daily BG-12 group and in 28% of the 3 times daily group. GI events occurred in 36% and 41%. Discontinuation due to GI events was 5% to 6% in the 2 BG-12 groups. Similar side effects were noted in the phase 2b study.[49] There were 2 deaths, both being the result of road accidents.

The mean white blood cell count and lymphocyte count decreased over the first year of treatment. No opportunistic infections and no serious infections were reported. The most common infections were nasopharyngitis, upper respiratory tract infections, urinary tract infection, and influenza. No malignancies were noted. Neoplasms and infections have not emerged as problems during the 2 decades of fumarate use for psoriasis.[47] No new or worsening safety signals were identified in the ENDORSE (A Dose-Blind, Multicenter, Extension Study to Determine the Long-Term Safety and Efficacy of Two Doses of BG00012 Monotherapy in Subjects with Relapsing-Remitting Multiple Sclerosis) trial, a 5-year extension study of the 2 phase 3 trials (DEFINE and CONFIRM).[50]

### Therapies Under FDA Review: Alemtuzamab

Alemtuzumab is a humanized monoclonal antibody against CD52, an antigen found on the surface of normal and malignant lymphocytes.[51] The monoclonal antibody was first constructed with the Cambridge pathology laboratories, leading to the name "Campath."[52] This antibody causes rapid complement-mediated lysis of almost all circulating lymphocytes by targeting the CD52 antigen, a low-molecular-weight glycoprotein present on the surface of most lymphocyte lineages, causing prolonged T-cell depletion.[52] The impact on T-cell depletion is also long lasting, with the median recovery time of CD4 lymphocytes to the lower limit of normal after 35 months.[53]

Alemtuzumab has been studied in several trials. Alemtuzumab was compared with interferon beta-1a 44 μg 3 times weekly in a randomized blinded phase 2 trial in previously untreated, early, relapsing-remitting MS.[54] A set of 334 patients in 49 centers across Europe and the United States were randomized. Eligibility requirements included an onset of symptoms no more than 36 months before the time of screening, at least 2 clinical episodes during the previous 2 years, a score of 3 or less on the EDSS, and 1 or more enhancing lesions on at least 1 of 4 monthly MRIs. Patients received 1:1:1 alemtuzumab, 12 mg/d, 24 mg/d, or interferon beta-1a. Alemtuzumab was given by intravenous infusion on 5 consecutive days during the first month and 3 consecutive days at months 12 and 24, and patients were premedicated with 1 g of methylprednisolone. The coprimary measures of efficacy were the time to sustained disability and the relapse rate. Secondary outcomes were the proportion of patients who did not have a relapse, changes in lesion burden (on T2), and brain volume.

Alemtuzumab reduced the risk of sustained disability by 71% compared with interferon beta-1a. There were no significant differences between the groups receiving 12 or 24 mg doses. In both alemtuzumab groups, the mean disability score on EDSS improved by 0.39 points, and it worsened by 0.38 points for those on interferon. Alemtuzumab reduced the rate of relapse by 74% compared with interferon. The ARR for the interferon group was 0.36 versus 0.10 for alemtuzumab. The proportion of patients who remained relapse free was 80% for alemtuzumab versus 52% for interferon. There was a reduction in the volume of lesions as seen on T2-weighted MRI in all 3 study groups, but it was more marked after treatment with alemtuzumab.

At 5-year follow-up, alemtuzumab reduced the risk of sustained disability by 72% and the rate of relapse by 69% compared with interferon.[55] The ARR from baseline to month 60 was 0.11 for alemtuzumab and 0.35 for interferon.

Alemtuzumab was investigated in 2 recent phase 3 clinical trials: CARE-MS I and CARE-MS II.[56,57] CARE-MS I (Comparison of Alemtuzumab and Rebif Efficacy in Multiple Sclerosis) recruited a population of previously untreated patients with early MS with low disability levels. CARE-MS II recruited patients with relapsing MS who had had disease activity while on immunomodulatory therapy with either interferon or glatiramer acetate.[58]

CARE-MS I patients were randomized 2:1 to alemtuzumab, 12 mg given once daily for five days and then once per day for 3 days 12 months later, or subcutaneous interferon beta-1a, 44 μg 3 times weekly. Coprimary end points were relapse rate and time to 6-month sustained accumulation of disability. About 40% of the patients in the interferon group showed relapsed compared with 22% of the alemtuzumab-treated patients, a 54.9% improvement. About 59% of the patients receiving interferon were relapse free compared with 78% of the alemtuzumab group and 11% of the interferon group had sustained disability compared with 8% of the alemtuzumab group. The results were similar to the phase 2 study that it replicated, demonstrating a profound impact on relapse rate. However, unlike the phase 2 study, it did not show an effect on worsening of impairment or disability compared with those treated with interferon.[58] Those treated with alemtuzumab had nearly identical rates of disability progression in the 2 trials, but the interferon group had a much lower rate in CARE-MS I (11%) than in the phase 2 study (26%).

CARE-MS II was a 2-year rater-masked randomized controlled phase 3 trial. This study enrolled patients with at least 1 relapse on an interferon or glatiramer acetate. Patients were randomized 1:2:2 to receive subcutaneous interferon beta-1a 3 times weekly, alemtuzumab, 12 mg, or alemtuzumab, 24 mg, (although the 24 mg group was discontinued to aid recruitment). Coprimary end points were relapse rate and time to 6-month sustained disability. About 51% of the interferon-treated patients showed relapse compared with 35% of the alemtuzumab-treated patients, a 49.4% improvement. About 47% of the interferon-treated patients were relapse free compared with 65% of the alemtuzumab patients and 20% of the interferon patients had sustained disability compared with 13% of the alemtuzumab-treated patients.[57] Patients had fewer new or enlarging T2 lesions and contrast-enhancing lesions but no significant advantage in brain volume.[58]

Acquired autoimmunity has been a common adverse effect of alemtuzumab. The phase 2 study was launched in December 2002 and stopped in September 2005 after reports of 3 cases of immune thrombocytopenic purpura (ITP), including 1 death.[54] About 30% of alemtuzumab-treated patients developed thyroid disorders over 5 years (compared with 4% of those treated with interferon), 2 patients developed papillary thyroid cancer, 3% had ITP, and 1 had Goodpasture syndrome.[52]

Mild-to-moderate infectious complications were also more common in those treated with alemtuzumab than in those treated with interferon (67% vs 46%). About 16% of treated patients developed herpes zoster, necessitating prophylactic treatment with acyclovir.[52]

Infusion reactions with alemtuzumab are common, occurring in nearly all patients (90% had infusion reactions in both phase 3 trials).[56,57] This reaction is thought to be a cytokine release phenomenon during the first infusion, which causes temporary neurologic deterioration in sites of preexisting demyelination. This reaction can often be managed with intravenous methylprednisolone pretreatment.[52]

### Updates on Existing Therapies: Risk Stratification with Natalizumab

Natalizumab (Tysabri) was initially FDA approved for the treatment of relapsing forms of MS in 2004, pulled off of the market in 2005, and reapproved in 2006. Natalizumab is an $\alpha_4$ integrin antagonist. $\alpha_4\beta_1$ integrin, a protein on the surface of lymphocytes, interacts with vascular cell adhesion molecule 1, which is expressed on the surface of vascular endothelial cells in the brain and spinal cord blood vessels, mediating the adhesion and migration of lymphocytes across the BBB.[59] Natalizumab blocks binding to endothelial receptors.

Natalizumab showed a profound effect on relapsing forms of MS in 2 separate clinical trials (AFFIRM [Natalizumab Safety and Efficacy in Relapsing Remitting Sclerosis] and SENTINEL [Safety and Efficacy of Natalizumab in Combination with Interferon Beta-1a in Patients with Relapsing Remitting Multiple Sclerosis]). Natalizumab reduced the rate of clinical relapses by 68% and led to an 83% reduction in the accumulation of new or enlarging T2 lesions. However, the great promise of natalizumab was tempered by the rare, but serious, occurrence of PML.

PML is a demyelinating disease of the CNS caused by JCV, a human polyomavirus. Primary asymptomatic infection occurs in childhood. The virus remains quiescent in the kidneys, bone marrow, and lymphoid tissue. Symptoms of treatment-related PML have included alterations in mental status, ataxia, myoclonus, seizures, and attention disorders. There have been no reported cases of ON or spinal cord involvement. Radiographic findings include multiple subcortical white matter lesions and lesions in the cerebellar peduncles. Unlike cases of "classical" (nontreatment related) PML, many patients have evidence of gadolinium enhancement on MRI. Diagnosis is made by confirmation of viral DNA in CSF or on brain biopsy.[60] The "typical" most frequent radiographic pattern of early natalizumab-related PML cases includes large, confluent, subcortical lesions with low signal on T1-weighted images and high signal on T2-weighted and diffusion-weighted images, often with contrast enhancement.[61]

Natalizumab has been definitively associated with PML. Several clear risk factors have emerged for the development of PML: duration of therapy, prior immunosuppressant use, and JCV antibody status. The risk of PML increased with increasing duration of treatment, with the greatest increase in risk occurring after 2 years of therapy with limited data beyond 4 years. The use of immunosuppressants before natalizumab use was also noted to increase the risk. Commonly used immunosuppressants included mitoxantrone (Novantrone), methotrexate, cyclophosphamide, azathioprine, and mycophenolate mofetil. Use of methylprednisolone, prednisone, and adrenocorticotropic hormone for the treatment of MS relapses is not considered "immunosuppressant use" and is not a risk factor for PML. About 42% of patients with natalizumab-related PML had prior immunosuppressive treatment; 20.3% of all natalizumab-treated patients had been exposed to immunosuppressive drugs.[62] No specific duration of immunosuppressant use or relation to the start of natalizumab was noted to be a known risk factor, in part due to great variability in both. Biogen Idec developed a two-step enzyme-linked immunosorbent assay for anti-JCV antibody, which was approved by the FDA. Gorelik and colleagues[63] reported a 53.6% incidence of anti-JCV antibodies in patients with MS with a 2.5% fall-negative rate. The prevalence of anti-JCV antibodies ("JCV positive") was found to be 54.9% in the STRATIFY-1 study. The prevalence increased with age and was lower among women.[64]

Antibody status is likely the most important risk factor because infection with JCV is required for the development of PML. The highest risk is in those who test positive for all 3 risk factors (duration of therapy more than 24 months, prior immunosuppressant use, and JCV-antibody-positive status) with 11.1 cases per 1000 patients. For those who test positive for JCV with prior immunosuppressant use on therapy with natalizumab for 1 to 24 months, the risk is 1.6 cases per 1000 patients. For those who test positive for JCV with no prior immunosuppressant use with more than 24 months of treatment, the risk is 4.6 per 1000 patients. For those who are test positive for JCV with no prior immunosuppressant use with less than 24 months of treatment, the risk is 0.56 cases per 1000 patients.[64] Fox and Rudick[62] estimated the risks for those with all 3 risk factors to be 1:85; for those who test positive for JCV antibody with history of immunosuppressant use with less than 24 months treatment, the risk was 1:454. For those who test positive for JCV antibody and have no history of immunosuppressant use, the risk at greater than 24 months was determined to be 1:241; up to 24 months of treatment, 1:1288. For those who test negative for JCV antibody with history of immunosuppressant use, the risk was 1:3396 after 24 months and 1:18,171 before that. For those who test negative for JCV antibody with no history of immunosuppressant use, the risk was 1:9629 after 24 months and 1:51,526 before that. There have been limited cases in which an individual tested negative for JCV and yet was later diagnosed with PML. No patient tested negative for JCV within 6 months of a confirmed PML diagnosis. JCV antibody testing is currently recommended every 6 months for those who remain antibody negative. Those who test positive are considered "always positive" and do not need to be retested.

The diagnosis of PML, although a serious one that can lead to death or significant disability, is not a universally "fatal" diagnosis, and the overall neurologic impact in those who are diagnosed quickly may be limited. Patients with MS with treatment-related PML have a 79% survival rate.[65] There is no accepted "standard of care" due to the limited number of cases. However, plasma exchange (PLEX) has been shown to rapidly clear natalizumab, reducing mean serum natalizumab concentrations by an average of 92% from baseline to 1 week after the final PLEX session.[66] PLEX was also shown to increase the ability of peripheral blood mononuclear cells from natalizumab recipients to cross the BBB, critical to the treatment of PML. Without PLEX it would take close to 2 months to fully clear natalizumab from the circulation with some residual effects up to 6 months.[67] Use of granulocyte colony-stimulating factor (G-CSF) has also been advocated.[68] G-CSF increases circulating lymphocytes, increases the adhesive properties of T cells independent of VLA (Very Late Activation Antigen)-4, and increases immune surveillance in the CNS, thereby likely accelerating the clearance of JCV.

Select patients with treatment-related PML may benefit from corticosteroid treatment of immune reconstitution inflammatory syndrome (IRIS). IRIS has been seen in almost all treatment-related PML cases.[65] IRIS is thought to be mediated by a brisk influx of JCV-specific T cells into the CNS.[69] Corticosteroids have been advocated for the treatment of IRIS, which can be associated with clinical worsening, profound contrast enhancement, and mass effect.[70] The optimal timing of corticosteroid treatment is not clear. Prophylactic treatment may not be beneficial because it may blunt the JCV-specific T-cell response and lead to unopposed progression of PML. Corticosteroids could possibly be reserved until there is clinical or MRI evidence of IRIS.[69]

What has perhaps become a greater challenge to clinicians is what to do with those who test positive for JCV antibody. A return to baseline disease activity, or perhaps a "rebound" effect beyond baseline activity, has been noted since the original phase 2 studies (the latter "rebound effect" being more controversial).[67] Some studies have argued that although there is a return to baseline disease activity over 4 to 7 months after natalizumab treatment interruption, disease activity does not exceed levels seen in placebo-treated subjects, arguing against a "rebound effect."[67] However, there are at least case reports of severe MS relapses after treatment cessation that seem consistent with inflammatory disease activity beyond a simple "return to baseline."[71,72]

### Complementary and Alternative Therapies

There has been considerable interest in nonpharmacologic treatment strategies for MS. Vitamin D supplementation is a specific treatment for which there is growing basic science and clinical research support. Vitamin D receptor is found on cells of the CNS, which may be a site of action, metabolism, and catabolism of vitamin D.[73] Vitamin D may inhibit the maturation of APCs and inflammatory cytokine production and promote an antiinflammatory profile.[73,74] The role of vitamin D as a possible contributing factor to the development of MS was suggested as early as the 1970s and may be one of the several factors that account for the striking geographic predilection of the disease.[75] Sun exposure and dietary sources of vitamin D during childhood and adolescence have been associated with a lower risk of developing MS.[76,77] Women who use supplemental vitamin D (largely from multivitamins) have been found to have a 40% lower risk of MS than women who do not use supplemental vitamin D.[77]

Vitamin D supplementation seems to largely be safe. Excessive vitamin D supplementation can lead to an increase in plasma calcium, hypercalcemia, reduced bone mineral density, and serious complications such as renal and heart failure.[73] However, these would be quite rare side effects with adequate vitamin D doses. Doses ranging from 400 international units (IUs) daily to 4000 IUs daily have been advocated, seem to be safe, and may possibly confer a treatment benefit to patients as part of their overall care.

There is less data in support of other dietary supplements as a component of the treatment of MS. Diet rich in polyunsaturated fats, omega fatty acids, and multivitamins have been advocated as potentially beneficial. To date, there is no convincing evidence that any of these have a major impact on disease progression or relapse rate.[78] However, available data are incomplete at best and there is clearly some dietary role in the management of MS.

## SUMMARY

Treatment of MS, long elusive despite the best (and worst) of intentions, has now become an area of rapidly increasing options for patients and physicians. While Lord Brain once quipped of the "treatments" for MS, "The multiplication of remedies is eloquent of their inefficacies", the increasing armamentarium is now reflective of increasing efficacy. It is telling that this article will likely be "outdated" shortly after it is published because of the rapid expansion of therapies such as laquinimod, daclizumab, ocrelizumab, which are currently being investigated. These are likely not the long-awaited "cures" for MS, but it would be truly sweet if they close in on the "whole loaf."

### Case study

A 26-year-old man presents for diplopia with left gaze. Symptoms developed over the course of 1 week and were associated with a generalized headache. He was evaluated by ophthalmology and referred for a contrast-enhanced cranial MRI. The MRI revealed a large (1-cm) right frontal GdE lesion, several perpendicularly oriented periventricular lesions, and at least 1 juxtacortical lesion. A contrast-enhanced cervical spinal cord MRI was normal. Results of laboratory studies including a comprehensive metabolic panel, complete blood cell count, vitamin B$_{12}$ level, and Lyme antibody titer were normal or negative. Spinal fluid analysis was notable for a normal white blood cell count and protein level, with the presence of more than 5 oligoclonal bands unique to the cerebrospinal fluid. He had a prompt clinical response to a course of high-dose intravenous methylprednisolone followed by an oral prednisone taper.

He returned to clinic at the end of the oral steroid taper, approximately 50 days after the initial development of symptoms. The diplopia for which he had initially sought medical attention had completely resolved. However, he had developed new onset numbness and gait difficulties over the past 48 hours. On examination, he was noted to have a sensory level to the midchest. Repeat cranial and cervical imaging revealed a new GdE lesion at C5 level spanning less than 1 vertebral level. His gait did not improve despite an additional course of high-dose methylprednisolone, and he was admitted for plasmapheresis.

The patient returned to clinic after his hospitalization to discuss treatment options. For the past 2 decades, the discussion largely would have resolved around 1 of 2 injectable treatment options: variously dosed interferon or once daily glatiramer acetate. However, the patient and his physician now had several new treatment options to discuss. The critical elements for the patient and physician to understand are the patient's potential risk from disease (his gender, short time interval between clinical relapses, and spinal cord involvement, making him a "high-risk" patient for further attacks and future disability), the side effects of the various medications in relation to his overall health status (which was fortunately otherwise completely healthy), risk stratification for serious side effects such as PML, the available long-term safety data (or lack thereof), and his personal preferences about dosing options and frequencies (oral, injectable or intravenous; daily, every other day, weekly, or monthly).

There is no "simple" therapeutic answer for the treatment of MS, no "one-size-fits-all" remedy to this notoriously heterogeneous disease. Multiple considerations must be made and understood. However, it is now at least some comfort that patients and their physicians have a rapidly expanding number of options at their disposal.

## REFERENCES

1. Compston A, Lassmann H, McDonald I. The Story of Multiple Sclerosis. In: Compston A, Confavreux C, Lassmann, et al, editors. McAlpine's Multiple Sclerosis. 4th Edition. Philadelphia: Elsevier; 2006. p. 1–68.

2. The IFNB Multiple Sclerosis Study Group. Interferon beta-1b is effective in relapsing-remitting multiple sclerosis: clinical results of a multicenter, randomized, double-blind, placebo-controlled trial. Neurology 1993;43:655–61.
3. Paty DW, Li DK. The IFNB Multiple Sclerosis Study Group. Interferon beta-1b is effective in relapsing-remitting multiple sclerosis: MRI results of a multicenter, randomized, double-blind, placebo-controlled trial. Neurology 1993;43:662–7.
4. Arnason BG. Interferon beta in multiple sclerosis. Neurology 1993;43:641–3.
5. Schumacher FA, Beeve GW, Kibler RF, et al. Problems of experimental trials of therapy in multiple sclerosis: report by the panel on the evaluation of experimental trials in multiple sclerosis. Ann N Y Acad Sci 1965;122:552–68.
6. Young IR, Hall AS, Pallis CA, et al. Nuclear magnetic resonance imaging of the brain in multiple sclerosis. Lancet 1981;8255:1063–6.
7. Poser CM, Paty DW, Schelenberg LC, et al. New diagnostic criteria for multiple sclerosis: guidelines for research protocols. Ann Neurol 1983;1:227–31.
8. McDonald WI, Compston A, Edan G, et al. Recommended diagnostic criteria for multiple sclerosis: guidelines from the International Panel on the diagnosis of multiple sclerosis. Ann Neurol 2001;50:121–7.
9. Polman CH, Reingold SC, Edan G, et al. Diagnostic criteria for multiple sclerosis: 2005 revisions to the "McDonald Criteria. Ann Neurol 2005;58:840–6.
10. Polman CH, Reingold SC, Banwell B, et al. Diagnostic criteria for multiple sclerosis: 2010 revisions to the McDonald criteria. Ann Neurol 2011;69:292–302.
11. Barkhof F, Filippi M, Miller DH, et al. Comparison of MRI imaging criteria at first presentation to predict conversion to clinically definite MS. Brain 1997;120:2059–69.
12. Tintore M, Rovira A, Martinez M, et al. Isolated demyelinating syndromes: comparison of different MR imaging criteria to predict conversion to clinically definite multiple sclerosis. AJNR Am J Neuroradiol 2000;21:702–6.
13. Swanton JK, Fernando K, Dalton CM, et al. Modification of MRI criteria for multiple sclerosis in patients with clinically isolated syndrome. J Neurol Neurosurg Psychiatry 2006;77:830–3.
14. Selchen D, Bhan V, Blevins G, et al. MS, MRI and the 2010 McDonald criteria: a Canadian expert commentary. Neurology 2012;79(Suppl 2):S1–13.
15. Uitdehaag BM, Barkof F, Coyle PK, et al. The changing face of multiple sclerosis clinical trial populations. Curr Med Res Opin 2011;27:1529–37.
16. Klawiter EC, Cross AH, Naismith RT. The present efficacy of multiple sclerosis therapeutics: is the new 66% just the old 33%? Neurology 2009;73:984–90.
17. Weiner HL. Multiple sclerosis is an inflammatory T-cell-mediated autoimmune disease. Arch Neurol 2004;61:1613–5.
18. Chaudhuri A, Behan PO. Multiple sclerosis is not an autoimmune disease. Arch Neurol 2004;61:1610–2.
19. Bar-Or A. The immunology of multiple sclerosis. Semin Neurol 2008;28:29–45.
20. Dhib-Jalbut S. Pathogenesis of myelin/oligodendrocyte damage in multiple sclerosis. Neurology 2007;68(Suppl 3):S13–21.
21. Racke MK. Update on the pathogenesis of multiple sclerosis. Adv Stud Med 2008;8(5):137–43.
22. Kowarick MC, Pellkofer HL, Cepok S, et al. Differential effects of fingolimod (FTY720) on immune cells in the CSF and blood of patients with MS. Neurology 2011;76:1214–21.
23. Mehling M, Johnson TA, Antel J, et al. Clinical immunology of the sphingosine 1-phosphate receptor modulator fingolimod (FTY720) in multiple sclerosis. Neurology 2011;76(Suppl 3):S20–7.

24. Kappos L, Radue EW, O'Connor P, et al, FREEDOMS Study Group. A placebo-controlled trial of oral fingolimod in relapsing multiple sclerosis. N Engl J Med 2010;362:387–401.

25. Cohen JA, Barkhof F, Comi G, et al, TRANSFORMS Study Group. Oral fingolimod or intramuscular interferon for relapsing multiple sclerosis. N Engl J Med 2010;362:402–15.

26. Efficacy and Safety of Fingolimod (FTY720) in Patients with Relapsing-remitting Multiple Sclerosis (FREEDOMS II). Available at: http://clinicaltrials.gov/ct2/show/results/NCT00355134?sect=X615#part. Accessed April 11, 2013.

27. Calabresi PA, Radue EW, Goodin D, et al. Efficacy and safety of fingolimod in patients with relapsing multiple sclerosis (RRMS): Results from an additional 24-month double-blind, placebo-controlled study (FREEDOMS II study). In: 64th American Academy of Neurology Annual Meeting. Emerging Science Session, New Orleans (LA) 2012. p. 015.

28. Hashmonay R, Kappos L, Cohen JA, et al. Consistent efficacy of fingolimod across clinical development program. In: 4th Corporation Meeting of the Consortium of Multiple Sclerosis Centers and Americas Committee for Treatment and Research in Multiple Sclorosis, San Diego (CA). 2012. p. DX68.

29. Jeffrey, S. PML Reported in MS Patient on Fingolimod. Available at: http://www.medscape.com/viewarticle/762039. Accessed April 16, 2013.

30. Cohen JA, O'Conner P, Caliolo T, et al. Long term safety of fingolimod in relapsing multiple sclerosis: update to integrated analyses of phase 2 and 3 studies and extension phases. In: 28th Congress of the European Treatment and Research in Multiple Sclerosis (ECTRIMS). Lyon, France. 2012. p. 983.

31. Schwab P, Zhou Y, Stemkowski S, et al. Analysis of first dose observation data for MS treatment with fingolimod. In: Fourth Cooperative Meeting of the Consortium of Multiple Sclerosis Centers (CMSC) and Americas Committee for Treatment and Research in Multiple Sclerosis (ACTRIMS). San Diego, CA 2012.

32. Samson K. Health officials launch investigation in death of patients taking fingolimod. Neurology Today 2012;12(4):27-28. Available at: http://www.aan.com/elibrary/neurologytoday/?event=home.showArticle&id=ovid.com:/bib/ovftdb/00132985-201202160-00001. Accessed April 11, 2013.

33. FDA Drug Safety Communication: Revised recommendations for cardiovascular monitoring and use of multiple sclerosis drug Gilenya (fingolimod). Available at: http://www.fda.gov/Drugs/DrugSafety/ucm303192.htm. Accessed April 11, 2013.

34. Jain N, Bhatti MT. Fingolimod-associated macular edema: incidence, detection, and management. Neurology 2012;78:672–80.

35. O'Connor P, Wolinsky J, Confavreux C, et al. Randomized trial of oral teriflunomide for relapsing multiple sclerosis. N Engl J Med 2011;365:1293–303.

36. Miller A, Turpault S, Menguy-Vacheron F. Rapid elimination procedure of teriflunomide with cholestyramine or activated charcoal. In: 17th Annual Meeting of the Americas Committee for Treatment and Research in Multiple Sclerosis. San Diego, CA: p. 10.

37. Results from second phase III study of teriflunomide show reduced relapse rate, slower progression of disability. Available at: http://www.businesswire.com/news/home/20121012005423/en/Genzyme-Presents-Phase-III-Study-Once-daily-Oral. Accessed April 16, 2013.

38. Phase III study with teriflunomide versus placebo in patients with first clinical symptom of multiple sclerosis (TOPIC). Available at: http://clinicaltrials.gov/ct2/show/results/NCT00622700. Accessed April 11, 2013.

39. Freedman MS, Confavreux C, Comi G, et al. Hair thinning associated with teriflunomide therapy is manageable. In: 17th Annual Meeting of the Americas Committee for Treatment and Research in Multiple Sclerosis. San Diego, CA June, 2012.

40. Chambers CD, Tutuncu ZN, Johnson D, et al. Human pregnancy safety for agents used to treat rheumatoid arthritis: adequacy of available information and strategies for developing post-marketing data. Arthritis Res Ther 2006;8: 225–35.

41. Chambers CD, Johnson DL, Robinson LK, et al. Birth outcomes in women who have taken leflunomide during pregnancy. Arthritis Rheum 2010;62:1494–503.

42. Cassina M, Johnson DL, Robinson LK, et al. Pregnancy outcome in women exposed to leflunomide before or during pregnancy. Arthritis Rheum 2012;64: 2085–94.

43. Kieseier B, Benamor M, Benzerdjeb H, et al. Pregnancy outcomes from the teriflunomide clinical development programme: retrospective analysis of the teriflunomide clinical trial database. In: 28th Congress of the European Committee for Treatment and Research in Multiple Sclerosis. Lyon, France. p. 737.

44. Genzyme reports top-line results for TENERE study of oral teriflunomide in relapsing multiple sclerosis. Available at: http://www.businesswire.com/news/home/20111219006550/en/Genzyme-Report-Top-line-Results-TENERE. Accessed April 11, 2013.

45. Gold R, Kappos L, Arnold DL, et al. Placebo-controlled phase 3 study of oral BG-12 for relapsing multiple sclerosis. N Engl J Med 2012;367:1098–107.

46. Kappos L, Gold R, Miller DH, et al. Efficacy and safety of oral fumarate in patients with relapsing remitting multiple sclerosis: a multicenter randomized double blind, placebo-controlled phase IIb study. Lancet 2008;367(12):1463–72.

47. Ropper AH. The "Poison Chair" Treatment for multiple sclerosis. N Engl J Med 2012;367:1149–50.

48. Fox RJ, Miller DH, Phillips JT, et al. Placebo-controlled phase 3 study of oral BG-12 or glatiramer acetate in multiple sclerosis. N Engl J Med 2012;367:1087–97.

49. Kappos L, Gold R, Miller DH. Effect of BG-12 on contrast-enhanced lesions in patients with relapsing-remitting multiple sclerosis: subgroup analyses from the phase 2b study. Mult Scler 2012;18(3):314–21.

50. Phillips JT, Fox RJ, Selmaj K, et al. Long-term safety and tolerability of oral BG-12 (dimethyl fumarate) in relapsing-remitting multiple sclerosis: interim results from ENDORSE. In: 28th Congress of the European Committee for Treatment and Research in Multiple Sclerosis. Lyon, France October, 2012. p. 1103.

51. Ford CC, Fox EJ. Assessing safety and potential risks of disease-modifying therapies for multiple sclerosis. The Science of MS Management 2012;2(3):3–13.

52. Robertson NP. Alemtuzumab for multiple sclerosis: a new age of immunotherapy. J Neurol 2013;260:343–5.

53. Hill-Cawthorne GA, Button T, Tuohy O, et al. Long term lymphocyte reconstitution after alemtuzumab treatment of multiple sclerosis. J Neurol Neurosurgery Psychiatry 2012;83:298–304.

54. Coles AJ, Compston DA, Selmaj KW, et al, The CAMMS223 Trial Investigators. Alemtuzumab vs interferon beta-1a in early multiple sclerosis. N Engl J Med 2008;359:1786–801.

55. Coles AJ. Alemtuzumab more effective than interferon beta-1a at 5-year follow up of CAMMS223 clinical trial. Neurology 2012;78:1069–78.

56. Cohen JA, Coles AJ, Arnold DL, et al, CARE-MS I Investigators. Alemtuzumab versus interferon beta-1a as first line treatment for patients with relapsing

multiple sclerosis after disease-modifying therapy: a randomised controlled phase 3 trial. Lancet 2012;380:1819–28.

57. Coles AJ, Twyman CL, Arnold DL, et al, CARE-MS II Investigators. Alemtuzumab for patients with relapsing multiple sclerosis after disease-modifying therapy: a randomised controlled phase 3 trial. Lancet 2012;380:1829–39.

58. Sprenger T, Kappos L. Alemtuzumab for multiple sclerosis: who and when to treat? Lancet 2012;380:1795–7.

59. Polman CH, O'Connor PW, Havrdova E, et al. A randomized, placebo-controlled trial of natalizumab for relapsing multiple sclerosis. N Engl J Med 2006;354: 899–910.

60. Tan CS, Koralnik IJ. Progressive multifocal leukoencephalopathy and other disorders caused by JC virus: clinical features and pathogenesis. Lancet Neurol 2010;9:425–37.

61. Yousry TA, Habil DM, Pelletier D, et al. Magnetic resonance imaging pattern in Natalizumab-associated progressive multifocal leukoencephalopathy. Ann Neurol 2012;72:779–87.

62. Fox RJ, Rudick RA. Risk stratification and patient counseling for natalizumab in multiple sclerosis. Neurology 2012;78:436–7.

63. Gorelik L, Lerner M, Bixler S, et al. Anti-JC virus antibodies: implications for PML risk stratification. Ann Neurol 2010;68:295–303.

64. Bloomgren G, Richman S, Hotermans C, et al. Risk of natalizumab-associated progressive multifocal leukoencephalopathy. N Engl J Med 2012;366:1870–80.

65. Vermersch P, Kappos L, Gold R, et al. Clinical outcomes of natalizumab-associated progressive multifocal leukoencephalopathy. Neurology 2011;76: 1697–704.

66. Khatri BO, Man S, Giovannoni G, et al. Effect of plasma exchange in accelerating natalizumab clearance and restoring leukocyte function. Neurology 2009;72:402–9.

67. O'Connor PW, Goodman A, Kappos L, et al. Disease activity return to baseline during natalizumab treatment interruption in patients with multiple sclerosis. Neurology 2011;76:1858–65.

68. Stefoski D, Balabanov R, Javed A, et al. Immunostimulatory effect of G-CSF is potentially beneficial In natalizumab-associated PML/IRIS. In: 28th Congress of the European Committee for Treatment and Research in Multiple Sclerosis. Lyon, France October, 2012.

69. Antoniol C, Jilek S, Schluep M, et al. Impairment of JCV-specific T-cell response by corticotherapy. Effect on PML-IRIS management? Neurology 2012;79:2258–64.

70. Clifford DB, De Luca A, Simpson DM, et al. Natalizumab-associated progressive multifocal leukoencephalopathy in patients with multiple sclerosis: lessons from 28 cases. Lancet Neurol 2010;9:438–46.

71. Lenhard T, Biller A, Mueller W, et al. Immune reconstitution inflammatory syndrome after withdrawal of Natalizumab? Neurology 2010;75:831–3.

72. Rigau V, Mania A, Befort P, et al. Lethal multiple sclerosis relapse after natalizumab withdrawal. Neurology 2012;79:2214–6.

73. Smolders J, Damoiseaux J, Menheere P, et al. Vitamin D as an immune modulator in multiple sclerosis, a review. J Neuroimmunol 2008;194:7–17.

74. Smolders J, Peelen E, Thewissen M, et al. Safety and T cell modulating effects of high dose vitamin D3 supplementation in multiple sclerosis. PLoS One 2010;5: e15235.

75. Cantorna MT. Vitamin D and multiple sclerosis: an update. Nutr Rev 2008; 66(Suppl 2):S135–8.

76. McDowell TY, Amr S, Culpepper WJ, et al. Sun exposure, Vitamin D and age at disease onset in relapsing multiple sclerosis. Neuroepidemiology 2011;36: 39–45.
77. Munger KL, Zhang SM, O'Reilly E, et al. Vitamin D intake and incidence of multiple sclerosis. Neurology 2004;62:60–5.
78. Farinotti M, Vacchi L, Simi S, et al. Dietary interventions for multiple sclerosis [review]. Cochrane Database Syst Rev 2012;(12):CD004192.

# Update in the Treatment of High-grade Gliomas

Rimas V. Lukas, MD[a],*, Martin Kelly Nicholas, MD, PhD[b]

## KEYWORDS

- Gliomas • Surgery • Radiation therapy • Chemotherapy

## KEY POINTS

- As with other malignancies, recent advances in molecular diagnostics have advanced our understanding of high-grade gliomas and will influence their therapeutic management in the future.
- The role of temozolomide and radiation are being better defined in elderly patients with high-grade astrocytomas.
- The role of combined chemoradiation in grade III oligodendroglial tumors is becoming more established.
- The anti–vascular endothelial growth factor antibody, bevacizumab, is an important new agent in the treatment of recurrent high-grade astrocytomas.
- A combined multimodality approach is central to the management of most high-grade gliomas.

## INTRODUCTION

This review focuses on updates of the treatment of high-grade gliomas, aggressive infiltrating neoplasms of the central nervous system (CNS). The authors highlight the key historical trials as well as other studies that represent important recent advances in the field. High-grade (grade III and IV) gliomas include both astrocytomas and oligodendrogliomas. A concerted multidisciplinary approach using several modalities in combination is often used in their treatment. This approach typically begins with a diagnostic and potentially therapeutic surgical procedure. Typically, this is followed by radiation therapy (RT) and often chemotherapy. The authors detail the specific approaches to each tumor subtype in the following sections.

Funding Sources: None.
Conflict of Interest: R.V. Lukas previously served on advisory board for Genentech. M.K. Nicholas previously served on advisory board for Genentech and Novocure.
[a] Department of Neurology, University of Chicago, 5841 South Maryland Avenue, MC 2030, Chicago, IL 60637, USA; [b] Section of Neurosurgery, Departments of Neurology and Radiation and Cellular Oncology, University of Chicago, 5841 South Maryland Avenue, MC 2030, Chicago, IL 60637, USA
* Corresponding author.
E-mail address: rlukas@neurology.bsd.uchicago.edu

Neurol Clin 31 (2013) 847–867
http://dx.doi.org/10.1016/j.ncl.2013.03.005

## PATIENT EVALUATION OVERVIEW
### Histology

Although molecular diagnostics for high-grade gliomas have undergone significant changes over the past few years, routine histology remains the gold standard of diagnosis. This point is reflected in updates to the most recent edition of the World Health Organization's (WHO) classification of CNS tumors.[1] Although many molecular details are discussed, they typically serve to refine rather than define a tumor by type. This review focuses on grade III and IV gliomas, but tumors of lower grade are mentioned when appropriate. This discussion is most important when comparing and contrasting the so-called secondary glioblastoma (GBM), high-grade tumors that arise in a stepwise fashion from tumors of lower grade, from the more common primary GBM, a tumor that begins as a high-grade neoplasm. The features that distinguish primary from secondary GBM are described by the WHO but, again, are not based on routine histology. This distinction is not routinely made but, as shown later, has become of more interest as molecular pathology further defines subtypes.

### Oligodendrogliomas

Oligodendrogliomas are infiltrating tumors with round or ovoid nuclei and perinuclear halos, artifacts of tissue preparation. Microcalcification, microcysts, and chicken-wire vasculature are seen in some but not all cases. Oligodendrogliomas have 2 pathologic grades: II and III (anaplastic oligodendrogliomas [AO]). AO tumors are defined by prominent mitotic activity on routine histologic stains but not the MIB-1 labeling index, an antibody-based test of Ki-67 protein expression that is important in cell proliferation. Both endothelial proliferation and focal areas of necrosis may be seen in AO. Although certain molecular diagnostic features are frequently encountered in oligodendrogliomas, they do not define the tumor by the WHO diagnostic criteria. These features are discussed further later.

### Astrocytomas

Astrocytomas typically share morphologic and histologic features characteristic of astrocytes, which may include immunohistochemical (IHC) staining for glial fibrillary acidic protein, a protein often expressed in reactive astrocytes. Infiltrating gliomas are of 3 pathologic grades: II, III, and IV. Anaplastic astrocytomas (AA), grade III, are distinguished from grade II astrocytomas by nuclear pleomorphism and the presence of mitoses. Although the WHO classification system allows for scant mitoses in grade II tumors, there is no clear cutoff distinguishing a grade II from a grade III tumor. Glioblastoma, previously termed *glioblastoma multiforme* by the WHO classification system, is a grade IV astrocytoma. It is differentiated from AA by the presence of either of the cardinal features of endothelial proliferation (often described as glomeruloid) and/or necrosis (often described as pseudopalisading). Gliosarcoma, large cell GBM, and gliofibroma are further subclassifications under the current classification system.

### Mixed oligoastrocytomas

At times the distinction between oligodendrogliomas and astrocytomas is unclear. Distinct cell populations resembling either tumor type can be seen admixed in the same tumor leading to a histologic diagnosis of a grade II oligoastrocytoma or grade III anaplastic oligoastrocytoma (AOA). A separate histologic entity, GBM with oligodendroglial features (WHO grade IV) is also described. This pleomorphism raises questions about the cells of origin in these tumors, making room for the current thinking about both neural stem cells and brain tumor stem cells in glioma.[2] The underlying molecular features, described later, that allow for this histologic subclassification may prove to be important in predicting both the natural history and response to treatment of a specific tumor.

## Molecular Diagnostics

Although molecular diagnostics are not currently used to define the pathologic diagnosis, they play an increasing role in classifying tumors into subcategories characterized by genetic and epigenetic features (**Table 1**). As we learn more of the behavior subserved by these molecular changes, we may find more personalized approaches to treatment. For example, analysis of data from The Cancer Genome Atlas (TCGA) project has identified 4 distinct subtypes of GBM: classic, neural, proneural, and mesenchymal. Each subtype demonstrates different patterns of gene expression, age at diagnosis, survival time, and responses to current therapies.[4] The classic GBM are associated with epidermal growth factor receptor (EGFR) overexpression and lack mutation of the *TP53* tumor suppressor gene. This subgroup is also associated with the longest survival following aggressive standard-of-care therapy. Tumors in the neural subgroup express many genes associated with normal neurons. People in this subgroup are older and respond less well to standard treatments. Thus, a molecular profile is now emerging that may underlie the long-known fact that advanced age is a negative prognostic factor in GBM. The proneural subgroup is associated with a higher rate of mutations of isocitrate dehydrogenase (*IDH*), *TP53*, and platelet-derived growth factor receptor alpha (*PDGFRα*) genes. These patients are typically younger and have a longer overall survival (OS), independent of treatment. The mesenchymal subtype is characterized by higher amounts of inflammation and necrosis. Like the classic subtype, patients with the mesenchymal subtype have reduced mortality following standard intensive treatment. This paragraph describes only some of the features that distinguish between subtypes. However, it sets the stage for some of the specific molecular characterizations discussed later. Because high-grade gliomas are characterized by dozens of molecular aberrations, the following discussion is limited to several examples. Each example typifies a common molecular mechanism involved in tumorigenesis: chromosome translocation, the metabolome, epigenetics, and signal transduction. Still more could be given, but these will serve to highlight the interactions between biologic pathways.

### 1p19q deletions

Codeletion of the short arm of chromosome 1 (1p) and the long arm of chromosome 19 (19q) is a cytogenetic aberration initially described in a large subset of oligodendrogliomas almost 20 years ago.[5] Similar codeletion patterns are found on occasion in other brain tumors, neurocytomas, for example, but most are found in tumors with oligodendroglial morphology.[6] Although both 1p and 19q can be deleted in isolation, 1p19q codeletion is associated both with a more favorable natural history and response to treatment, discussed further later.[7,8] Eventually, an unbalanced translocation resulting in a derivative 1p/19q chromosome was found that may explain the concurrent 1p19q loss.[9] A fusion protein resulting from this translocation that might account for the unique response of these tumors to DNA-damaging agents has not been found. Overexpression of the neuronal intermediate filament, alpha-internexin protein (INA), is known to be associated with 1p19q codeleted tumors.[10] However, because it is located on chromosome 10, it is not a candidate product of the 1p/19q derivative chromosome. The mechanism underlying increased INA expression in these tumors remains unknown. Another protein, capicua homolog (Drosphila), is encoded by the *CIC* gene, which is located on chromosome 19q. Mutations in this gene are common in 1p/19q codeleted oligodendrogliomas but not other glial

**Table 1**
The most common genetic, epigenetic, and chromosomal alterations in the high-grade gliomas discussed in this review

| Genetic Category | Anaplastic Oligodendroglioma | Secondary GBM | Primary GBM |
|---|---|---|---|
| Oncogene | EGFR<br>Amplification<br>Overexpression[a]<br><br>PDGF/PDGFR<br>Overexpression[a] | EGFR<br>Amplification<br>Overexpression[a]<br><br>PDGF/PDGFR<br>Overexpression[a]<br>Amplification<br>MDM2<br>Amplification | EGFR<br>Amplification<br>Overexpression<br>Mutation<br><br><br><br>MDM2<br>Amplification<br>Overexpression<br>CDK4<br>Amplification |
| Tumor Suppressor Gene | TP53<br>Mutation<br>PTEN<br>Loss<br>CDKN2A<br>Loss or mutation<br>RB<br>Mutation | TP53<br>Mutation[a]<br>PTEN<br>Mutation[b]<br>CDKN2A<br>Loss or mutation[b]<br>RB<br>Mutation[c]<br>NF1<br>Loss or mutation<br>DCC<br>Loss or mutation | <br><br>PTEN<br>Mutation[b]<br>CNKN2A<br>Loss or mutation[b]<br>RB<br>Mutation[c]<br>NF1<br>Loss or mutation |
| Metabolome | IDH1 and 2<br>Mutation[a] | IDH1 and 2<br>Mutation[a,c] | IDH1 and 2<br>Mutation[c] |
| Genomic Region | del 1p[a], 19q[a]<br>del 9p, 10q | del 10q, 11p[a]<br>del 19q[a] | del 9p, 10q<br>12 q amplicon |
| Epigenetic | MGMT promoter<br>Hypermethylation | MGMT promoter<br>Hypermethylation[c] | MGMT promoter<br>Hypermethylation |

Only those occurring with a frequency of more than 10% are listed (others, less frequent, may be found in reference[3]).

*Abbreviations:* CDKN2A, cyclin-dependent kinase inhibitor 2A and its 3 common transcript variants; DCC, deleted in colon cancer gene; del, deletion of a chromosome segment; EGFR, epidermal growth factor receptor gene; IDH 1 and 2, isocitrate dehydrogenase genes 1 and 2; MDM2, murine double minute 2 gene; MGMT, methyl guanine methyl DNA transferase gene; NF1, neurofibromatosis type 1 gene; PDGF, platelet-derived growth factor gene; PDGFR, platelet-derived growth factor receptor gene; PTEN, phosphatase and tensin homolog gene; RB, retinoblastoma gene; TP53, p53 tumor suppressor gene.

[a] Indicates abnormalities that occur upstream in tumors of lower grade that progress to form high-grade gliomas.
[b] Indicates those more common in primary than in secondary GBM.
[c] Indicates abnormalities that are more common in secondary than in primary GBM.

neoplasms.[11] Again, any evidence that the derivative 1p/19q chromosome is driving expression of the mutant protein is lacking. Of interest, however, is the strong association between CIC and IDH mutations in these tumors (see later discussion).

### IDH mutations
IDH is an enzyme involved in oxidative metabolism. It occurs in 2 forms, IDH1 and IDH2, expressed in the cytoplasm and mitochondria, respectively. Mutations in either

the *IDH1* or *IDH2* genes are common in leukemia and gliomas.[12] *IDH1* mutations are more common in glioma, whereas *IDH2* mutations predominate in leukemias. Discovered first in leukemia, their presence in glioma came as a surprise in a high-throughput sequencing study of GBM, where *IDH1* mutations were first discovered.[13] A subsequent screen of a larger cohort of malignant gliomas revealed both *IDH1* and *IDH2* mutations in a variety of histologies.[14] In general, IDH mutations are more common in tumors of lower grade and may be present in astrocytomas, oligodendrogliomas, and tumors of mixed phenotype. Mutations in either of these genes are associated with a more favorable prognosis. Most *IDH1* mutations in gliomas are caused by a single point mutation in which histidine is substituted for arginine at codon 132 (denoted R132H). This can now be determined by IHC. There is a close correlation between the presence of *IDH* mutation and 1p19q codeletion in oliodenrogliomas.[15] *IDH* mutations are more common in low-grade glial tumors, but when found in GBM, confer a better prognosis. This may reflect their origin from the so-called secondary GBM. The presence of *IDH* mutations can be used to in an effort to distinguish between low-grade infiltrating gliomas (WHO grade II), where they are often present, and pilocytic astrocytomas (WHO grade I), where they are not. Similarly, the presence of *IDH* mutations can aid in distinguishing tumor cells from normal and gliotic brain tissue, both of which lack *IDH* mutations.[14]

The discovery of *IDH* mutations in glioma has expanded the field to include cell metabolism and its relation to tumorigenesis. Although much remains to be learned, it is clear from the work to date that the mutant IDH proteins affect cellular metabolism in ways that alter histone interactions; the epigenetic regulation of gene expression; and, through downstream effects on hypoxia inducible factor-1a, proangiogenic factors.[12]

### Methylguanine-DNA methyltransferase promoter methylation

Methylation of the promoter for the methylguanine-DNA methyltransferase gene (*MGMT*) is an epigenetic phenomenon with both prognostic and predictive significance in malignant glioma.[16] MGMT is a DNA repair enzyme that removes the methyl groups added by temozolomide (TMZ) to the $O^6$ position of guanine. Although not the only site of DNA methylation by TMZ, the presence of $O^6$ methylation on guanine preferentially affects cell fate. MGMT expression is downregulated by methylation of its promoter. Reduced MGMT expression leads to increased net DNA damage and, in turn, greater antitumor effects. Because MGMT is often linked to TMZ effects, it is important to recognize the distinction between TMZ-mediated methylation of DNA residues (a direct effect of TMZ exposure) and DNA promoter methylation (a basic biologic mechanism for the regulation of gene expression). MGMT function in a tumor can be evaluated by several methods, including enzyme activity, protein expression as seen on IHC, MGMT mRNA expression, and *MGMT* promoter methylation assays. These techniques can result in conflicting information if they are applied to the same tumor sample.[17] Reasons for this include variation in MGMT expression within tumor samples. Methylation-specific polymerase chain reaction (MSP) is most commonly used in clinical trials, and standardized clinical laboratory tests are available.

MGMT promoter methylation is but one example of epigenetic factors at work in malignant glioma. The TCGA, as part of its comprehensive analysis of GBM, identified distinct methylation patterns in GBM. Of note, the data distinguished 2 GBM subsets. Those with the better prognosis by methylation profile resembled secondary GBM, whereas those with the less favorable prognosis resembled the primary GBM.[18] Clinicians are yet to use these findings to therapeutic advantage, but several potential drug targets have been identified as a result of this effort.

## EGFR

EGFR is a receptor tyrosine kinase that acts at many levels in growth and development, including the brain. EGFR is one of a family of proteins that interact with each other and with a variety of ligands to achieve their pleomorphic effects (reviewed in reference[19]). It also plays a role in gliomagenesis and is often overexpressed and/or mutated in GBM. These abnormalities were once thought to be a principal feature of the so-called primary GBM. Results from the TCGA analysis have shown that these features characterize most of the classic molecular subtype. Of note, GBM with EGFR abnormalities are distinct from those with IDH mutations and 1p19q codeletion.[4] EGFR has been evaluated as a target in several clinical trials without success in most patients.[20] This finding can be explained by the number of potentially activating mutations in the diverse intracellular signaling pathways that lie downstream of the EGFR.[3] This situation may also be the case in glioma stem cells whereby, in addition, compensatory activation of other EGFR-family proteins may mediate drug resistance.[21]

### Molecular Features: Convergence or Divergence?

It is clear from the examples cited earlier that patterns emerge as we learn of the varieties of molecular pathologies in malignant glioma. Some, like IDH mutations, seem surprising and take the field in new directions. Others, like redundancy in oncogenic mutations in EGFR-mediated signaling pathways, challenge the notion of a magic bullet ever being designed for these tumors. Perhaps most striking is the cosegregation of key findings into prognostic subsets. Why, for example, are 1p19q codeletion, IDH mutation, and MGMT promoter methylation so often closely linked in tumors? It is hope that continued study will provide answers and reveal mechanisms that suggest improved treatment outcomes.

## PHARMACOLOGIC TREATMENT OPTIONS
## TMZ

### TMZ for astrocytic tumors

---

**Case study**

A 48-year-old man developed new-onset headaches 4 weeks before presentation. These headaches were present on first awakening in the morning. Their intensity increased over time, leading to evaluation with imaging. Magnetic resonance imaging (MRI) revealed a left temporal heterogeneously enhancing lesion (**Fig. 1A**). The patient underwent a craniotomy with extensive resection of tumor (see **Fig. 1B**). Pathology revealed GBM. He was treated with RT with concomitant TMZ followed by adjuvant TMZ. He had clinical and radiographic progression after 5 cycles (see **Fig. 1C**). His regimen was then changed to single-agent bevacizumab. His first imaging study after initiating bevacizumab (BEV) demonstrated stable disease, with subsequent imaging revealing a partial radiographic response (see **Fig. 1D**). He subsequently progressed after approximately 6 months on this regimen. Despite progression, the patient maintained a good performance status. He was treated with several subsequent salvage regimens but finally died approximately 2 years after his initial diagnosis.

---

TMZ, an alkylating agent that exerts its antiproliferative effects through the covalent bonding of methyl groups to the $O^6$ and $N^7$ positions of guanine, received accelerated approval by the US Food and Drug Administration (FDA) in 1999 as a single agent for recurrent AA. In 2005, this was followed by its approval, combined with and following RT, for newly diagnosed GBM. Approval for recurrent AA was based on results from a

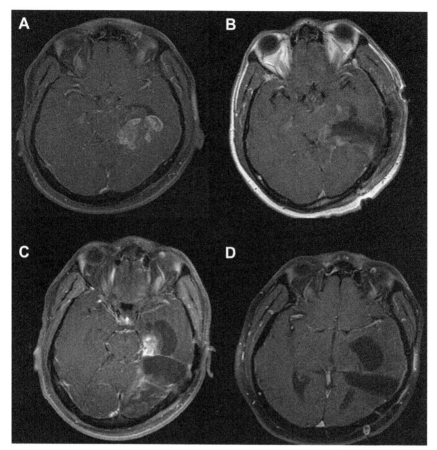

Fig. 1. Axial T1 postcontrast MRIs. (A) Preoperative image of a left temporal GBM. (B) Post-operative image revealing extensive subtotal resection. (C) Radiographic progression of GBM during treatment with TMZ. New enhancement in the right medial temporal lobe anterior to the resection cavity is noted. (D) Marked radiographic response is noted after initiation of Bevacizumab.

single-arm phase II trial in recurrent AA or AOA using TMZ (150–200 mg/m$^2$ for 5 out of 28 days), which demonstrated a 6-month progression-free survival (PFS6) of 46%, median PFS of 5.4 months, 35% objective radiographic response rate (RR), and median OS of 13.6 months.[22] Although there is a lack of class I evidence to support the use of TMZ in patients with *newly* diagnosed AA, there is prospective data suggestive of improved outcomes with TMZ either alone or with RT in this setting.[23] Many neuro-oncologists use the same treatment regimen for newly diagnosed AA as they do for newly diagnosed GBM for which there is a greater body of evidence in its support. A randomized phase III European Organization for Research and Treatment of Cancer/National Cancer Institute of Canada (EORTC/NCIC)–sponsored clinical trail comparing RT with concomitant daily TMZ (75 mg/m$^2$) followed by 6 additional cycles of TMZ (150–200 mg/m$^2$ on a 5 out of 28 day schedule) compared with RT alone demonstrated an improvement in median OS from 12.1 months to 14.6 months in the TMZ-treated arm. At 2 years, the survival improved from 10.4% to 26.5%.[24] At 5 years, the survival was 1.9% in the control arm (RT alone) and 9.8% for those receiving additional TMZ.[25] Patients with MGMT promoter methylation as assessed by MSP had an improved survival compared with those without *MGMT* promoter methylation. The difference in survival was most pronounced in the TMZ-treated patients.[16] Of note, although patients with *MGMT* promoter methylation had the best outcomes at 5 years, those with unmethylated promoters also saw a benefit to the addition of TMZ. This finding suggests that although the status of MGMT expression is important, other factors also influence chemotherapy response.

This pivotal phase III clinical trial that still defines the standard of care for newly diagnosed GBM demonstrated that prolonged exposure to TMZ provided a distinct benefit. Because TMZ is generally well tolerated, the following question quickly emerged: would more TMZ result in even better responses? In an attempt to determine this, the Radiation Therapy Oncology Group (RTOG) 0525 trial randomized patients to either the standard TMZ dosing schedule (150–200 mg/m$^2$ for 5 out of 28 days) or to a dose-dense regimen (75–100 mg/m$^2$ for 21 out of 28 days) for adjuvant TMZ following RT with concomitant TMZ. All patients were expected to receive 12 (rather than 6) adjuvant TMZ cycles, provided toxicity did not preclude it. No significant improvement in PFS or OS was noted between groups. However, OS was longer in the RTOG 0525 study compared with the EORTC/NCIC pivotal trial. It is possible that subsequent salvage regimens received by patients in the RTOG study may have influenced this. Echoing the findings in the pivotal trial, *MGMT* promoter methylation status again demonstrated an important prognostic marker.[26]

Age at diagnosis continues to be an important prognostic factor in response to treatment of malignant glioma. Both the very young and the elderly have worse prognoses. Radiation exposure in young children continues to limit treatment options for them. In addition, there is evidence that malignant gliomas in the pediatric population differ at the molecular level from adults.[27] Although brain tumors, as a whole, are the commonest solid tumors in children, malignant gliomas remain rare. Their discussion lies beyond the scope of this article. However, because these tumors are more common with advancing age and life expectancy continues to improve, it is important to determine the optimal treatment regimen for this age group. The pivotal trial that resulted in approval of TMZ in newly diagnosed GBM limited enrollment to patients aged 18 to 65 years.[24] The optimal management regimen for elderly patients with GBM and other high-grade astrocytomas, a poorer prognostic group, remains uncertain.[28,29] However, several challenges present themselves. These challenges include, but are not limited to, defining *the elderly* and the effects of comorbidities on treatment-related toxicities and survival. Recent clinical trials have attempted to shed light on these issues. Strategies have ranged from reducing total RT doses, with or without the use of TMZ, to the elimination of RT altogether in favor of single-agent TMZ. These studies are outlined in **Table 2**. Defining an optimal treatment strategy for the elderly remains an elusive goal. Retrospective studies have demonstrated improved outcomes in elderly patients treated with combination RT/TMZ compared with RT alone.[36] In all of the studies described earlier, the incidence of hematologic toxicities was greater than that seen in the younger patient populations. At this time, there is no defined standard of care for elderly patients with high-grade astrocytomas, and management should be tailored to the individual patient. Various approaches to RT in this patient population are discussed later.

### TMZ for oligodendroglial tumors

TMZ has been best studied in astrocytic tumors; however, it also has activity in the treatment of oligodendroglial tumors. Although a regimen of procarbazine, lomustine (CCNU), and vincristine (PCV) was demonstrated to be of benefit in the treatment of oligodendrogliomas before the development of TMZ,[37] the greater tolerability

**Table 2**
**Glioma clinical trials**

| Authors | Phase | Age | PS | Histology | Treatment | OS |
|---|---|---|---|---|---|---|
| Wick et al,[30] 2012 | III | >65 | KPS ≥60 | AA, GBM | RT 60 Gy over 6 wk vs TMZ (100 mg/m²) 7 d on/7 d off | 9.6 mo vs 8.6 mo |
| Malmstrom et al,[31] 2012 | III | >60 | WHO ≥2 | GBM | TMZ (200 mg/m²) 5 of 28 d vs RT 34 Gy over 2 wk vs RT 60 Gy over 6 wk | 8.3 mo vs 7.5 mo vs 6.0 mo |
| Perez-Larraya et al,[32] 2011 | II | >70 | KPS <70% | GBM | TMZ 5 of 28 d | 25 wk |
| Minnitti et al,[33] 2012 | II | ≥70 | KPS ≥60 | GBM | RT 40 Gy over 3 wk with daily TMZ (75 mg/m²) followed by TMZ (150–200 mg/m²) 5 of 28 d × 12 cycles | 12.4 mo |
| Roa et al,[34] 2004 | III | ≥60 | ≥60 | GBM | RT 60 Gy over 6 wk vs 40 Gy over 3 wk | 5.6 mo vs 5.1 mo |
| Keime-Guibert et al,[35] 2007 | III | ≥70 | ≥70 | AA, GBM | RT 54 Gy over 6 wk vs supportive care | 29.1 wk vs 16.1 wk |

*Abbreviations:* KPS, Karnofsky performance status; OS, media overall survival; PS, performance status.

of TMZ and its efficacy in astrocytic tumors led to an increase in its use in oligodendrogliomas. Evidence from phase II trials using TMZ as initial chemotherapy for oligodendrogliomas of various grades further demonstrated both its tolerability and effectiveness.[38–40] The role for TMZ in treating oligodendrogliomas, either alone or in combination with RT, is evolving. Studies comparing different combinations are underway. As discussed later, it is clear from large randomized studies that RT followed by PCV chemotherapy is superior to RT alone for newly diagnosed anaplastic gliomas harboring the 1p19q codeletion. How these data, 17 years in the making, will influence the future use of TMZ in these tumors is to be determined.

### Procarbazine, CCNU, and PCV Chemotherapy

#### PCV for astrocytic tumors
The PCV chemotherapy regimen, administered in six 6-week cycles, has been used in the treatment of malignant gliomas for more than 3 decades. Its use expanded following the publication of the final results of a cooperative group study demonstrating the superiority of PCV over single-agent carmustine (BCNU) in the adjuvant treatment of anaplastic gliomas.[41] The design of this study has been criticized for its histologic grading scheme that may have allowed inclusion of tumors deemed less than anaplastic by competing grading systems. PCV then went on to become the standard against which other regimens study would be tested in anaplastic glioma studies. Several subsequent single-arm phase II clinical trials assessed the effects of adding PCV after RT for newly diagnosed AA and GBM.[42,43] However, studying a large cohort of AA retrospectively, Prados and colleagues[44] found that OS rates were the same if patients received CCNU alone or PCV in combination. These findings, coincident with the development of TMZ and its improved safety profile, resulted in less PCV use for astrocytomas of all grades. That said, PCV or its components (CCNU or procarbazine) are still commonly used as salvage regimens when TMZ fails.[45,46]

### PCV for oligodendroglial tumors

PCV has had an important role in the treatment of oligodendroglial tumors. An early phase II study of newly diagnosed and recurrent contrast-enhancing AO treated with up to 6 cycles of PCV demonstrated a response rate (RR) of 75%. In this study, similarly impressive RRs were noted in those newly diagnosed and progressing after RT.[37] It was demonstrated early on that tumors with oligodendroglial histology and 1p19q codeletions had durable responses to chemotherapy with PCV.[8] A large retrospective study of more than 1000 patients with AO demonstrated an improved time to progression in patients with 1p19q codeletions treated with PCV alone (7.6 years) versus TMZ alone (3.3 years).[47] This finding has raised again the question of the optimal chemotherapy regimen for these patients. The long-term follow-up results of 2 randomized phase III trials demonstrated a benefit in median OS with the addition of PCV to RT for AO, particularly for the tumors with a 1p19q codeletion. RTOG 9402 randomized patients with newly diagnosed AO or AOA to four 6-week cycles of PCV followed by RT versus RT alone. Although there was no difference in OS between the two arms for the cohort of patients, patients with 1p19q codeletion has a significant improvement in median OS (14.7 years vs 7.3 years).[48] The EORTC Brain Tumor Group Study 26 951 randomized patients with newly diagnosed AO to RT (59.4 Gy) followed by 6 cycles of PCV versus RT (59.4 Gy) alone. The median OS was significantly improved in the chemoradiation arm (306.0 months vs 42.3 months). In patients with a 1p19q codeletion, there was a trend in improved OS (median OS not yet reached vs 112 months) with chemoradiation compared with the RT-only arm.[49] These results argue strongly in favor of combined modality therapy for AO with 1p19q codeletions. Because earlier reports from each of these studies had failed to show a benefit for adjuvant PCV in AO, an international multi-arm study (CODEL, NCT00887146) evaluating the role of TMZ alone or in combination with RT was underway in 1p19q codeleted anaplastic gliomas.[50,51] The future of this study is now in question as debate continues on the role of PCV in this patient population.

### BEV

Neoangiogenesis is a hallmark histologic feature of GBM, manifested on routine histologic specimens as endothelial proliferation. Vascular endothelial growth factor (VEGF) is a potent proangiogenic factor and is expressed by GBM in high concentrations.[52] BEV, a humanized monoclonal antibody directed against VEGF, received accelerated FDA approval in the treatment of progressive GBM in 2009. This approval was based on the results of 2 phase II trials of this antiangiogenic agent. The larger of these two studies (n = 167) randomized patients with recurrent GBM to receive either BEV alone or in combination with irinotecan, a topoisomerase inhibitor.[53] Those patients on single-agent BEV could cross over to receive BEV with irinotecan at progression. Improvements of both PFS and RR were noted when compared with historical controls. Although noncomparative, there was no difference in these endpoints between the treatment groups. Toxicities were higher in those receiving irinotecan. Another phase II trial in recurrent GBM used BEV followed by BEV and irinotecan. Similar results were noted in this study. No additional benefit was noted to adding irinotecan after progression on BEV.[54] The marked improvement in RR compared with previously evaluated regimens is caused, at least in part, by BEV's effect on the permeability of the blood-brain barrier (BBB). This decrease in BBB permeability is associated with reduced gadolinium enhancement, previously the gold standard for measurement of a drug's activity on GBM.[55] Another consequence of BEV's action at the BBB is a marked reduction in cerebral edema, which is associated with a reduced need for steroids and an improvement in measures of life quality.[56,57]

The earlier-referenced studies have led to the widespread use of BEV for recurrent high-grade astrocytomas. In a single-arm phase II study that added BEV to the standard of care in newly diagnosed GBM, significant improvements were noted in PFS, a radiologic endpoint, but not OS.[58] Additional phase II trials have explored variations on the timing and dosing schedule of BEV in similar patient populations.[59,60] Two phase III randomized, placebo-controlled, clinical trials are underway to evaluate the role for BEV in the newly diagnosed GBM population (NCT00884741, NCT00943825). The results of these studies should clarify the role for BEV in the adjuvant setting for GBM.[61]

## NONPHARMACOLOGIC TREATMENT OPTIONS
### RT

RT has long formed a cornerstone in the management of high-grade gliomas. The role of RT in high-grade gliomas has been recently reviewed and the authors refer readers to these articles for additional details.[62,63] A few terms merit definition. A *radiation-absorbed dose* (rad) is equivalent to a centigray. Doses used in glioma treatment are usually referred to in either centigray (for fraction size) or gray (for total dose). A dose prescription defines the number of fractions delivered over a length of time. Attempts to deliver larger doses in smaller fractions are referred to as *hypofractionation* schedules. Those aimed at using more frequent, smaller fractions are called *hyperfractionation* schemes. An RT dose/survival relationship has been established in high-grade gliomas for some time. In newly diagnosed nonelderly patients with AA and GBM, 60 Gy delivered over 6 weeks in 200-cGY fractions is the most frequently used dosing regimen. The addition of stereotactic radiosurgery (SRS) followed by standard RT plus BCNU did not demonstrate any benefit in the RTOG 9305 phase III clinical trial when compared with standard RT plus BCNU without SRS.[64] This evidence argues against adding an SRS boost to standard RT in the newly diagnosed setting. Attempts to deliver higher cumulative dose of 70.4 Gy using hyperfractionation schemes also failed to show a survival advantage.[65]

As noted earlier, the elderly have a poorer prognosis. They also suffer greater morbidity of treatment. Attempts have been made to reduce toxicity without negatively impacting survival. Several studies have demonstrated that lower cumulative doses delivered in a variety of fractionation schemes results in similar survival rates but with reduced toxicity. These schemes are outlined in **Table 1**. In the elderly patient population with newly diagnosed high-grade gliomas, specifically in patients with astrocytic tumors, there is evidence that either an abbreviated course of RT, substitution of chemotherapy for RT, or a combination of these approaches may all be reasonable therapeutic considerations. Trials demonstrating relative comparability of 5 out of 28 days or week on/week off TMZ over standard dose RT have been discussed earlier as has a single-arm study combining low-dose RT with TMZ.[30,31,33] A benefit has been demonstrated using RT (50 Gy in 1.8-Gy fractions) in patients with AA and GBM aged 70 years or older with a Karnofsky performance status (KPS) of 70 or greater when compared with supportive care alone. The median OS was 29.1 weeks versus 16.9 weeks.[35] Short-course RT in place of standard RT has been shown to be comparable in an elderly patient population (aged $\geq$60 years, KPS $\geq$60) with GBM. Similar outcomes (OS 5.1 months vs 5.6 months, $P = .57$; 6-month survival 44.7% vs 41.7%) were seen in patients treated with standard RT (60 Gy in 30 fractions) when compared with short-course RT (40 Gy in 15 fractions).[34] At this time, there are several management options for elderly patients with high-grade gliomas, and treatment should be tailored to the individual patient.

The role of RT in recurrent high-grade gliomas is less clearly defined. Potential benefits from additional RT have been tempered by concerns for RT-related toxicity, particularly radiation necrosis. Various techniques have been used in an attempt to limit the toxicity of reirradiation. Hypofractionated SRS has been shown to correlate with improved survival in large retrospective studies as well as smaller prospective studies, particularly in patients with smaller tumor volumes. Somewhat surprisingly, even patients with only a short interval before progression after their initial RT had improved OS with the addition of hypofractionated SRS.[66,67]

Although photons are the most common source of radiation used, including in all of the studies discussed earlier, there has been growing interest in the potential role of other radiation sources. Carbon ions and protons are two that have been studied. The ability of these sources to create tight delivery fields with limited exit trajectories conceivably increases the dose to desired targets while limiting collateral injury to normal brain and surrounding tissues. Prospective data in using these modalities in both the newly diagnosed and recurrent settings, particularly in conjunction with current standard chemotherapeutics, are limited and further study is warranted.[68,69]

## COMBINATION THERAPIES

Combination treatment with surgery, RT, and chemotherapy is central to the management of high-grade gliomas today and defines the standard of care. This topic is discussed earlier. At this time, results of large phase III trials support the use of RT and chemotherapy as the standard of care for GBM and AO with 1p19q codeletion.[24,48,49] The optimal management of AA and AO and AOA without 1p19q codeletion has not yet been fully established, although a multimodality approach is often used. Recurrent disease can be treated with any combination of approaches. Clinical trials for recurrent disease often limit treatment to a single modality, chemotherapy, for instance, because their goal is to study the safety and efficacy of previously untested agents.

### Role of Resection

Surgery has long played a role in both the diagnosis and treatment of high-grade gliomas. National Comprehensive Cancer Network's guidelines advocate for the maximum safe surgical resection of high-grade gliomas.[70] The influence of the extent of resection on important clinical endpoints is not completely clear. Most studies have been retrospective and have emphasized a single but important endpoint, OS. There is, however, prospective data suggesting an improved long-term quality of life in patients with high-grade glioma who have undergone more extensive resection.[71] Selection bias must be rigorously controlled in such studies because tumor location often dictates the degree of impairment and resectability of these tumors. Although the evidence is limited, there is a general trend in favor of attempts at extensive resection when possible.[72]

### Advanced Surgical Techniques

Continued advances in neurosurgical techniques have been investigated. In this subsection, the authors focus on recent techniques used to improve the extent of resection. The mapping of motor and language areas of the brain has allowed for more aggressive resections of high-grade gliomas by minimizing the risk of potential deficits. A trend in cortical mapping has been the shift from defining functionally active (positive) areas to relatively inactive (negative) areas, in turn leading to limited cortical exposure and more efficient surgeries.[73] The use of intraoperative imaging to increase the extent of surgical resection has been growing. Nonrandomized studies of intraoperative MRI have suggested the achievement of more extensive resections when adding this modality.[74] Intraoperative use of 5-aminolevulinic acid to cause fluorescence of tumoral tissue to assist in more extensive tumor resection has also been studied in nonrandomized trials.[75]

As stated earlier, the evidence for a benefit caused by more extensive resections has not yet been completely established. The use of the modalities described earlier may increase over time as additional data regarding safety and efficacy are accumulated. Obtaining class I evidence with regard to the extent of resection remains an elusive goal because randomized studies designed to evaluate such endpoints are challenging to design and accrue to.

### Surgery as Delivery Method for Other Therapies

The use of polifeprosan 20 wafers impregnated with the nitrosourea BCNU (Gliadel) was FDA approved in 1997 for patients with recurrent GBM for whom re-resection was indicated. In the phase III trial, the median OS was increased in the Gliadel arm (13.9 months vs 11.6 months). All patients received conventional RT. No patients received systemic chemotherapy because the goal of the study included avoidance of systemic toxicity. There was, however, an increased risk of cerebrospinal fluid leak (5.0% vs 0.8%) and intracranial hypertension (9.1% vs 1.7%) in the Gliadel arm.[76] The Gliadel wafer was subsequently approved for newly diagnosed GBM. Gliadel remains a treatment option for patients with resectable tumors. Convection-enhanced delivery (CED) remains another promising drug delivery strategy.[77] However, 2 phase III trials in recurrent GBM using CED to deliver 2 different agents, interleukin 13 (IL-13) pseudomonas exotoxin (cintredekin besudotox) and diphtheria toxin, failed to demonstrate a benefit.[78] CED and other neurosurgical delivery techniques are being actively investigated as methods of delivery of various novel therapeutics for high-grade gliomas.

## TREATMENT RESISTANCE/COMPLICATIONS
### TMZ Resistance

Given the importance of *MGMT* promoter methylation status on response to chemotherapy in malignant glioma, attempts have been made to reduce this DNA repair enzyme's activity in brain tumors. This resistance may be innate or acquired, the latter seen following initial responses to chemotherapy followed by tumor regrowth of chemotherapy-resistant cells. The literature is confusing in this regard because MGMT is also known as O(6)-alkylguanine DNA alkyltransferase (AGT); this came about when MGMT was found to remove alkyl groups, albeit less efficiently, as well as methyl groups from DNA residues.[79] In this review, the authors consistently use the term MGMT to refer to this enzyme, although references cited may use AGT in its stead.

The compound O(6)-benzylguanine (O6BG) is substrate for MGMT. As such, it competes with methylated guanine residues. It follows that the addition of O6BG to chemotherapies that work through guanine adduct formation might increase their antitumor effects. Phase I studies that examined the dose of O6BG required to suppress MGMT activity in peripheral blood mononuclear cells (PBMNC) and brain tumor tissue reached significantly different conclusions.[80,81] Although 40 $mg/m^2$ was sufficient to eliminate MGMT activity in PBMNC, 120 $mg/m^2$ was required to achieve the same effects in brain tumor tissue. Because of synergistic effects on myelosuppression, the doses of chemotherapy (either nitrosoureas or TMZ) needed to be substantially reduced. The phase III clinical trial evaluating O6BG with a nitrosourea was stopped early when interim analyses showed no benefit.[82,83]

MGMT must be resynthesized once it has interacted with a DNA adduct. For this reason, its activity might be reduced by continuous exposure to relevant chemotherapies. Strategies to exhaust the MGMT available in a given tumor cell include alternate dosing regimens with TMZ, a drug with a relatively low toxicity profile. These schedules include 21 of every 28 days, 7 days on followed by 7 days off, and daily low-dose TMZ. This rationale was implicit in the design of the RTOG 0525 study, referenced earlier, whereby patients received either additional cycles of the conventional regimen or a so-called dose-dense regimen at first diagnosis (RTOG 0525). Although the results of this study were not significant, smaller, nonrandomized studies using alternate TMZ dosing at disease recurrence have demonstrated a modest benefit to this approach.[84] The enzyme poly (ADP-ribose) polymerase (PARP) facilitates the repair of single-strand DNA breaks that, if unrepaired, can lead to double-strand breaks during DNA replication.[85] PARP inhibitors impair this process and have been shown in preclinical models to synergize with chemotherapy in select tumor subsets.[86] Clinical trials comparing the effects of chemotherapy with or without PARP inhibitors are underway for high-grade gliomas (NCT00994071, NCT01390571).

### BEV Resistance

Recurrent GBM is one of the few tumors for which BEV is approved for use as a single agent. More often, it is combined with either cytotoxic or targeted chemotherapy. As mentioned, BEV has dramatic effects on the MRI appearance of malignant gliomas, casting further doubt on the validity of our interpretive assumptions. A variety of MRI changes may be seen following BEV administration, ranging from complete radiographic responses to the presence of diffusely infiltrating nonenhancing tumor. This latter finding has prompted debate about the role of BEV in promoting a phenotypic shift in GBM whereby cells become more invasive and migratory. Although it is not clear that BEV drives this phenotypic shift, there is evidence that molecular subtypes of GBM demonstrate distinct patterns of growth on antiangiogenic agents at the time of progression.[87] Not all patients who receive BEV demonstrate this pattern of change on MRI. For example, in the larger of the phase II trials that led to its accelerated FDA approval, only 16% of patients treated on the BEV-alone arm had a conversion from local tumor to diffuse tumor spread at time of progression. This percentage was higher (39%) in the combination arm.[88] These findings raise important questions about patterns of recurrence when antiangiogenic agents are used alone or in combination and warn of still further confusion as we move forward with clinical trials.

In an attempt to more fully use imaging capabilities in determining response (favorable and unfavorable) to BEV, several studies are worth mentioning. There is growing evidence supporting the use of pretreatment apparent diffusion coefficient (ADC) volume as a predictor for OS and PFS for BEV-treated patients in this setting.[89] This use may prove to have broad clinical applicability because ADC sequences are a component of most standard MRIs. Additional investigations of nonstandard correlative studies, such as 3'-deoxy-3'-[18F]fluorothymidine ([18]F-FLT)-positron emission tomography (PET) and 3,4-dihydroxy-6-[18F]-fluoro-l-phenylalanine ([18]F-FDOPA)-PET have demonstrated that a decrease in tracer uptake after the initiation of BEV correlates with improved PFS ([18]F-FLT, [18]F-FDOPA) and improved OS ([18]F-FDOPA).[90]

It is one thing to recognize changes in imaging that suggest a change in tumor behavior and another to understand the biologic features that drive this behavior. Many questions remain to be answered. For example, are inherent and acquired resistance mediated by the same mechanisms? What changes in which molecular pathways mediate these responses? Some clues are emerging. As noted earlier, distinct gene expression profiles emerge from enhancing and nonenhancing portions of malignant glioma following exposure to BEV.[87] Several molecular pathways, long known to mediate glioma growth and invasion, are also implicated in these changes in behavior following exposure to BEV. For example, in animal models using human GBM xenografts, expression of c-Met (a protein involved in tumor invasion and metastasis) is upregulated following exposure to BEV.[91] Similarly, in both patient samples and GBM xenograft models, BEV exposure has been shown to result in the upregulation of signal transducer and activator of transcription 3 pathway[92] Other pathways are under investigation and an understanding of their roles in mediating tumor behavior will be critical to treatment strategies in the future.

## EVALUATION OF OUTCOME AND LONG-TERM RECOMMENDATIONS
### Clinical Trial Endpoints

The authors have implied through out this review that radiographic clinical trial endpoints in neuro-oncology studies are vulnerable to biologic effects of RT, antiangiogenic agents, and immune therapies. Post hoc analyses of radiographic endpoints have often shown them to be valid. Clinical trial endpoints for high-grade gliomas have recently been reviewed.[93] PFS, PFS6, and RR will rely on the definitions used for radiographic progression. Defining progression and regression is complicated by the well-described phenomena of pseudoprogression and pseudoregression. Recent efforts to refine the response criteria have led to the Radiology Assessment in Neuro-Oncology (RANO) criteria, which are replacing the longstanding MacDonald criteria in glioma clinical trials. Unique features of the RANO criteria include an attempt to address the issues of pseudoprogression after RT and include the assessment of non-enhancing tumor. The RANO criteria preclude the diagnosing progression less than 12 weeks after chemoradiotherapy unless progression occurs outside of the RT field or there is histologic diagnosis of progressive tumor. RANO also takes into account significant changes on T2/fluid-attenuated inversion recovery sequences for patients on antiangiogenic therapies and stable or increasing doses of steroids. The investigators also note caution in noting regression in patients on antiangiogenic therapies (pseudoregression) because of their mechanism of action. Persistence of radiographic improvement is necessary for at least 4 weeks for scans to qualify as true responses.[55] OS, long the gold standard outcome measure in glioma clinical trials, has always been influenced by factors such as age and performance status. Now, as we develop more significant salvage therapies, subsequent treatment may also have an impact on this important outcome measure.

Less traditional clinical trial endpoints, such as quality of life and performance on neuropsychiatric assessments, have been playing a growing role in the design of clinical trials. These endpoints will likely only grow further in their importance.[94]

### Long-term Follow-up

Long-term follow-up for patients with high-grade gliomas and either complete responses or stable disease no longer on active therapy typically involves regular clinical and radiographic follow-up. Over time, the interval between reevaluations is expanded. If patients develop new or worsening signs or symptoms before the scheduled follow-up, earlier evaluation is often warranted.

## SUMMARY/DISCUSSION

The authors discuss recent updates to the standard of care for high-grade gliomas and attempt to provide an understanding of areas where the optimal management is not yet fully elucidated. In general, a multidisciplinary approach carefully considering the role of surgery, RT, and chemotherapy is used to optimize patient survival and quality of life. The authors attempt, through the use of several examples, to demonstrate how advances in our understanding of these tumors at the molecular level is influencing approaches to treatment. To date, none of these has significantly influenced the standard of care. Properties to CNS tissue confound our interpretation of imaging, and the authors attempt to demonstrate the ways in which this has influenced trial design and outcomes. The CNS is a small, complex, and vulnerable tissue; and advances in treating rumors that arise within it are the result of sustained efforts on the parts of individuals and cooperative groups. However, we seem poised, after decades of persistence, to advance the field in meaningful ways.

## REFERENCES

1. Louis DN, Ohgaki H, Wiestler OD, et al, editors. WHO classification of tumors of the central nervous system. 4th edition. Lyon (France): International Agency for Research on Cancer; 2007.
2. Ohgaki H, Kleihues P. Genetic profile of astrocytic and oligodendroglial gliomas. Brain Tumor Pathol 2011;28:177–83.
3. Nicholas MK, Lukas RV, Chmura S, et al. Molecular heterogeneity in glioblastoma: therapeutic opportunities and challenges. Semin Oncol 2011;38: 243–53.
4. Verhaak RG, Hoadley KA, Purdom E, et al. Integrated genomic analysis identifies clinically relevant subtypes of glioblastoma characterized by abnormalities in PDGFRA, IDH1, EGFR, and NF1. Cancer Cell 2010;17:98–110.
5. Cairncross JG, Ueke K, Zlatescu MC, et al. Specific genetic predictors of chemotherapeutic response and survival in patients with anaplastic oligodendrogliomas. J Natl Cancer Inst 1998;90:1473–9.
6. Horbinski C, Miller CR, Perry A. Gone FISHing: clinical lessons learned in brain tumor molecular diagnostics over the last decade. Brain Pathol 2011;21:57–73.
7. Smith JS, Perry A, Borell TJ, et al. Alterations of chromosome arms 1p and 19q as predictors of survival in oligodendrogliomas, astrocytomas, and mixed oligoastrocytomas. J Clin Oncol 2000;18:636–45.
8. Ino Y, Betensky RA, Zlatescu MC, et al. Molecular subtypes of anaplastic oligodendroglioma: implications for patient management at diagnosis. Clin Cancer Res 2001;7:839–45.
9. Griffin CA, Burger P, Morsberger L, et al. Identification of der(1;19)(q10;p10) in five oligodendrogliomas suggests mechanism of concurrent 1p and 19q loss. J Neuropathol Exp Neurol 2006;65:988–94.
10. Mokhtari K, Ducray F, Kros JM, et al. Alpha-internexin expression predicts outcome in anaplastic oligodendroglial tumors and may positively impact the efficacy of chemotherapy: European organization for research and treatment of cancer trial 26951. Cancer 2011;117:3014–26.
11. Yip S, Butterfield YS, Morozova O, et al. Concurrent CIC mutations, IDH mutations, and 1p/19q loss distinguish oligodendrogliomas from other cancers. J Pathol 2012;226:7–16.
12. Prensner JR, Chinnaiyan AM. Metabolism unhinged: IDH mutations in cancer. Nat Med 2011;17:291–3.
13. Parsons DW, Jones S, Zhang X, et al. An integrated genomic analysis of human glioblastoma multiforme. Science 2008;321:1807–12.
14. Yan H, Parsons DW, Jin G, et al. IDH1 and IDH2 mutations in gliomas. N Engl J Med 2009;360:765–73.

15. Labussiere M, Idbaih A, Wang XW, et al. All the 1p19q codeleted gliomas are mutated on IDH1 or IDH2. Neurology 2010;74:1886–90.
16. Hegi ME, Diserens AC, Gorlia T, et al. MGMT gene silencing and benefit from temozolomide in glioblastoma. N Engl J Med 2005;352:997–1003.
17. Weller M, Stupp R, Reifenberger G, et al. MGMT promoter methylation in malignant gliomas: ready for personalized medicine? Nat Rev Neurol 2010;6:39–51.
18. Noushmehr H, Weisenberger DJ, Diefes K, et al. Identification of a CpG island methylator phenotype that defines a distinct subgroup of glioma. Cancer Cell 2010;17:510–22.
19. Nicholas MK, Lukas RV, Jafri NF, et al. Epidermal growth factor receptor-mediated signal transduction in the development and therapy of gliomas. Clin Cancer Res 2006;12:7261–70.
20. Siebert DM, Shakur SF, Pytel P, et al. EGFR as a therapeutic target in glioblastoma. Rev Health Care 2012;3:35–51.
21. Clark PA, Iida M, Treisman DM, et al. Activation of multiple ERBB family receptors mediates glioblastoma cancer stem-like cell resistance to EGFR- targeted inhibition. Neoplasia 2012;14:420–8.
22. Yung WK, Prados MD, Yaya-Tur R, et al. Multicenter phase II trial of temozolomide in patients with anaplastic astrocytoma or anaplastic oligoastrocytoma at first relapse. Temodal Brain Tumor Group. J Clin Oncol 1999;17:2762–71.
23. Wick W, Hartmann C, Engel C, et al. NOA-04 randomized phase III trial of sequential radiochemotherapy of anaplastic glioma with procarbazine, lomustine, and vincristine or temozolomide. J Clin Oncol 2009;27:5874–80.
24. Stupp R, Mason WP, van den Bent MJ, et al. Radiotherapy plus concomitant and adjuvant temozolomide for glioblastoma. N Engl J Med 2005;352:987–96.
25. Stupp R, Hegi ME, Mason WP, et al. Effects of radiotherapy with concomitant and adjuvant temozolomide versus radiotherapy alone on survival in glioblastoma in a randomised phase III study: 5-year analysis of the EORTC-NCIC trial. Lancet Oncol 2009;10:459–66.
26. Ahluwahlia MS. 2010 Society for Neuro-Oncology Annual Meeting: a report of selected studies. Expert Rev Anticancer Ther 2011;11:161–3.
27. Byeon SJ, Myung JK, Kim SH, et al. Distinct genetic alterations in pediatric glioblastomas. Childs Nerv Syst 2012;28:1025–32.
28. Curran WJ Jr, Scott CB, Horton J, et al. Recursive partitioning analysis of prognostic factors in three Radiation Therapy Oncology Group malignant glioma trials. J Natl Cancer Inst 1993;85:704–10.
29. Fisher JL, Schwartzbaum JA, Wrensch M, et al. Epidemiology of brain tumors. Neurol Clin 2007;25:867–90.
30. Wick W, Platten M, Meisner C, et al. Temozolomide therapy alone versus radiotherapy alone for malignant astrocytoma in the elderly: the NOA-08 randomised, phase III trial. Lancet Oncol 2012;13:707–15.
31. Malmstrom A, Gronberg H, Marosi C, et al. Temozolomide versus standard 6-week radiotherapy versus hypofractionated radiotherapy in patients older than 60 years with glioblastoma: the Nordic randomised, phase III trial. Lancet Oncol 2012;13:916–26.
32. Gallego Perez-Larraya J, Ducray F, Chinot O, et al. Temozolomide in elderly patients with newly diagnosed glioblastoma and poor performance status: an ANOCEF phase II trial. J Clin Oncol 2011;29:3050–5.
33. Minnitti G, Lanzetta G, Scaringi C, et al. Phase II study of short-course radiotherapy plus concomitant and adjuvant temozolomide in elderly patients with glioblastoma. Int J Radiat Oncol Biol Phys 2012;83:93–9.

34. Roa W, Brasher PM, Bauman G, et al. Abbreviated course of radiation therapy in older patients with glioblastoma multiforme: a prospective randomized clinical trial. J Clin Oncol 2004;22:1583–8.

35. Keime-Guibert F, Chinot O, Taillandier L, et al. Radiotherapy for glioblastoma in the elderly. N Engl J Med 2007;56:1527–35.

36. Barker CA, Chang M, Chou JF, et al. Radiotherapy and concomitant temozolomide may improve survival elderly patients with glioblastoma. J Neurooncol 2012;109:391–7.

37. Cairncross G, Macdonald D, Ludwin S, et al. Chemotherapy for anaplastic oligodendroglioma. National Cancer Institute of Canada Clinical Trials Group. J Clin Oncol 1994;12:2013–21.

38. van den Bent MJ, Taphoorn MJ, Brandes AA, et al. Phase II study of first-line chemotherapy with temozolomide in recurrent oligodendroglial tumors: the European Organization for Research and treatment of Cancer Brain Tumor Group Study 26971. J Clin Oncol 2003;21:2525–8.

39. Mikkelsen T, Doyle T, Anderson J, et al. Temozolomide single-agent chemotherapy for newly diagnosed anaplastic oligodendroglioma. J Neurooncol 2009;92:57–63.

40. Gan HK, Rosenthal MA, Dowling A, et al. A phase II trial of primary temozolomide in patients with grade III oligodendroglial brain tumors. Neuro Oncol 2010;12:500–7.

41. Levin VA, Silver P, Hannigan J, et al. Superiority of post-radiotherapy adjuvant chemotherapy with CCNU, procarbazine, vincristine (PCV) over BCNU for anaplastic gliomas: NCOG 6G61 final report. Int J Radiat Oncol Biol Phys 1990;18:321–4.

42. Ron IG, Gal O, Vishne TH, et al. Long-term follow-up in managing anaplastic astrocytoma by multimodality approach with surgery followed by postoperative radiotherapy and PCV-chemotherapy: phase II trial. Am J Clin Oncol 2002;25: 296–302.

43. Murphy C, Pickles T, Knowling M, et al. Concurrent modified PCV chemotherapy and radiotherapy in newly diagnosed grade IV astrocytoma. J Neurooncol 2002; 57:215–20.

44. Prados MD, Scott C, Curran WJ Jr, et al. Procarbazine, lomustine, and vincristine (PCV) chemotherapy for anaplastic astrocytoma: a retrospective review of radiation therapy oncology group protocols comparing survival with carmustine or PCV adjuvant chemotherapy. J Clin Oncol 1999;17:3389–95.

45. Kappelle AC, Postma TJ, Taphoorn MJ, et al. PCV chemotherapy for recurrent glioblastoma multiforme. Neurology 2001;56:118–20.

46. Schmidt F, Fisher J, Herrlinger U, et al. PCV chemotherapy for recurrent glioblastoma. Neurology 2006;66:587–9.

47. Lassman AB, Iwamoto FM, Cloughesy TF, et al. International retrospective study of over 1000 adults with anaplastic oligodendroglial tumors. Neuro Oncol 2011; 13:649–59.

48. Cairncross G, Wang M, Shaw E, et al. Phase III trial of chemoradiotherapy for anaplastic oligodendroglioma: long-term results of RTOG 9402. J Clin Oncol 2013;31:337–43.

49. van den Bent MJ, Brandes AA, Taphoorn MJ, et al. Adjuvant procarbazine, lomustine, and vincristine chemotherapy in newly diagnosed anaplastic oligodendroglioma: long-term follow up of EORTC brain tumor group study 26951. J Clin Oncol 2013;31:344–50.

50. Cairncross G, Berkey B, Shaw E, et al. Phase III trial of chemotherapy plus radiotherapy versus radiotherapy alone for pure and mixed anaplastic oligodendroglioma (RTOG 9402): Intergroup Radiation Therapy Oncology Group trial 9402. J Clin Oncol 2006;24:2707–14.

51. van den Bent MJ, Carpentier AF, Brandes AA, et al. Adjuvant PCV improves progression free survival but not overall survival in newly diagnosed anaplastic oligodendrogliomas and oligoastrocytomas: a randomized European Organization for Research and Treatment of Cancer phase III trial. J Clin Oncol 2006;24: 2715–22.

52. Robles Irrizary L, Hambardzumyan D, Nakano I, et al. Therapeutic targeting of VEGF in the treatment of glioblastoma. Expert Opin Ther Targets 2012;16: 973–84.

53. Friedman HS, Prados MD, Wen PY, et al. Bevacizumab alone and in combination with irinotecan in recurrent glioblastoma. J Clin Oncol 2009;27:4733–40.

54. Kreisl TN, Kim L, Moore K, et al. Phase II trial of single agent bevacizumab followed by bevacizumab plus irinotecan at tumor progression in recurrent glioblastoma. J Clin Oncol 2009;27:740–5.

55. Wen PY, Macdonald DR, Reardon DA, et al. Updated response assessment criteria for high-grade gliomas: response assessment in neuro-oncology working group. J Clin Oncol 2010;28:1963–72.

56. Vredenburgh JJ, Cloughesy T, Samant M, et al. Corticosteroid use in patients with glioblastoma at first or second relapse treated with bevacizumab in the BRAIN study. Oncologist 2010;15:1329–34.

57. Wefel JS, Cloughesy T, Zazzali JL, et al. Neurocognitive function in patients with recurrent glioblastoma treated with bevacizumab. Neuro Oncol 2011;13:660–8.

58. Lai A, Tran A, Nghiemphu PL, et al. Phase II study of bevacizumab plus temozolomide during and after radiation therapy for patients with newly diagnosed glioblastoma multiforme. J Clin Oncol 2011;29:142–8.

59. Narayana A, Gruber D, Kunnakkat S, et al. A clinical trial of bevacizumab, temozolomide, and radiation for newly diagnosed glioblastoma. J Neurosurg 2012; 116:341–5.

60. Vredenburgh JJ, Desjardins A, Kirkpatrick JP, et al. Addition of bevacizumab to standard radiation therapy and daily temozolomide is associated with minimal toxicity in newly diagnosed glioblastoma multiforme. Int J Radiat Oncol Biol Phys 2012;82:58–66.

61. Chinot OL, de La Mott Rouge T, Moore N, et al. AVAglio: phase III trial of bevacizumab plus temozolomide and radiotherapy in newly diagnosed glioblastoma multiforme. Adv Ther 2011;28:334–40.

62. Taw BB, Gorgulho AA, Selch MT, et al. Radiation options for high-grade gliomas. Neurosurg Clin N Am 2012;23:259–67.

63. Niyazi M, Siefert A, Schwartz SB, et al. Therapeutic options for recurrent malignant glioma. Radiother Oncol 2011;98:1–14.

64. Souhami L, Seiferheld W, Brachman D, et al. Randomized comparison of stereotactic radiosurgery followed by conventional radiotherapy followed by conventional radiotherapy with carmustine to conventional radiotherapy with carmustine for patients with glioblastoma multiforme: report of Radiation Therapy Oncology Group 93-05 protocol. Int J Radiat Oncol Biol Phys 2004;60: 853–60.

65. Prados MD, Wara WM, Sneed PK, et al. Phase III trial of accelerated hyperfractionation with or without difluromethylornithine (DMFO) versus standard

fractionated radiotherapy with or without DMFO for newly diagnosed patients with glioblastoma multiforme. Int J Radiat Oncol Biol Phys 2001;49:71–7.

66. Fogh SE, Andrews DW, Glass J, et al. Hypofractionated stereotactic radiation therapy: an effective therapy for recurrent high-grade gliomas. J Clin Oncol 2010;28:3048–53.

67. Ernst-Steken A, Ganslandt O, Lambrecht U, et al. Survival and quality of life after hypofractionated stereotactic radiotherapy for recurrent malignant glioma. J Neurooncol 2007;81:287–94.

68. Mizumoto M, Tsuboi K, Igaki H, et al. Phase I/II trial of concomitant boost proton radiotherapy for supratentorial glioblastoma multiforme. Int J Radiat Oncol Biol Phys 2010;77:98–105.

69. Fitzek MM, Thorton AF, Rabinov JD, et al. Accelerated fractionated proton/ photon irradiaton to 90 cobalt gray equivalent for glioblastoma multiforme: results of a phase II prospective trial. J Neurosurg 1999;91:251–60.

70. NCCN Clinical Practice Guidelines in Oncology. Central Nervous System Cancers. Version 1.2013. Available at: http://www.nccn.org/professionals/physician_gls/pdf/cns.pdf. Accessed February 18, 2013.

71. Brown PD, Maurer MJ, Rummans TA, et al. A prospective study of quality of life in adults of newly diagnosed high-grade gliomas: the impact of the extent of resection on quality of life on survival. Neurosurgery 2005;57:495–504.

72. Hardesty DA, Sanai N. The value of glioma extent of resection in the modern neurosurgical era. Front Neurol 2012;3:140.

73. Sanai N, Berger MS. Recent surgical management of gliomas. Adv Exp Med Biol 2012;746:12–25.

74. Kuhnt D, Becker A, Ganslandt O, et al. Correlation of the extent of tumor volume resection and patient survival in surgery of glioblastoma multiforme with high-field intraoperative MRI guidance. Neuro Oncol 2011;13:1339–48.

75. Nabavi A, Thurm H, Zountsas B, et al. Five-aminolevulinic acid for fluorescence-guided resection of recurrent malignant gliomas: a phase ii study. Neurosurgery 2009;65:1070–6.

76. Westphal M, Hilt DC, Bortey E, et al. A phase 3 trial of local chemotherapy with biodegradable carmustine (BCNU) wafers (Gliadel wafers) in patients with primary malignant glioma. Neuro Oncol 2003;5:79–88.

77. Ferguson S, Lesniak MS. Convection enhanced drug delivery of novel therapeutic agents to malignant brain tumors. Curr Drug Deliv 2007;4:169–80.

78. Kunwar S, Chang S, Westphal M, et al. Phase III randomized trial of CED of IL13-PE38QQR vs Gliadel wafers for recurrent glioblastoma. Neuro Oncol 2010;12:871–81.

79. Dolan ME, Pegg AE, Hora NK, et al. Effect of O6-methylguanine on DNA interstrand cross-link formation on chloroethylnitrosoureas and 2-chloroethyl(methylsulfonyl)methanesulfonate. Cancer Res 1988;48:3603–6.

80. Schilsky RL, Dolan ME, Bertucci D, et al. Phase I clinical and pharmacological study of O6-benzylguanine followed by carmustine in patients with advanced cancer. Clin Cancer Res 2000;6:3025–31.

81. Friedman HS, Kokkinakis DM, Pluda J, et al. Phase I trial of O6-benzylguanine for patients undergoing surgery for malignant gliomas. J Clin Oncol 1998;16:3570–5.

82. Quinn JA, Jiang SX, Reardon DA, et al. Phase I trial of temozolomide plus irinotecan plus O6-benzylguanine in adults with recurrent malignant glioma. Cancer 2009;115:2964–70.

83. Blumenthal DT, Spence AM, Stelzer KJ, et al. A phase III study of radiation therapy (RT) and O6-benzylguanine (O6-BG) plus BCNU versus RT and BCNU alone

for newly diagnose glioblastoma (GBM) and gliosarcoma. SWOG S0001. Available at: http://swog.org/Visitors/ViewProtocolDetails.asp?ProtocolID=1852.

84. Perry JR, Belanger K, Mason WP, et al. Phase II trial of continuous dose-intense temozolomide in recurrent malignant glioma: RESCUE study. J Clin Oncol 2010; 28:2051–7.

85. Basu B, Sandhu SK, de Bono JS. PAPR inhibitors: mechanism of action and their potential role in the prevention and treatment of cancer. Drugs 2012;72: 1579–90.

86. McEllin B, Camacho CV, Mukherjee B, et al. PTEN loss compromises homologous recombination repair in astrocytes: implications for glioblastoma therapy with temozolomide or ploy(ADP ribose) polymerase inhibitors. Cancer Res 2010;70:5457–64.

87. DeLay M, Jahangiri A, Carbonell WS, et al. Microarray analysis verifies two distinct phenotypes of glioblastomas resistant to antiangiogenic therapy. Clin Cancer Res 2012;18:2930–42.

88. Pope WB, Xia Q, Patton VE, et al. Patterns of progression in patients with recurrent glioblastoma treated with bevacizumab. Neurology 2011;76:432–7.

89. Pope WB, Qiao XJ, Kim HJ, et al. Apparent diffusion coefficient histogram analysis stratifies progression-free and overall survival in patients with recurrent GBM treated with bevacizumab: a multi-center study. J Neurooncol 2012;108: 491–8.

90. Harris RJ, Cloughesy TF, Pope WB, et al. 18F-FDOPA and 18F-FLT positron emission tomography parametric response maps predict response in recurrent malignant gliomas treated with bevacizumab. Neuro Oncol 2012;14:1079–89.

91. Jahangiri A, De Lay M, Miller LM, et al. Gene expression profile identifies tyrosine kinase c-Met as a targetable inhibitor of antiangiogenic therapy resistance. Clin Cancer Res 2013. [Epub ahead of print]. http://dx.doi.org/10.1158/1078-0432.CCR-12-1281.

92. De Groot J, Liang J, Kong LY, et al. Modulating antiangiogenic resistance by inhibiting the signal transducer and activator of transcription 3 pathway in glioblastoma. Oncotarget 2012;3:1036–48.

93. Reardon DA, Galanis E, DeGroot JF, et al. Clinical trial endpoints for high-grade gliomas: the evolving landscape. Neuro Oncol 2010;13:353–61.

94. Jalali R, Dutta D. Factors influencing quality of life in adult patients with primary brain tumors. Neuro Oncol 2012;14(Suppl 4):iv8–16.

# Immunotherapy for Alzheimer's Disease

Martin R. Farlow, MD*, Jared R. Brosch, MD

## KEYWORDS

- Alzheimer disease • β-amyloid • Immunotherapy

## KEY POINTS

- The amyloid hypothesis, which proposes β-amyloid deposition is the initiating factor for Alzheimer disease (AD), has been a major target for treatment trials.
- Transgenic mouse model studies suggest immunotherapy approach with either vaccination or monoclonal antibody administration may decrease β-amyloid plaques in the brain.
- Amyloid imaging-related abnormalities (vasogenic edema and microhemorrhages) are potentially serious adverse events related to immunotherapy for AD.
- Disappointing results from immunotherapy trials in Alzheimer dementia suggest treatment may need to be started earlier in Mild Cognitive Impairment (MCI) or asymptomatic stages.

## INTRODUCTION

Immunotherapy as used in this summary refers to vaccination stimulating a relevant response targeting Alzheimer disease (AD) pathology (amyloid deposits) or peripherally administered monoclonal antibodies targeting amyloid β (Aβ) protein, or polyclonal antibodies naturally present in intravenously administered immunoglobulins used to target Aβ protein. These approaches should be distinguished from immunosuppressive therapies (eg, steroids, nonsteroidal anti-inflammatory drugs). Epidemiologic studies have suggested these drugs might have a useful therapeutic role, but large double-blind clinical trials have been, to date, unfortunately negative.[1]

The key experiment motivating directly or indirectly all of recent immunotherapy approaches to removing amyloid plaques from the brains of patients with AD was enabled by availability of the PDAPP mouse transgenic model for AD, which overexpresses human APP with mutation at codon 717 substituting phenylalanine for valine and develops many of the neuropathological manifestations of AD in an age-dependent and brain-dependent regional manner also similar to the human illness.[2] Schenk and colleagues[3] vaccinated these transgenic mice with synthetic human

Department of Neurology, Indiana University School of Medicine, 355 West 16th Street, Suite 4700, Indianapolis, IN 46202, USA
* Corresponding author.
*E-mail address:* mfarlow@iupui.edu

Neurol Clin 31 (2013) 869–878
http://dx.doi.org/10.1016/j.ncl.2013.03.012
0733-8619/13/$ – see front matter © 2013 Elsevier Inc. All rights reserved.

$A\beta_{42}$ protein at 6 weeks, before pathology would have typically developed and also separately in mice older than 11 months when cortical plaques and gliosis are typically present. They demonstrated immunized mice produced high titers of antibody against $A\beta$ proteins and that younger mice never developed plaques, whereas in older mice amyloid plaque burden and gliosis were significantly reduced. Similar results have since been widely reproduced in several different transgenic models with various amyloid fragments and injection schedules. These experiments have suggested the potential utility of immunotherapy for both prevention of the illness and therapy for AD and provided the preclinical preliminary data supporting initial immunization studies by investigators at Elan Pharmaceuticals, Dublin, Ireland as therapy for AD.

## ACTIVE IMMUNE THERAPY FOR AD (VACCINATION)
### AN-1792

Immunologic therapy for human AD has its origins in the vaccine called AN-1792 (Elan Pharmaceuticals). The vaccine involved is an active immunization with an $A\beta_{1-42}$ peptide that provokes both a Th1-cell and Th2-cell response with subsequent B-cell response against amyloid. The first phase I clinical trial with 24 patients established initial evidence for tolerability. A second phase Ib randomized, placebo-controlled trial enrolled 80 patients and involved several dosages (50 or 225 µg plus 50 or 100 µg of adjuvant QS21) and multiple doses (up to 8 total injections) after an extension phase.[4] The major result of the phase Ib trial was again that there were no major safety concerns. One patient was found at autopsy to have sequelae of a meningoencephalitic process after dying of a pulmonary embolism nearly 1 year after the last injection. Antibodies to amyloid $A\beta$ were found at a level of greater than or equal to 1:1000 in 77% of the high-dose groups and 40% of the low-dose groups. The phase Ib trial was not powered to detect cognitive or functional outcomes from the vaccination and showed no difference compared with placebo in all measures except for Caregiver Disability Assessment for Dementia scale, which showed a slower rate of decline in the treatment group. Based on the results of the phase Ib trial, the higher dose 225 µg + 50 µg of adjuvant QS21 were chosen for subsequent trials.

The next phase IIa trial, which terminated early, was a randomized, placebo-controlled, double-blind clinical study that enrolled patients at 28 sites in Europe and the United States.[5] A total of 372 patients were randomized, and received 1 to 3 injections based before early termination of the study, although they were originally scheduled to receive 4 to 6 injections (4 for nonresponders, and 6 for responders: those with antibody titers >1:2200 after any of the first 4 injections). Although only 1 to 3 injections were given, 20% of the study population developed antibody titers greater than 1:2200. Within the short follow-up period there was no difference between the placebo group and the treatment group in any of the cognitive or disability scores. However, there was a trend toward statistically significant difference in the neuropsychological test battery: the treatment group showed less worsening in many of the battery scores with statistical significance in the memory segment. At least one study following a subset of these patients for a longer period showed decreased rate of decline in several standard measures.[6] Finally, a very small subset of patients with pretreatment and posttreatment cerebrospinal fluid (CSF) analysis showed a decrease in tau in the treatment group compared with the placebo group.

Significant adverse events led to the premature cessation of the phase IIa clinical trial. Meningoencephalitis occurred in 6% of the treatment group.[7] Of those who developed meningoencephalitis, 72% were in the responder group and development occurred within 70 days of the last injection. Onset was noted with confusion, headache, and lethargy. The severity of the meningoencephalitis varied quite substantially, with 66% having complete resolution within weeks and the remainder going on to have persistent cognitive decline and/or permanent focal neurologic sequelae. The mechanism for the meningoencephalitis is poorly understood; however, there is speculation that the addition of the polysorbate-80 stabilizer may have been the instigating factor in the development of this adverse side effect. In retrospect, the one patient from the phase Ib trial who was later found to have meningoencephalitis sequelae on autopsy after death likely had symptoms 6 weeks after the last injection. Subsequent analysis has shown that there was significant T-cell response in the autopsied brains of those with meningoencephalitis, implicating that the immunization that activates both Th1 cells and Th2 cells may lead to an unwanted cellular inflammatory response against amyloid in addition to the desired B-cell response leading to antibody creation.

One year after the completion of the phase Ib trial, a follow-up study commenced that tracked the survivors and analyzed autopsy data over the subsequent 3 years.[8] The follow-up study consisted of 36 patients who consented to regular follow-up. A total of 9 patients (2 of whom had died before the follow-up study commencement) underwent brain autopsy. Overall, the immunizations did not have a long-term clinical or survival benefit. The autopsy results showed a decreased Aβ load (both quantitatively and qualitatively based on histology) compared with age-matched nonimmunized AD controls. The degree of amyloid removal was variable; however, the 2 patients with nearly complete removal of plaques had the highest antibody titers during the treatment phase and also survived the longest after immunization (implying that amyloid removal may take long periods of time). Despite the nearly 100% removal of extracellular Aβ plaques, the neurodegenerative cascade continued in these patients. The conclusion from the follow-up is that amyloid removal may not be enough to combat the neurodegenerative process, however, with caveats that more time may be required for the benefits to be seen, as well as finding treatment approaches that do not invoke a cellular Th1 response. After the field had appropriately analyzed data from the failed AN-1792 trial, a number of approaches to preventing cellular response and/or maximizing humoral response to Aβ protein fragments were developed and were or are in further early-stage phase I trials (**Table 1**).

| Table 1 AD vaccination studies | | | |
|---|---|---|---|
| **Drug** | **Studies** | **Companies** | **Development** |
| AN-1792 | Elan | Elan | Halted |
| Merck | V950 | Merck | Ongoing |
| CAD106 | Novartis | Novartis | Ongoing |

*Data from* U.S. National Institutes of Health. Available at: Clinicaltrials.gov. Accessed March 13, 2013.

## PASSIVE IMMUNE THERAPY FOR AD (MONOCLONALS)
### Bapineuzumab

Bapineuzumab is a humanized monoclonal antibody that targets the N-terminus of Aβ. It binds Aβ extracellularly in aggregated fibrillary proteinaceous plaques (senile plaques). When infused intravenously, the drug acts as passive immunotherapy against

Aβ plaques. The drug was studied through several clinical trials to review safety and efficacy.

An initial phase II trial took place at 30 sites in the United States.[9] The trial involved 6 intravenous infusions of bapineuzumab every 13 weeks and used 4 different doses (122 patients) versus placebo infusions (107 patients). The trial showed no statistically significant outcomes but did show trends toward efficacy on the Alzheimer's Disease Assessment Scale–Cognitive subscale (ADAS-Cog) and the Disability Assessment for Dementia (DAD). The presence of vasogenic edema, as a part of amyloid-related imaging abnormalities (ARIA), was a major adverse effect from the drug treatment, occurring in 10% of the treated patients.[10] There seemed to be a dose dependence in the incidence of vasogenic edema with 11 of the 12 cases occurring with doses greater than 1.0 mg/kg. Also, apolipoprotein ε4 (APOE4) carriers accounted for 10 of the 12 cases. The hypothesis behind the generation of vasogenic edema was that it was attributable to permeability changes owing to removal of intravascular Aβ deposits. Later studies showed that asymptomatic patients with ARIA may remain asymptomatic even if treatment is continued. Based on these results, phase III trials were developed that studied APOE4 carriers separately from noncarriers.

These phase III trials' intent-to-treat populations involved 658 patients in the treatment group (0.5 mg/kg infused 6 times every 13 weeks) and 432 patients in the placebo group for the APOE4 carrier group; for the APOE4 noncarrier group, there were 621 patients in the treatment group (0.5 mg/kg or 1.0 mg/kg infused 6 times every 13 weeks; patients were divided equally among these 2 doses) and 493 patients in the placebo group. Results of these studies showed no clinical improvement in ADAS-Cog or DAD for both the APOE4 carrier and noncarrier groups.[11,12] There was a measurable difference between the treatment and placebo groups in global amyloid burden and reduction of CSF tau protein in the APOE4 carrier group and a reduction in CSF tau protein in the high-dose APOE4 noncarrier group; otherwise, there were no other improvements noted, including no change in brain volume loss. Vasogenic edema occurred in 15% of patients in the APOE4 carrier group and in 9% and 4% of the high-dose and low-dose APOE4 noncarrier treatment groups respectively. The edema was symptomatic in approximately 2% of those who developed it.

Although bapineuzumab showed targeting of relevant pathologic substrates in the brain and downstream biomarker changes, it failed to show clinical improvement or disease-modifying outcomes. Based on the results of the Phase III clinical trials, Pfizer and Johnson & Johnson, New Brunswick, NJ, USA announced in late July/early August 2012 that clinical development of bapineuzumab would be halted.

## SOLANEUZUMAB

Solaneuzumab is a humanized monoclonal antibody that targets Aβ in the central region of the peptide. In contrast to bapineuzumab, solaneuzumab targets soluble Aβ as opposed to deposited Aβ aggregates. Solaneuzumab has been evaluated in several clinical trials for safety and efficacy.

The initial Phase II trial (randomized, double-blinded, placebo-controlled) took place from May 2006 to May 2008 at 6 sites in the United States.[13] The Phase II trial involved 12 intravenous infusions of solaneuzumab or placebo delivered at 2 different dosages (100 mg or 400 mg) either weekly or every 4 weeks yielding 4 treatment groups and 1 placebo group (total of 52 patients randomized with 10 or 11 in each group). There was no significant difference in the ADAS-Cog scores between the treatment and placebo groups; however, these measurements were made at only 4 intervals up to 112 days. Plasma and CSF Aβ (1–40 and 1–42) were measured and found to have statistically significant increases with solaneuzumab compared with placebo. There was a dose-dependent response in the magnitude of increase of these levels. These biomarkers were felt to reflect peripheral binding of soluble Aβ with those proteins potentially being drawn from the cortex to a "peripheral sink." The drug was tolerated well and had no increased side effects compared with placebo, including a lack of vasogenic edema, meningitis, or signs of inflammatory response.

The Phase III trial was conducted in 2 separate randomized, double-blind, placebo-controlled trials with different primary outcomes (Expedition 1 and 2). Both trials involved patients with mild-moderate AD. Both trials used 400 mg every 4 weeks and combined represented close to 800 patients in the treatment group and 800 in the placebo group. Results for cognitive scores (ADAS11 and ADAS14), as well as functional scores (ADCS-ADL and ADCS-iADL), were reported for each trial at 80 weeks.[14] After the results of Expedition 1 suggested greater benefit in the mild sub-group, the Expedition 2 analysis plan was modified, with ADAS-Cog 14 in the mild-stage subgroup being the only principal outcome measure. Overall, there was no change in cognitive loss compared with placebo. When patients with mild AD were analyzed separately there was a statistically significant benefit in functional scores in Expedition 2 and in the pooled data. The conclusion from the trial was that the effect of solaneuzumab is likely small, takes months before effects are apparent, and may be more prominent in patients with mild AD. AD monoclonal antibodies in development are listed in **Table 2**.

| Table 2 AD monoclonal antibody studies | | | |
|---|---|---|---|
| **Drug** | **Studies** | **Company** | **Development** |
| Bapineuzumab AAB-001 | Phase III Negative | Elan Pharmaceuticals, Dublin, Ireland | Halted |
| Solaneuzumab | Phase III Negative but signal present in mild stage. Dominantly Inherited Alzheimer Network, presymptomatic and new phase III studies planned | Eli Lilly & Company, Indianapolis, IN, USA | Ongoing |
| Gantenerumab | Phase II/III | Roche, Nutley, NJ, USA | Ongoing |
| Crenezumab | Phase III/II | Genentech, San Francisco, CA, USA | Ongoing |
| Biogen BIIB037 | Phase I | Biogen, Berkshire, United Kingdom | Ongoing |

*Data from* U.S. National Institutes of Health. Available at: Clinicaltrials.gov. Accessed March 13, 2013.

## INTRAVENOUS IMMUNOGLOBULINS
### Phase I Studies

Intravenous immunoglobulin (IVIG) is a product produced from whole blood by frac-tionation that has been used for various immunodeficiency syndromes as well as in the treatment of myasthenia gravis and Guillian-Barré syndrome. IVIG naturally con-tains polyclonal antibodies that target oligoclonal as well as fibrillar Aβ proteins, and at least 2 studies have suggested these polyclonal antibodies are reduced in patients with AD. Two uncontrolled trials of 5 and 8 patients respectively suggested that 0.2 g or 0.4 g/kg of IVIG administered monthly, respectively, stabilized cognitive functioning in patients with mild-to-moderate AD for a period of 6 months.[15,16] Biomarker studies suggested amyloid $\beta_{1-40}$ proteins were reduced in CSF and increased in plasma as compared with baseline. These results were independently confirmed in another 8-patient trial in which Mini-Mental State Examination (MMSE) scores were actually improved by 2.5 points versus baseline at 6 months.[17] Based on these data, a placebo-controlled trial of either 0.4 g/kg or 0.8 g/kg IVIG per month administered either on a 2-week or every 4-week schedule lasting 6 months was undertaken in 24 patients with mild-to-moderate stage AD.[18] Although not published in this study in detail; IVIG has been reported to have had similar positive effects on stabilizing cognition, preventing brain atrophy on magnetic resonance imaging (MRI), and exhibiting similar patterns of change on plasma and CSF A$\beta$ protein assessments versus baseline. Four of these patients have been followed under open-label conditions for more than 4 years with apparently slowed disease progression (but with the major caveat of the potential selection bias that those patients seeing benefit may be more likely to remain on therapy).

## OCTAPHARMA IVIG
### Phase II Study

A double-blind, randomized, placebo-controlled, multicenter trial in the United States and Germany assessed different dosage and frequency regimens in patients with mild-to-moderate stage AD (MMSE 16–26 at baseline) in a Phase II trial of 6 months' duration.[19] Dosage arms included 0.2 g/kg, 0.5 g/kg, 0.8 g/kg, and placebo with 0.9% isotonic NaCl every 4 weeks or half these doses every 2 weeks. A total of 58 patients were randomized (15 to placebo and 43 patients to IVIG groups) with 55 patients having at least one post baseline assessment and 49 patients completing the protocol. The principal outcome for this study was change in area under the curve (AUC) value for plasma A$\beta_{1-40}$ from baseline versus placebo. There was a significant decrease in AUC value for A$\beta_{1-42}$ for the 0.5 g and 0.8 g week groups versus placebo, but not for the others. When all the IVIG groups were pooled, plasma A$\beta_{1-42}$ levels were significantly decreased versus placebo. Overall differences observed did not appear to be significant. There were no changes in any of the cognitive or functional outcomes (ADAS-Cog, MMSE, alzheimer's disease cooperative studies - activities of daily living [ACDS-ADL], or clinical dementia rating - sum of boxes [CDR-SOB]).

Neither MRI whole brain volumes nor hippocampal atrophy rates showed difference in change versus baseline as compared with placebo in any of the treatment groups. 18-Fluoro-deoxyglucose positron emission tomography (FDG-PET) revealed decrease in glucose metabolism in bilateral hippocampal mesial temporal brain regions, but with significantly less reduction in IVIG-treated groups as compared with placebo. Adverse events were similar between the groups. With regard to safety, one patient receiving IVIG had an ischemic stroke in the MCA (middle cerebral artery) territory. With regard to ARIA abnormalities, vasogenic edema was not observed, but a total of 6 of 43 IVIG-treated patients had new incident microbleeds, with new hemorrhages being most common in subjects with preexisting microbleeds at baseline. All newly incident microbleeds were asymptomatic and the treatment schedules were not altered.

In summary, this study failed to demonstrate plasma or CSF A$\beta$ protein level changes indicating target engagement, or showed evidence of any benefit on structural MRI or by cognitive assessments. Some decrease in rate of deterioration of metabolism was seen in FDG-PET results versus placebo, but without corresponding positive clinical correlates. It was concluded that longer studies would be necessary to determine whether IVIG is associated with significant clinical benefit.

## ADCS-BAXTER IVIG
### Phase II/III Studies

This 24-patient phase II trial provided preliminary data to support an ongoing double-blind placebo-controlled IVIG treatment trial in 390 patients with mild-to-moderate stage AD of 18 months' duration being conducted by the Alzheimer Disease Cooperative Study Group and the Baxter Corporation.[20] Results of this large multicenter trial with extensive biomarker assessments should be available later this year (2013) and will have the statistical power to more definitely determine whether IVIG as a treatment modality for AD has clinical utility.

## SUMMARY

Clinical trials of immunotherapies to stabilize or aid removal of amyloid plaques in patients with AD have not as yet yielded relevant clinical benefits and have caused significant adverse events in some patients. The initial vaccination study in patients with mild-to-moderate stage AD with AN-1792 caused encephalitis in 8% of patients and had to be halted. After long investigation, the primary cause was thought to be activation of cellular, in addition to humoral, immunity causing deleterious inflammatory effects in the brain. With the vaccination approach, it has also proved very difficult in elderly subjects to raise significant antibody titers, a finding that also has been found in similar later studies. Vaccination studies, which have followed, have modified the injected immunogens to limit stimulation of cellular immunity and similarly there has been modification of formulation to use more efficient adjuvants and carrier proteins for the immunogens in an attempt to raise higher titers of antibodies in a greater percentage of AD patients. Results of vaccination studies since have been mixed with generally better safety, variable effects on antibody production, and biomarker engagement, but no convincing evidence, yet of an effect on clinical symptoms.

With regard to passive immunization approaches, data from large phase III trials with bapineuzumab targeting fibrillar amyloid and with solaneuzumab targeting oligoclonal Aβ proteins, have both failed to show significant beneficial effects with regard to clinical disease progression. There are a number of potential explanations for these failures, including that the amyloid hypothesis is incorrect and that deposition of fibrillar amyloid in particular is a marker of AD but not a driving force in overall disease progression. With regard to bapineuzumab, ARIA events limit dosing and it may be that insufficient antibody can be given to mobilize removal of amyloid by this antibody. Solaneuzumab does not target fibrillar amyloid and the proposed peripheral sink hypothesis, which suggests its engagement with peripheral Aβ drawing Aβ from plaques in the brain may simply be wrong.

For both of these antibodies, the amyloid-related target may simply be wrong. Finally, soluble or fibrillar Aβ may be correct targets but by the biological disease stage that patients with AD have significant clinical symptoms, the illness is too advanced with too many cortical neurofibrillary tangles (NFT), disrupted synapses, inflammation, oxidative damage, and so forth for removal of amyloid by these antibodies to make any difference regarding clinical symptoms. For this reason there has been a major shift in populations being targeted in AD clinical trials, with many studies now focused on MCI or early-stage AD confirmed by biomarker as the potentially most responsive disease stage for immunotherapy.

Further, these studies (**Table 3**) have moved to primary prevention, seeking to treat asymptomatic patients with genetically inherited disease-causing genes, treating patients for up to 15 years before estimated clinical onset of AD symptoms.[21] Similarly in the A4 trial, asymptomatic elderly patients with cortical amyloid deposits but normal cognitive function will be treated with a monoclonal antibody targeting these amyloid deposits.

**Table 3**
**Prevention studies in patients at risk for Alzheimer disease**

| | | |
|---|---|---|
| Alzheimer Prevention Initiative (API) | Crenezumab Monoclonal AG to Aβ | 5 y – 300 |
| Dominantly Inherited Alzheimer Network Treatment Trial (DIAN TT) | Solaneuzumab – Lilly Gantenerumab – Roche B-secretase inhibitor – Lilly | 5 y – 160 |
| A4 – Anti-amyloid treatment in patients with normal cognition and brain amyloid deposits | Antibody therapy | 3 y – 1000 |

In conclusion, immunotherapy approaches to remove amyloid and/or delay disease progression in patients at risk for or with clinical symptoms have not been successful. Nevertheless, better understanding of the potential consequences associated with amyloid deposition at different disease stages in the future should improve chances for more targeted therapeutic approaches with better odds for success in the near future.

**Potential case study**

A 73-year-old white woman, high school educated, is referred to you for progressive difficulties with short-term memory and personal hygiene issues. The patient lives with her husband, who tries to help with the patient's toileting, bathing, and food preparation, but he is limited by his own many medical problems. The patient is accompanied by her daughter who claims that her mother has lost 15 pounds over the past 6 months and she was found last week lost in the neighbor's fenced-in backyard, soiled, and obviously had not bathed for several days.

On neurologic examination, there was lack of cooperation, but motor strength and tone, sensory, and cerebellar functions were all symmetric and normal as was her gait. Mental status testing revealed her to be alert, if somewhat disoriented and confused, repeating past experiences obsessively, while having difficulty responding to questions regarding her health and functioning in activities of daily living. Her MMSE score was 16 of 30. A computed tomography scan of her head was normal and she had a normal vitamin B12, thyroid-stimulating hormone, and basic metabolic panel. You conclude the most likely diagnosis is Alzheimer dementia in the moderate stage. The daughter states that she read on the Internet that using nonsteroidal anti-inflammatory drugs delays progression of Alzheimer dementia. She asks your opinion if this is true and also wonders what other drugs may be available to help with her symptoms.

**REFERENCES**

1. Jaturapatporn D, Isaac MG, McCleery J, et al. Aspirin, steroidal and non-steroidal anti-inflammatory drugs for the treatment of Alzheimer's disease. Cochrane Database Syst Rev 2012;(2):CD006378.
2. Games D, Adams D, Alessandrini R, et al. Alzheimer-type neuropathology in transgenic mice overexpressing V717F beta-amyloid precursor protein. Nature 1995;373(6514):523–7.

3. Schenk D, Barbour R, Dunn W, et al. Immunization with amyloid-β attenuates Alzheimer-disease-like pathology in the PDAPP mouse. Nature 1999;400:173–7.
4. Bayer AJ, Bullock R, Jones RW, et al. Evaluation of the safety and immunogenicity of synthetic AB42 (AN1792) in patients with AD. Neurology 2005;64:94–101.
5. Gilman S, Koller M, Black RS, et al. Clinical effects of A(beta) immunization (AN1792) in patients with AD in an interrupted trial. Neurology 2005;64:1553–62.
6. Vellas B, Black R, Thal LJ, et al. AN1792 (QS-21)-251 Study Team. Long-term follow-up of patients immunized with AN1792: reduced functional decline in antibody responders. Curr Alzheimer Res 2009;6(2):144–51.
7. Orgogozo JM, Gilman S, Dartigues JF, et al. Subacute meningoencephalitis in a subset of patients with AD after A(beta)42 immunization. Neurology 2003;61: 46–54.
8. Holmes C, Boche D, Wilkinson D, et al. Long-term effects of Abeta42 immunisation in Alzheimer's disease: follow-up of a randomised, placebo-controlled phase I trial. Lancet 2008;372(9634):216–23.
9. Salloway S, Sperling R, Gilman S, et al. A phase 2 multiple ascending dose trial of bapineuzumab in mild to moderate Alzheimer disease. Neurology 2009;73: 2061–70.
10. Sperling R, Salloway S, Brooks DJ, et al. Amyloid-related imaging abnormalities in patients with Alzheimer's disease treated with bapineuzumab: a retrospective analysis. Lancet Neurol 2012;11:241–9.
11. Salloway S, Sperling R, Honig LS, et al. A randomized, double-blind, placebo-controlled clinical trial of intravenous bapineuzumab in patients with mild to moderate Alzheimer's disease who are apolipoprotein e ε4 non-carriers. Stockholm (Sweden): European Federation of Neurological Societies; 2012.
12. Sperling R, Salloway S, Raskind M, et al. A randomized, double-blind, placebo-controlled clinical trial of intravenous bapineuzumab in patients with mild to moderate Alzheimer's disease who are apolipoprotein e ε4 carriers. Stockholm (Sweden): European Federation of Neurological Societies; 2012.
13. Farlow M, Arnold SE, Van Dyck CH, et al. Safety and biomarker effects of solanezumab in patients with Alzheimer's disease. Alzheimers Dement 2012;8:261–71.
14. Doody RS. Phase 3 studies of solanezumab for mild to moderate Alzheimer's disease. Boston (MA): American Neurological Association; 2012.
15. Kountouris D. Therapeutic effects of piracetam combined with intravenous immunoglobulin premature of Alzheimer type. J Neural Transm 2000;107(5):18.
16. Dodel, R, Rominger A, Bartenstein P, et al. Intravenous immunoglobulin for treatment of mild-to-moderate Alzheimer's disease: a phase 2, randomised, double-blind, placebo-controlled, dose-finding trial. The Lancet online January 31, 2013. Available at: http://dx.doi.org/10.1016/S1474-4422(13)70014-0.
17. Relkin NR, Szabo P, Adamiak B, et al. 18-month study of intravenous immunoglobulin for treatment of mild Alzheimer's disease. Neurobiol Aging 2009; 30(11):1328–36.
18. Relkin N, Tsakanikas DI, Adamiak B, et al. A double-blind, placebo-controlled, phase II clinical trial of intravenous immunoglobulin (IVIG) for treatment of Alzheimer's disease [abstract]. Neurology 2008;70(11):A393.
19. Farlow MR, Dodel R, Jessen F, et al. A randomized, double-blind, placebo-controlled dose-finding trial of intravenous immunoglobulin (Octapharma AG) in patients with Alzheimer's disease (GAM10-04). 63rd Annual Meeting of the American Academy of Neurology. Honolulu, April 10–15, 2011. P07.224, p. A620.
20. A phase 3 study evaluating safety and effectiveness of immune globulin intravenous (IGIV 10%) for the treatment of mild to moderate Alzheimer's disease.

[Clinicaltrials.gov identifier NCT00818662]. US National Institutes of Health; 2009. Available at: ClinicalTrials.gov. Accessed March 13, 2013.

21. Reiman EM, Langbaum JB, Fleisher AS, et al. Alzheimer's prevention initiative: a plan to accelerate the evaluation of presymptomatic treatments. J Alzheimers Dis 2011;26(Suppl 3):321–9.

# Index

*Note:* Page numbers of article titles are in **boldface** type.

### A

Acute ischemic stroke
    endovascular recanalization of, **705–719**. *See also* Endovascular recanalization, of acute
        ischemic stroke
    thrombolytic therapy for
        unanswered questions in, **677–704**. *See also* Thrombolytic therapy, for acute
            ischemic stroke, unanswered questions in
ADCS-Baxter IVIG
    for Alzheimer's disease, 875
AEDs. *See* Antiepileptic drugs (AEDs)
Alemtuzamab
    in MS management, 835–837
Alzheimer's disease
    immunotherapy for, **869–878**
        active, 870–871
        ADCS-Baxter IVIG, 875
        AN-1792, 870–871
        bapineuzumab, 871–872
        intravenous immunoglobulins, 873–874
        introduction, 869–870
        octapharma IBIG, 874–875
        passive, 871–872
        solaneuzumab, 872–873
AN-1792
    for Alzheimer's disease, 870–871
Aneurysm(s)
    intracranial
        unruptured
            flow diverters for, **737–747**. *See also* Flow diverters, for unruptured intracranial
                aneurysms
Anticoagulant(s)
    in CVT management, 776–777
    in ICH management, 725
    for stroke prevention in atrial fibrillation, **659–675**. *See also* specific agents and Atrial
        fibrillation, stroke prevention in, anticoagulants for
Antiepileptic drugs (AEDs), **785–798**
    ezogabine/retigabine, 789–791
    lacosamide, 787–788
    new agents, 787–793
    perampanel, 791–793
    rufinamide, 788–789

Neurol Clin 31 (2013) 879–889
http://dx.doi.org/10.1016/S0733-8619(13)00069-8
0733-8619/13/$ – see front matter © 2013 Elsevier Inc. All rights reserved.

**neurologic.theclinics.com**

Antiplatelet agents
    described, 633
    in stroke prevention, **633–657**
        aspirin, 634–644
        aspirin + extended release dypiridamole, 647–648
        cangrelor, 649
        cilostazol, 646–647
        clopidogrel, 634–646
        mechanism of action of, 634–648
        novel agents, 648–650
        ongoing clinical trials of, 650–651
        prasugrel, 649
        sarpogrelate, 650
        ticagrelor, 648
        triflusal, 649–650
        vorapaxar and atopaxar, 650
Apixaban
    for stroke prevention in atrial fibrillation, 666–667
Arteriovenous malformations (AVMs)
    of the brain, **749–763**
        biology of, 749–750
        cerebral
            management of, 754–759
        clinical presentation of, 751–753
            headache, 752–753
            hemorrhage, 751–752
            neurologic deficits, 753
            seizures, 752
        diagnosis of, 753–754
        future directions in, 760
        natural history of, 750–751
        pathophysiology of, 749–750
Aspirin
    in stroke prevention, 634–644
Aspirin + extended release dypiridamole, 647–648
Astrocytomas
    evaluation of, 848
Atopaxar and vorapaxar
    in stroke prevention, 650
Atrial fibrillation
    stroke prevention in
        anticoagulants for, **659–675**
            apixaban, 666–667
            case study, 660
            complications of, 670–673
            dabigatran, 663–666
            edoxaban, 667–670
            introduction, 660–661
            patient evaluation, 662–663
            rivaroxaban, 666
AVMs. *see* Arteriovenous malformations (AVMs)

**B**

Bapineuzumab
    for Alzheimer's disease, 871–872
BEV
    in high-grade glioma management, 856–857
BG-12
    in MS management, 834–835
Brain
    AVMs of, **749–763**. *see also* Arteriovenous malformations (AVMs), of the brain


**C**

Cangrelor
    in stroke prevention, 649
CCNU
    in high-grade glioma management, 855–856
Cerebral edema
    in CVT
        management of, 774
Cerebral venous thrombosis (CVT), **765–783**
    clinical findings in, 766–767
    diagnostic dilemmas related to, 771
    introduction, 765–766
    management of, 772–777
        acute treatment in, 772–773
        in adults
            clinical outcomes of, 777
        cerebral edema–related, 774
        in children, 777–780
        long-term anticoagulation in, 776–777
        mechanical thrombectomy in, 773
        seizure-related, 774–776
        setting of, 772
        thrombolysis in, 773
    neuroimaging of, 767–769
    risk factors for, 768–770
Children
    CVT in
        management of, 777–780
Cilostazol
    in stroke prevention, 646–647
Clopidogrel
    in stroke prevention, 634–646
Clot removal with MERCI or aspiration with penumbra
    in endovascular recanalization of acute ischemic stroke, 708–711
Complementary and alternative therapies
    in MS management, 839
CVT. *See* Cerebral venous thrombosis (CVT)

**D**

Dabigatran
    for stroke prevention in atrial fibrillation, 663–666
DBS. *See* Deep brain stimulation (DBS)
Deep brain stimulation (DBS)
    in nonparkinsonian movement disorders, **809–826**
        introduction, 809–811
        patient overview and management goals, 812–815
            dystonia, 813–815
            ET, 812–813
            GTS, 815
        patient selection issues in, 811–812
        research and innovation related to, 817–820
        surgical targets and operative nuances, 815–817
    in Parkinson disease management
        complications of, 804
        early *vs.* late treatment with, 804
Dypiridamole
    extended release
        aspirin +
            in stroke prevention, 647–648
Dystonia
    DBS in
        patient overview and management goals, 813–815


**E**

Edoxaban
    for stroke prevention in atrial fibrillation, 667–670
EGFR. *See* Epidermal growth factor receptor (EGFR)
Electrical stimulation of anterior nucleus of thalamus
    in epilepsy management, 793
Endovascular angioplasty and stenting
    in endovascular recanalization of acute ischemic stroke, 707–708
Endovascular recanalization
    of acute ischemic stroke
        future directions in, 715–717
        new strategies for, **705–719**
            clot removal with MERCI or aspiration with penumbra, 708–711
            endovascular angioplasty and stenting, 707–708
            IA thrombolysis, 706–707
            introduction, 705–706
            IV-OA tPA ultrasound, 707
            in neurothrombectomy era, 708–713
            stent-based thrombectomy, 711–713
            tandem occlusions, 713
            trials of
                results assessment, 713–714
Endovascular thrombectomy
    for acute ischemic stroke, 692

Epidermal growth factor receptor (EGFR)
    in high-grade glioma evaluation, 852
Epilepsy, **785–798**
    incidence of, 785
    introduction, 785–787
    management of
        AEDs in, **785–798**. *See also* Antiepileptic drugs (AEDs)
        neurostimulation in, 786, 793–795. *See also* Neurostimulation, in epilepsy
            management
Essential tremor (ET)
    DBS in
        patient overview and management goals, 812–813
ET. *See* Essential tremor (ET)
External trigeminal stimulation
    in epilepsy management, 794–795
Ezogabine/retigabine
    in epilepsy management, 789–791


F

Fingolimod
    in MS management, 830–832
Flow diversion
    intravascular, 745–746
    for unruptured intracranial aneurysms
        contraindications to, 738
        indications for, 738
Flow diverters
    for unruptured intracranial aneurysms, **737–747**
        controversies in use of, 740–741
        future directions in, 741–745
        initial experience with, 738–740
        introduction, 737–738
        limitations of, 740–741
        ongoing studies, 741–745


G

Gilles de la Tourette syndrome (GTS)
    DBS in
        patient overview and management goals, 815
Glioma(s)
    high-grade, **847–867**. *See also* High-grade gliomas
GTS. *See* Gilles de la Tourette syndrome (GTS)


H

Headache(s)
    brain AVMs and, 752–753
Hemorrhage
    brain AVMs and, 751–752
    intracerebral. *See* Intracerebral hemorrhage (ICH)

Hemostatic therapy
    in ICH management, 724
High-grade gliomas
    evaluation of, 848–852
        astrocytomas, 848
        convergence *vs.* divergence in, 852
        EGFR in, 852
        histology in, 848
        IDH mutations in, 850–851
        MGMT promoter methylation in, 851
        mixed oligoastrocytomas, 848–849
        molecular diagnostics in, 849–852
        oligodendrogliomas, 848
        1p19q deletions in, 849–850
    treatment of, **847–867**
        BEV in, 856–857
        CCNU in, 855–856
        combination therapies in, 858–859
        complications of, 859–861
        introduction, 847
        nonpharmacologic, 857–858
        outcome of
            evaluation of, 861
            long-term recommendations related to, 861
        PCV in, 855–856
        pharmacologic, 852–857
        procarbazine in, 855–856
        radiation therapy in, 857–858
        resistance to, 859–861
        TMZ in, 852–855
        update on, **847–867**


I

IA thrombolysis
    in endovascular recanalization of acute ischemic stroke, 706–707
ICH. *See* Intracerebral hemorrhage (ICH)
IDH mutations
    in high-grade glioma evaluation, 850–851
Immunoglobulin(s)
    intravenous
        for Alzheimer's disease, 873–874
Immunotherapy
    for Alzheimer's disease, **869–878**. *See also* Alzheimer's disease, immunotherapy for
Intracerebral hemorrhage (ICH)
    treatment of
        anticoagulants in, 725
        hemostatic therapy in, 724
        ICU management in, 722–724
        medical management in, 722–728
        minimally invasive strategies in, 729–731

neuroprotective strategies in, 725–728

new developments in, **721–735**

   case report, 722

   introduction, 721

open craniotomy in, 728–729

surgical management in, 728–731

Intracranial aneurysms

  unruptured

    flow diverters for, **737–747**. *See also* Flow diverters, for unruptured intracranial aneurysms

Intravenous immunoglobulins

  for Alzheimer's disease, 873–874

Ischemic stroke

  acute

    endovascular recanalization of, **705–719**. *See also* Endovascular recanalization, of acute ischemic stroke

    thrombolytic therapy for

      unanswered questions in, **677–704**. *See also* Thrombolytic therapy, for acute ischemic stroke, unanswered questions in

IV-IA tPA ultrasound

  in endovascular recanalization of acute ischemic stroke, 707

IV tPA thrombolysis

  for acute ischemic stroke

    unanswered questions in

      defining therapeutic time windows for, 683–687

      landmark studies and 3-hour time window for, 681–683


**L**

Lacosamide

  in epilepsy management, 787–788

Lomustine (CCNU)

  in high-grade glioma management, 855–856


**M**

Mechanical thrombectomy

  in CVT management, 773

Methylguanine-DNA methyltransferase (MGMT) promoter methylation

  in high-grade glioma evaluation, 851

MGMT promoter methylation. *See* Methylguanine-DNA methyltransferase (MGMT) promoter methylation

Mixed oligoastrocytomas

  evaluation of, 848–849

MS. *See* Multiple sclerosis (MS)

Multiple sclerosis (MS)

  described, 827

  diagnostic criteria for

    update on, 828–829

  introduction, 827–828

  pathogenesis of, 829–830

Multiple (*continued*)
    therapeutic options for, **827–845**
        alemtuzamab, 835–837
        complementary and alternative therapies, 839
        under FDA review, 835–837
        fingolimod, 830–832
        natalizumab
            risk stratification with, 837–839
        recently approved therapies, 830–835
        tecfidera, 834–835
        teriflunomide, 832–834
        update on, **827–845**


N

Natalizumab
    in MS management
        risk stratification with, 837–839
Neurologic deficits
    brain AVMs and, 753
Neuroprotective strategies
    in ICH management, 725–728
Neurostimulation
    in epilepsy management, 786, 793–795
        electrical stimulation of anterior nucleus of thalamus, 793
        external trigeminal stimulation, 794–795
        responsive neurostimulation, 793–794
Nonparkinsonian movement disorders
    DBS in, **809–826**. *See also* Deep brain stimulation (DBS), in nonparkinsonian
        movement disorders


O

Octapharma IBIG
    for Alzheimer's disease, 874–875
Oligoastrocytomas
    mixed
        evaluation of, 848–849
Oligodendrogliomas
    evaluation of, 848
1p19q deletions
    in high-grade glioma evaluation, 849–850
Open craniotomy
    in ICH management, 728–729


P

Parkinson disease
    axial features of, 804
    surgical treatment of, **799–808**
        DBS complications related to, 804
        emerging concepts in, 804–805
        intermediate-frequency stimulation in, 805

introduction, 799–800
    operative procedure, 802–803
    outcomes of, 803
    patient selection for, 800–802
    postoperative programming, 803
    rate *vs.* pattern of neuronal firing in, 805
    target selection in, 802
PCV. *See* Vincristine (PCV)
Perampanel
    in epilepsy management, 791–793
Platelet antiaggregants. *See* Antiplatelet agents
Prasugrel
    in stroke prevention, 649
Procarbazine
    in high-grade glioma management, 855–856

**R**

Radiation therapy
    in high-grade glioma management, 857–858
Responsive neurostimulation
    in epilepsy management, 793–794
Rivaroxaban
    for stroke prevention in atrial fibrillation, 666
Rufinamide
    in epilepsy management, 788–789

**S**

Sarpogrelate
    in stroke prevention, 650
Seizure(s)
    brain AVMs and, 752
    in CVT
        management of, 774–776
Solaneuzumab
    for Alzheimer's disease, 872–873
Sonothrombolysis
    for acute ischemic stroke, 692
Stent-based thrombectomy
    in endovascular recanalization of acute ischemic stroke, 711–713
Stroke
    ischemic
        acute. *See* Acute ischemic stroke
    prevention of
        antiplatelet agents in, **633–657**. *See also* Antiplatelet agents, in stroke prevention

**T**

Tecfidera
    in MS management, 834–835
Temozolomide (TMZ)
    in high-grade glioma management, 852–855

Teriflunomide
  in MS management, 832–834
Thrombectomy
  endovascular
    for acute ischemic stroke, 692
  mechanical
    in CVT management, 773
  stent-based
    in endovascular recanalization of acute ischemic stroke, 711–713
Thrombolysis
  in CVT management, 773
  IA
    in endovascular recanalization of acute ischemic stroke, 706–707
  IV tPA
    for acute ischemic stroke, 681–687
Thrombolytic therapy
  for acute ischemic stroke
    unanswered questions in, **677–704**
      concomitant therapies, 692–694
      endovascular thrombectomy vs. IV thrombolysis, 690–692
      IA thrombolysis vs. IV thrombolysis, 687–689
      introduction, 677–679
      IV tPA thrombolysis
        defining therapeutic time windows for, 683–687
        landmark studies and 3-hour time window for, 681–683
      outcome determinants, 694–699
        collaterals, 697
        imaging modalities, 695–696
        in older patients, 699
        stroke location, 697–698
        wake-up strokes, 698–699
      patient evaluation, 679–681
      PROACT-II and IMS-III trials, 687–689
      sonothrombolysis, 692
      surgical/nonpharmacologic treatment options, 690–692
Thrombosis
  cerebral venous. See Cerebral venous thrombosis (CVT)
Ticagrelor
  in stroke prevention, 648
TMZ. See Temozolomide (TMZ)
Tremor(s)
  essential
    DBS in
      patient overview and management goals, 812–813
Triflusal
  in stroke prevention, 649–650

U

Ultrasound
  IV-IA tPA
    in endovascular recanalization of acute ischemic stroke, 707

## V

Vincristine (PCV)
  in high-grade glioma management, 855–856
Vorapaxar and atopaxar
  in stroke prevention, 650

Printed and bound by CPI Group (UK) Ltd, Croydon, CR0 4YY

08/06/2025

01896875-0003